EXERCISE MEDICINE
Physiological Principles
and Clinical Applications

EXERCISE MEDICINE

Physiological Principles
and Clinical Applications

Edited by

Alfred A. Bove

*Cardiovascular Division
and Department of Physiology
Mayo Foundation
Rochester, Minnesota*

David T. Lowenthal

*The Likoff Cardiovascular Institute
Hahnemann University School of Medicine
Philadelphia, Pennsylvania*

 ACADEMIC PRESS, INC.

(Harcourt Brace Jovanovich, Publishers)

**Orlando   San Diego   New York   London
Toronto   Montreal   Sydney   Tokyo**

ACADEMIC PRESS, INC.
Orlando, Florida 32887

United Kingdom Edition published by
ACADEMIC PRESS, INC. (LONDON) LTD.
24/28 Oval Road, London NW1 7DX

Library of Congress Cataloging in Publication Data

Main entry under title:

Exercise medicine.

    Bibliography: p.
    Includes index.
    1. Sports medicine. 2. Exercise--Physiological
aspects. 3. Exercise therapy. I. Bove, Alfred A.
II. Lowenthal, David T. [DNLM: 1. Exertion
2. Sports medicine. WE 103 M489]
RC1210.E94   1983   613.7'0880814   83-7095
ISBN 0-12-119720-4

PRINTED IN THE UNITED STATES OF AMERICA

85 86 87 88   9 8 7 6 5 4 3 2

*To those
who have taught us
and to those
whom we have taught*

Contents

I
Physiological Aspects of Sports and Exercise

1. Structure and Functional Organization of Skeletal Muscle
KENNETH M. BALDWIN

2. Cardiovascular Physiology of Exercise
RUSSELL T. DOWELL

II
Women, Youth, and the Elderly

7. Gynecological and Obstetrical Aspects of Exercise

MONA M. SHANGOLD

8. Exercise in the Young

BONITA FALKNER

9. Exercise in the Elderly

ALFRED A. BOVE

III
Medical Aspects of Sports and Exercise

18. Medical Aspects of Diving

ALFRED A. BOVE AND OTTO APPENZELLER

19. Prescribing Exercise Programs

ALBERT M. PAOLONE

Contributors

OTTO APPENZELLER (185, 347), Department of Neurology, University of New Mexico School of Medicine, Albuquerque, New Mexico 87131

RUTH ATKINSON (185), Department of Neurology, University of New Mexico School of Medicine, Albuquerque, New Mexico 87131

KENNETH M. BALDWIN (3), Department of Physiology, University of California, Irvine, California 92717

ALFRED A. BOVE (174, 230, 347), Cardiovascular Division and Department of Physiology, Mayo Foundation, Rochester, Minnesota 55905

SUSAN J. BRODERMAN (291, 321), The William Likoff Cardiovascular Institute, Hahnemann University School of Medicine, Philadelphia, Pennsylvania 19102

RITA A. CAREY (113), Smith Kline and French Laboratories, Philadelphia, Pennsylvania 19130

RUSSELL T. DOWELL (19), Department of Physiology, University of Kansas Medical Center, Kansas City, Kansas 66103

DANIEL C. DuPONT (29, 259), Division of Pulmonary Diseases, Hahnemann University School of Medicine, Philadelphia, Pennsylvania 19102

BONITA FALKNER (163), Department of Pediatrics, Hahnemann University School of Medicine, Philadelphia, Pennsylvania 19102

PHILIP FELIG (305), Department of Medicine, Yale University School of Medicine, New Haven, Connecticut 06510

ALLAN P. FREEDMAN (29, 259), Division of Pulmonary Diseases, Hahnemann University School of Medicine, Philadelphia, Pennsylvania 19102

RONALD M. LAWRENCE (335), Department of Psychiatry, University of California School of Medicine, Los Angeles, California 90024

STANLEY H. LORBER (279), Department of Medicine, Temple University Medical School, Philadelphia, Pennsylvania 19140

DAVID T. LOWENTHAL (291, 321), The William Likoff Cardiovascular Institute, Hahnemann University School of Medicine, Philadelphia, Pennsylvania 19102

GABE MIRKIN (89), Department of Physical Education, University of Maryland, College Park, Maryland 20740

PAUL A. MOLÉ (43), Department of Physical Education, Human Performance Laboratory, University of California, Davis, California 95616

ALBERT M. PAOLONE (361), Department of Physical Education, Temple University, Philadelphia, Pennsylvania 19122

MONA M. SHANGOLD (145), Department of Obstetrics and Gynecology, Cornell University Medical College, New York, New York 10021

Preface

Although much attention has been given to athletes and their medical problems and to exercise in the cardiac patient, little attention has been directed toward the exercise-related problems confronting the average person or those who might have a chronic illness and wish to exercise. Our clinical experience indeed was forcing us to deal more and more with chronically ill patients who wanted to improve their physical condition. Much of our approach to dealing with hypertension, congenital heart disease, chronic renal disease, various endocrine disorders, and neurologic disorders has been empirical since few data have been available specifically addressing exercise in these diseases. Since the majority of the exercising population are casual athletes, we found the need for a book addressing the interaction of exercise and common problems found in most medical practice. This work provides a spectrum of information ranging from basic exercise physiology to how to deal with geriatric patients who exercise. The basic exercise physiology is provided so that clinical judgments can be based on physiologic principles. Since it is impossible to cover every medical problem, solutions to uncommon problems can be deduced from a knowledge of basic exercise physiology. Mirkin's chapter on nutrition reflects his extensive experience with a multitude of sport and exercise problems. He has provided useful insight into nutritional misconceptions and problems that arise in certain sports. Two chapters on women and exercise are included because of the pressing need by female athletes for advice. Carey's chapter on physiology and Shangold's clinical chapter should provide answers to most questions that arise concerning women and exercise. The series of clinical chapters reflects the experiences of each author in dealing with aspects of sports and exercise by medical specialty.

The chapters on youth and the elderly have been included because of the frequent questions that arise when people at the extremes of life become involved with exercise. The recent developments in physiological aspects of exercise are considered in Chapter 17. A chapter on diving medicine is included because there are a number of unique problems associated with the sport of diving, and several important and potentially lethal combinations of chronic illness and diving that are often overlooked by the physician not familiar with this sport. Treatment of the neurological injuries associated with diving requires special facilities, and an understanding of these disorders will avoid mistreatment of the occasional diving injury one may encounter.

We included a final chapter on developing exercise programs and providing prescriptions for exercise so that specific information could be provided for those who wish to exercise. The guidelines set forth in this chapter are well established and have been found to be safe for patients with a variety of diseases and for persons of any age.

We have not included the orthopedic aspects of sports medicine because this topic has received considerable attention in the past, and we have not discussed cardiac rehabilitation because of numerous books, papers, and reports available on this subject. The guidelines of Chapter 19, however, are applicable to the cardiac patient and are used for cardiac rehabilitation.

This book will provide physicians and others involved in exercise programs with a reference for advising patients and well persons about exercise. The current trend in exercise dictates that we should not deny an individual the opportunity to exercise but, instead, should tailor an exercise program to fit individual capacity and preferences. With this approach, many patients will become active and functional and well persons may reduce their risk for cardiovascular disease.

ALFRED A. BOVE
DAVID T. LOWENTHAL

I

Physiological Aspects of Sports and Exercise

CHAPTER 1

Structural and Functional Organization of Skeletal Muscle

KENNETH M. BALDWIN

Department of Physiology
University of California
Irvine, California

I. INTRODUCTION

Muscles are biological machines that convert chemical energy, derived from the reaction between food substrate and oxygen, into force production and me-

Exercise Medicine: Physiological Principles
and Clinical Applications

chanical work. The goal of this chapter is to discuss some fundamental structural, biochemical, and physiological properties of contracting skeletal muscle which will form a background for the various topics presented in subsequent chapters. The material in this chapter is organized into seven major topics: (1) mechanical properties of skeletal muscle; (2) architectural features of skeletal muscle; (3) the role of subcellular organelles in regulating the contraction process; (4) organization of key metabolic pathways involved in energy production; (5) functional organization of skeletal muscle fibers; (6) normal recruitment of muscle fiber types; and (7) the adaptability of muscle fibers in response to physical activity and inactivity.

II. MECHANICAL PROPERTIES OF SKELETAL MUSCLE

In examining the physiological properties of skeletal muscle during contraction, it is important at the outset to distinguish between two fundamentally important, yet distinctly different properties, namely strength and endurance. The strength of a muscle refers to its ability to generate force or tension when stimulated to contract. Although the factors that regulate the force output of a muscle during a given contraction are complex, the maximal force production (P_0) of a muscle is related to its physiological cross section of contractile material. Endurance, on the other hand, refers to the ability of a muscle to sustain a given amount of contractile output (force), or to repeat contractions over and over, regardless of the magnitude of force being generated. Generally, a muscle's endurance capacity is related to its effectiveness in maintaining energy to support the mechanical process of contraction. These two properties ultimately dictate one's performance capacity for most activities. Consequently, any program of physical conditioning designed to improve the performance capacity of muscle must consider these two properties.

The mechanical properties of skeletal muscle are expressed in terms of both its force and contractile speed generating capability. The force (tension) output of a muscle can be varied in two primary ways. The first involves stimulating a given fiber at different frequencies. As stimulation frequency increases, force production increases until the muscle fiber attains its peak tetanic tension (P_0) (11,13). Fast-twitch muscles (described in more detail later) achieve peak tetanic force at high stimulation frequencies, whereas slow-twitch muscles reach tetanic tension at low stimulating frequencies (11,13). However, both fast-twitch and slow-twitch muscles attain similar peak tetanic tensions when normalized for cross-sectional area (13). The different tetanic tension patterns generated by fast and slow contracting muscles are thought to relate to differences in (1) the kinetic properties of the sarcoplasmic reticulum for releasing and sequestering calcium, and (2) myosin ATPase in these types of muscle. Calcium levels in the cytoplasm are responsible for regulating the contraction response. Under most physiological conditions, skeletal muscles contract tetanically rather than in twitch fashion.

A second way that a muscle can increase its force production is to recruit more fibers for a given response (3,14). For most activities, not all the fibers comprising a given muscle are stimulated to contract. The proportion of fibers recruited will depend on the degree that various neurons innervating the fibers are activated via the nervous system (3). The process of activating neurons is complex and will be discussed later.

The speed of muscle contraction refers to the length of time it takes the muscle to develop tension when contracting isometrically (defined as tension generation without fiber shortening) or to shorten isotonically (defined as fiber shortening against a load). The most fundamental mechanical property of skeletal muscle is its force–velocity relationship, which describes the muscle's ability to shorten as a function of the force it generates during a given isotonic contraction (13). As shown in Fig. 1, this relationship is hyperbolic for both fast-twitch and slow-twitch muscles. Note that as the load increases, shortening velocity decreases and vice versa. Also, at any given relative load below P_0, fast-twitch muscles can generate greater shortening velocities than slow-twitch muscles. Stated another way, if both muscle types were to contract at the same velocity, the fast-twitch muscle can generate greater relative amounts of force than the slow-twitch muscle. These factors are important when considering the use of the different types of muscles for performing activities requiring different power requirements. In subsequent sections, fast-twitch and slow-twitch muscles will be characterized further regarding their biochemical, metabolic, and physiological properties.

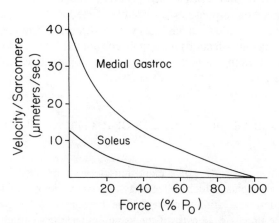

Fig. 1. Plot of force–velocity relationship of fast-twitch (medial gastroc) and slow-twitch (soleus) muscle. The V_{max} of shortening is correlated with the myosin ATPase activity. Note that the soleus generates much slower rates of shortening for any given relative work load.

III. GROSS MORPHOLOGY AND FIBER ARCHITECTURE

In man, muscle constitutes approximately 40% of body mass. A typical human muscle is comprised of tens of thousands of fibers of cylindrical shape and of varying length. A typical fiber in adult man may have a diameter of 50–70 μm and a length varying from a few millimeters to tens of centimeters. In comparing one muscle to another, both the fiber length and the fiber length/muscle length ratio will differ (13). Moreover, the orientation of the fibers relative to the long axis of the muscle's tendon will vary from muscle to muscle. This fiber angulation (called pinnation) allows for varying numbers of fibers to attach along the length of the tendon. The differences in angle of pinnation that exist between two muscles may account, in part, for their differences in physiological cross-sectional area and, hence, force-generating capability (13). Muscles with greater angles of pinnation generally contain more fibers and thus can exert greater total force. In contrast, a muscle containing fibers with little angle of pinnation generally benefits from a more effective transmission of force at the muscle tendon. Muscles with small angles of pinnation generally are suited energetically for sustaining force output. For example, the slow-twitch soleus muscle, which has a high metabolic efficiency for maintaining isometric tension, has a parallel arrangement of its fibers, whereas the fast-twitch medial gastrocnemius muscle, noted for its power output, has a pinnate fiber arrangement (13).

The gross architecture of a muscle can also affect its shortening properties. Generally, the longer a given muscle and the more parallel the alignment of its fibers, the greater its capacity for distance of shortening and shortening velocity (see Fig. 1). This occurs primarily because there are more functional units (sarcomeres) arranged in series to the direction of movement (13). These factors affect the contraction response independently of the biochemical properties regulating certain contractile mechanics, as will be discussed below. Consequently, a muscle's architectural features need to be considered when evaluating its functional role in performing various activities. These important features are summarized in Table I.

IV. SUBCELLULAR ORGANIZATION OF A TYPICAL MUSCLE FIBER

The mechanical properties of skeletal muscle are controlled by a number of subcellular components, which collectively regulate various aspects of the excitation–contraction–relaxation sequence. The primary cellular components involved in these processes consist of the sarcolemma, the sarcotubular network, and the myofibril complex. These cellular components are shown in Fig. 2 and their functional role during contraction is listed in Table II.

TABLE I

Effect of Fiber Architecture on Mechanical Properties of Skeletal Muscle

Orientation to tendon	Functional advantage	Types of muscles involved
Parallel arrangement (angle of pinnation < 10°)	1. More effective translation of produced force at tendon 2. Greater extent and speed[a] of shortening 3. Greater economy of maintaining tension	Predominantly slow-twitch muscle (soleus)
Pinnate arrangement (angle of pinnation > 20°)	Greater physiological cross-sectional area to enhance force and power output	Predominantly fast-twitch muscle (gastrocnemius)

[a] This property is primarily fiber-length and fiber-type dependent. Muscles with fibers arranged in parallel generally have longer fiber lengths.

A. Sarcolemma

This structure consists predominantly of a lipoprotein membrane that defines the boundary between intracellular and extracellular spaces. Portions of the extracellular space are carried into the interior of the cell via tiny openings in the sarcolemma called transverse or T tubules (8). The primary function of the sarcolemma is to propagate the action potential along the fiber surface and into

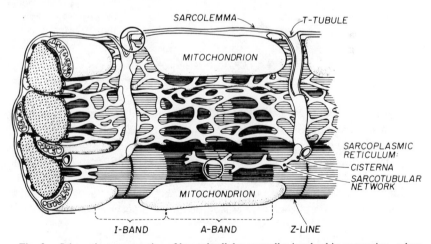

Fig. 2. Schematic representation of key subcellular organelles involved in contraction–relaxation and energy production processes in skeletal muscle cells. See text and Table II for discussion of the function of the various components.

TABLE II

Location and Primary Function of Subcellular Components Involved in Excitation–Contraction–Relaxation Processes in Skeletal Muscle

Subcellular component	Primary location	Primary function
Sarcolemma	Cell membrane	Propagation of action potential
Transverse tubules	Invagination into cell at selected sites along membrane	Conduct action potential to cell interior (terminal cisternae)
Terminal cisternae	Subsarcolemmal; adjacent to T tubules	Release Ca^{2+} to initiate contraction
Sarcoplasmic reticulum (longitudinal)	Surrounds myofibrils	Sequester calcium to cause relaxation
Myosin	Thick filament of A band of sarcomere	Catalyze ATP degradation; interacts with actin to produce force and shortening
Actin	Thin filament of I band region of sarcomere	Interacts with myosin to produce force and shortening
Tropomyosin	Situated along "groove" of double stranded actin molecules	Normally obstructs actin sites from binding myosin
Troponin	At specified regions along actin molecule	Regulator protein complex (1) binds to both actin and tropomyosin; (2) binds calcium and initiates transformation in tropomyosin–actin protein alignment to enable actin to interact with myosin

the fiber interior along the T tubules so that the contractile process can be turned on. A secondary function of the sarcolemma is to control ion fluxes across the cell membrane in order to maintain intracellular and extracellular ionic composition. The membrane components of the sarcolemma making up the T tubule system are located at specified sites along the surface. These invaginations provide a means for the inward spread of the action potential to ensure that subsequent activation of the contractile structures can occur rapidly.

B. Sarcoplasmic Reticulum

This subcellular component consists of a series of tubules arranged longitudinally in the interior of the muscle cell (Fig. 2). The sarcoplasmic recticulum can be divided into two functional components. The first, called the subsarcolemmal cisternae, is located beneath the sarcolemma adjacent to the end of a T tubule. This region where the cisternae reside adjacent to a T tubule is called a triad (two cisternae and one T tubule). The cisternae are the sites from which calcium is released to initiate contraction. The second component, the longitudinal sarcotubular network, consists of a network of vesicles surrounding the contractile proteins. The longitudinal portion functions to sequester calcium (by an active process) from the contractile system to bring about muscle relaxation.

C. Myofibrils

Myofibrils constitute the contractile system, which consists of four complex proteins: myosin, actin, tropomyosin, and troponin. These four proteins are arranged into a functional unit called a sarcomere (see Fig. 2). The sarcomere consists of two overlapping bands called the anisotropic or A band and the isotropic or I band. Each I band is bisected by a narrow darkly staining Z line. Also, a broad dense M zone or band is formed in the center of the A band. The sarcomere is defined as the region between two Z lines and thus consists of a single A band plus two adjacent half-I bands.

The A band is comprised of thick filaments consisting primarily of the protein myosin. The two half-I bands at either side of the A bands contain thin filaments, which extend into the A band in the center of the sarcomere from their origin at the Z lines. The thin filaments consist largely of actin and the regulatory proteins tropomyosin and troponin. A brief outline of the location and function of the various contractile proteins is presented in both Fig. 3 and Table II.

D. Summary of Events Involved in Contraction

The electrical signal of membrane depolarization is transmitted along the fiber surface (sarcolemma) and inward along the transverse tubule network. Subse-

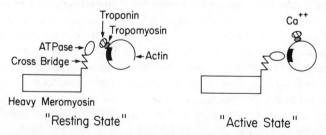

Fig. 3. Schematic representation of the alignment of the essential proteins during rest and during contraction in which calcium binds to troponin and changes the ultrastructural alignment of the proteins. Not shown is the energy transformation process in which ATP is degraded to provide free energy for contraction.

quent depolarization of the terminal cisternae of the triad region of the sarcosplasmic reticulum leads to the release of calcium to the contractile machinery. The concentration of cytosolic calcium is raised from a resting level of approximately 10^{-7} M to approximately 10^{-5} M, which is sufficient to saturate the troponin-c binding sites on the actin filament (Table II) (8). The calcium binding to troponin causes a transformational change in the tropomyosin–actin conformation which enables actin to interact with the head region of the myosin (Fig. 3). This latter site normally is in a so-called ''activated'' Mg^{2+}-ATP state. The interaction of actin with myosin is manifested by an energy transformation process in which the mechanical process of contraction occurs such that force development and/or shortening is made possible by the free energy released from ATP conversion to ADP and P_i. This is catalyzed by the myosin ATPase. A number of transformational changes in the cross bridge structure of the myosin molecule are postulated to cause the actin to slide by the myosin (sliding filament theory) to produce shortening of the sarcomere. The sarcomere shortens for both isometric and isotonic contraction because there are elastic elements residing in the contractile machinery which must be overcome for the actual manifestation of tension development and shortening to occur. Relaxation involves the sequestering of calcium by the sarcoplasmic reticulum (longitudinal portion). Recall that this is also an energy-dependent process, in that one ATP molecule is used to pump two molecules of calcium. Also, an ''activated'' Mg-ATP–myosin complex must be restored. This is accomplished by resynthesis of ATP via metabolic processes, and requires a complex series of reactions occurring in both the cytoplasm and mitochondria, which will be discussed in Section V.

V. ENERGY PRODUCTION IN SKELETAL MUSCLE

A. High Energy Stores

Skeletal muscles contain only small amounts of ATP (5-7 μmoles/g), which is the chemical substrate used for both contraction and relaxation. Therefore, ATP must be continually regenerated as rapidly as it is used during contraction. Muscle also contains another high energy phosphate compound, phosphocreatine, which can react with ADP, the product of ATP breakdown, to immediately regenerate ATP (Table III). This reaction is catalyzed by the enzyme, creatine phosphokinase, which is in great abundance in most skeletal muscle fibers. However, skeletal muscle contains limited amounts of phosphocreatine (15–20 μmoles/g); consequently, chemical reactions that involve the metabolism of food substrate (primarily carbohydrates and fatty acids) are necessary if sufficient energy is to be provided to maintain contractile activity for extended periods (minutes to hours).

B. Substrate Energy Storage and Metabolism

The primary muscle substrate immediately available for ATP synthesis is glycogen. Human skeletal muscle can store varying amounts of glycogen (10–25 mg/g) depending on one's dietary and activity patterns. During contraction, key regulatory enzymes (phosphorylase and phosphofructokinase) are activated to metabolize glycogen to pyruvic acid. These transformations allow for small but rapid yields of ATP (Table III) for the maintenance of contraction. The generated pyruvate can be further metabolized to carbon dioxide with an additional yield of relatively large amounts of ATP (Table III). These reactions occur in the mitochondria, which are the sites where metabolism of substrates occurs in a complex series of reactions ultimately linked to the reduction of molecular oxygen to water. The capacity for oxidation of pyruvate is primarily dependent on the number of mitochondria present in a given fiber. In some fibers, the capacity for glycogenolysis is much greater than the capacity of the mitochondria to metabolize pyruvate. Under these conditions, the pyruvate is converted to lactate in the cytoplasm so that glycogenolysis can continue. In those fibers in which lactate is readily produced, the fiber is thought to be primarily an anaerobic functioning fiber, i.e., relying heavily on glycogen breakdown to lactate. In addition to glycogen, most fibers also utilize exogenous glucose, which is provided via the blood supply. However, in skeletal muscle, the uptake rate of glucose is relatively low compared to the rate of glycogen breakdown. The regulation of carbohydrate metabolism during exercise will be discussed in greater detail in subsequent chapters.

TABLE III

Summary of Metabolic Stoichiometry of ATP Synthesis and Degradation in Skeletal Muscle

I. Chief ATP utilization reactions:

$$ATP \xrightarrow{\substack{\text{myosin} \\ \text{sarcoplasmic} \\ \text{reticulum ATPase}}} ADP + P_i \text{ (free energy release)}$$

II. Anaerobic pathways for ATP synthesis:

$$ADP + phosphocreatine \xrightarrow{\substack{\text{creatine} \\ \text{phosphokinase}}} ATP + creatine$$

$$2 ADP \xrightarrow{\text{myokinase}} ATP + AMP$$

$$Glycogen^a + 3 ADP \longrightarrow 2 \text{ Pyruvate} + 3 ATP$$

III. Chief mitochondrial reaction schemes for ATP synthesis:

$$2 \text{ Pyruvate} + 6 O_2 + 36 ADP \longrightarrow 6 CO_2 + 6 H_2O + 36 ATP$$

$$Palmitate + 23 O_2 + 130 ADP \longrightarrow 16 CO_2 + 16 H_2O + 130 ATP$$

_a_ This is considered as a glucosyl unit. Note that one glucosyl molecule derives two pyruvate molecules. Subsequent metabolism of pyruvate is considered in terms of the glucosyl unit.

In addition to metabolizing carbohydrate, skeletal muscles can also metabolize fatty acids. There are two primary sources of fatty acids available to the muscle. The first source involves endogeneous triglycerides stored in the muscle fibers. The second involves the storage of fatty acids in triglyceride form in adipose tissue. These latter sources are released into the blood and transported to the muscles for utilization. The mobilization and oxidation of fatty acids are complex, and the key reactions involved in these processes will be discussed elsewhere in this volume. Moreover, as will be discussed in Section VI, different types of skeletal muscle fibers possess varying capacity for performing both anaerobic and aerobic metabolism of food substrate. The endurance property of a given muscle fiber is largely dependent on its capacity to sustain oxidative metabolic processes because these reactions provide for the greatest yield of ATP per unit of substrate metabolized. These points are summarized in Table III.

VI. ORGANIZATION OF MUSCLE FIBERS INTO FUNCTIONAL UNITS

The functional unit of skeletal muscle is called a motor unit. It consists of a single motor neuron innervating varying numbers of fibers of similar biochemical and physiological properties. At least three distinct types of motor units have been characterized in most mammalian muscles, including those of humans (3). They are briefly described below and outlined in Table IV.

A. Slow-Oxidative (Type I)

Muscle fibers comprising this motor unit have slow contraction properties, i.e., long contraction times and slow shortening velocities. These properties are thought to result from the slow calcium release and sequestering kinetics of the sarcoplasmic reticulum and from the low ATPase myosin isoenzyme, respectively, present in these fibers. Slow-twitch muscle fibers have a relatively high capacity to oxidize substrates such as pyruvate, palmitate, and ketones (2). These oxidative properties have been shown to correlate well with blood flow capacity during contraction. However, this type of motor unit has a low glycogenolytic capacity or a low capacity for anaerobic metabolism. The physiological and biochemical properties of this type of motor unit make it suited for sustaining the constant tension output that might be required for postural control at rest and during sustained locomotion. Slow-twitch fibers are fatigue resistant.

B. Fast-Oxidative-Glycogenolytic (Type IIa)

Fibers comprising this motor unit have fast contractile properties, which are correlated with the calcium uptake properties of the sarcoplasmic reticulum and

TABLE IV

Physiological and Biochemical Properties of Motor Units

Nomenclature	Fast-oxidative-glycogenolytic (Type IIa)	Fast-glycogenolytic (Type IIb)	Slow-oxidative (Type I)
Myosin ATPase	High	High	Low
Sarcoplasmic reticulum calcium sequestering	High	High	Low
Shortening velocity	High	High	Low
Contraction times (isometric)	Fast	Fast	Slow
Oxidative enzymes	High	Low	Moderate–High
Peak blood flow capacity	High	Low	Moderate–High
Glycogenolytic capacity	Moderate–High	High	Low
Relative number of fibers/motor unit	Moderate	High	Low
Tension output/motor unit	Moderate	High	Low
Recruitment pattern relative to work intensity	Low → high intensity	High intensity	Rest → low → high intensity

high ATPase activity of the fast-myosin isoenzyme. These fibers have both a high oxidative and a high glycogenolytic capacity. Consequently, they are suited for both aerobic and anaerobic energy requirements. Available evidence suggests that the fast-oxidative units are suited primarily for prolonged locomotor activities that may require moderate degrees of power output of the muscle (3,14).

C. Fast-Glycogenolytic (Type IIb)

Fibers comprising this unit are similar to the fast-oxidative-glycogenolytic fibers, with the exception that they have low concentrations of mitochondria. Thus, they rely more heavily on glycogen for energy. Available evidence also suggests that these fast fibers are somewhat larger than the oxidative types. Also, the number of fibers per individual motor unit is known to be high (3,14). Consequently, when these units are recruited, there is considerable enhancement of the force production and power output of the muscle (3,14). However, unlike the oxidative types, the fast-glycogenolytic type of motor unit is readily fatigable.

Each skeletal muscle is thought to contain hundreds to thousands of these three different units depending on its size. In many muscles, there is a roughly equal proportion of fast-twitch and slow-twitch units. With regard to fast-twitch types, there appears to be a spectrum of high and low oxidative fibers. Available evidence suggests that the proportion of fast- and slow-twitch types is genetically fixed. However, this may not always hold true. Studies on animal models, in which the functional role of the muscle is altered through surgical manipulation, suggest that certain properties in the fiber types can be transformed, i.e., fast myosin converted to slow myosin (1). In this context, it has been observed that elite endurance athletes contain a predominance of slow-twitch fibers, whereas elite sprinters or weight lifters contain a predominance of fast-twitch fibers (5). Although these properties may be largely genetically determined, the potential for conversion of fiber types in human muscle is still unresolved.

D. Motor Unit Recruitment

Studies performed on both animals and humans indicate that the slow-twitch units are preferentially used during resting conditions for maintaining postural support (3,14). Although the slow-twitch units continue to function during locomotor activities, as the intensity and power requirements become increased, the fast-twitch units are progressively recruited (14). The low oxidative units are probably not utilized until the intensity is either quite high or there is fatigue occurring in the oxidative types. Interestingly, there is some evidence to suggest that during certain ballistic movements, as in rapid limb movement, the recruitment of slow units may be inhibited (13). This is thought to occur because the limb velocity may require shortening velocities in excess of the slow units.

The biochemical properties of these fiber types, as outlined in Table IV, to a large extent determine the physiological capabilities of the muscle under a variety of conditions. Consequently, it is not surprising that most low intensity tasks can be sustained for long durations, because the motor units participating in the activities have a high resistance to fatigue. On the other hand, during conditions of high intensity exercise, endurance capacity frequently suffers because these activities require the participation of the fatigue labile, low oxidative motor units.

VII. EFFECTS OF ALTERED MUSCULAR ACTIVITY ON SKELETAL MUSCLE

Skeletal muscle has the capacity to adapt its morphological, biochemical, and functional properties in accordance with the functional demands imposed on it. The adaptive potential of skeletal muscle in response to various types of activities is discussed below and summarized in Table V.

A. Endurance Exercise

Studies involving both human and animal models indicate that regularly performed endurance exercise (running, cycling, swimming, etc.) enhances the

TABLE V

Summary of Effects of Altered Muscular Activity on Skeletal Muscle Metabolic and Functional Properties

Activity	Primary stimulus	Primary adaptations	Impact on muscle function
Endurance exercise	Repetitive contractions of relatively low force output	1. Increase in mitochondria 2. Relatively little change in anaerobic pathways 3. Relatively little hypertrophy	1. Increased endurance 2. Glycogen sparing during exercise 3. Reduced lactate production during work
Strength training (heavy resistance)	Intermittent increase in force requirements per cross-sectional area	1. Increased fiber cross-sectional area 2. Possible dilution of mitochondrial pool 3. No change in fiber typing	1. Increased strength and power 2. Possible reduction in endurance
Compensatory overload	Chronic increase in force requirements per cross-sectional area	1. Fiber enlargement 2. Fast- to slow-twitch fiber conversion 3. Maintenance of oxidative capacity	1. Increased mechanical function 2. Increased efficiency for maintaining tension 3. Increased fatigue resistance
Limb immobilization	Decrease in force requirements per cross-sectional area Decrease in contractile frequency	1. Muscle atrophy 2. Reductions in oxidative enzymes 3. Possible conversion of slow to fast-twitch fibers	Reduced strength and endurance

oxidative capacity of skeletal muscle (2,7,12). This adaptation is both intensity and duration specific. The intensity factor is important for inducing the adaptation in a large spectrum of motor units. Generally, those motor units utilized more frequently during the exercise program respond with the greatest change in oxidative enzymes. The metabolic significance of this adaptation most likely involves the muscle fibers becoming more effective in metabolizing alternative substrates (fatty acids, ketones) to replace, in part, carbohydrate (blood glucose and muscle glycogen) as the major source of energy for maintaining prolonged contractile activity (2,7,12). The functional significance of these changes is that the trained muscle has more endurance to enable the individual to perform work for longer duration.

Additional research suggests that there is little change in the capacity of muscle to perform anaerobic metabolism (2). Also, there is relatively little evidence to suggest that the biochemical components of the muscle regulating its contractile properties undergo change. In this context, it is important to emphasize that most endurance activities require a relatively low level of force output by the participating muscles (less than 30% of the maximal voluntary capacity). Consequently, the stimulus intensity for muscular enlargement and for changing the contractile properties and/or fiber-typing of a large portion of the muscle probably is insufficient.

B. Strength Training

This form of conditioning consists of subjecting skeletal muscle to repetitive contractions requiring a high force production. Contractions can be isometric (force generation without fiber shortening), isotonic (force generation plus fiber shortening), and eccentric (force generation plus fiber lengthening). Programs that involve "weight lifting" automatically incorporate both isotonic and eccentric contractions as the conditioning stimulus. Although the programs vary, most muscle groups are conditioned by three sets of contractions with ten individual contractions performed in each set. Generally, maximal force output is not a necessary conditioning factor in order to induce changes in muscle strength.

Strength training programs primarily result in increased muscle strength. This results from both better neural regulation of the contractile process and an increase in muscle mass. The best available evidence suggests that the fibers undergo hypertrophy rather than hyperplasia (6). However, the hypertrophied fibers may undergo a reduction in oxidative enzymes (mitochondria) as a result of selective enlargement of other cellular components. The evidence for this dilution in mitochondria is based primarily on ultrastructural analyses (9). Interestingly, when comparisons are made among different groups of athletes, weight lifters have the lowest levels of skeletal muscle oxidative enzymes and the lowest capacity for maximum oxygen uptake when normalized for body weight (5). Consequently, this form of training, while enhancing strength, may reduce muscle endurance. However, this possibility needs to be more thoroughly examined.

C. Compensatory Hypertrophy

There are situations in which a muscle or muscle group may have to take over the functional responsibility of another muscle (or muscle group) that might have become permanently damaged or impaired. Under these so-called conditions of "compensatory usage" or overload, the muscle becomes chronically stressed and undergoes enlargement. Although this type of model has not been explored extensively in humans, experiments performed on animals show that muscles enlarged by a compensatory process undergo changes in functional, metabolic, and biochemical propeties (1). Available evidence suggests that the oxidative capacity of the overloaded muscle changes in parallel to the enlargement, i.e., there is no dilution of the mitochondria. Histochemical and biochemical findings also show that the relative percentage of slow-twitch muscle fibers is increased (1). This may enable the muscle to become more effective in meeting the increased functional demand placed upon it. These studies have also provided information to suggest that a relatively high degree of mechanical stress is necessary for inducing fiber-type transformations.

D. Limb Immobilization

If a limb is placed in a cast or if the daily functional requirements of the muscles are reduced, as in chronic bed rest, the limb muscles undergo atrophy, or a reduction in size. This reduction in muscle size is manifest at the gross level in terms of muscle girth and at the cellular level in terms of fiber cross-sectional area. It does not appear that the fiber-typing is altered dramatically (slow-twitch conversion to fast-twitch) in human subjects; however, there is some evidence of conversion of slow-twitch to fast-twitch fibers in the antigravity muscle of experimental animals. Further studies involving cord transections strongly suggest that limiting the functional requirements of the muscle (chronic force output) may transform slow-twitch fibers to fast-twitch fibers. These results need to be extended further into human subjects. Of particular interest are the findings that suggest that the oxidative capacity of skeletal muscle is impaired as a result of limb immobilization (10,12). These observations collectively suggest that both the strength and endurance capacity of the immobilized muscles are impaired. Studies performed on animals and humans indicate that the atrophy process can be reversed through conditioning programs designed to enhance both the strength and endurance of the muscle (12).

REFERENCES

1. Baldwin, K. M., Valdez, V., Herrick, R. E., MacIntosh, A. M., and Roy, R. R. (1982). Biochemical properties of overloaded fast-twitch skeletal muscle. *J. Appl. Physiol.: Respir. Environ. Exercise Physiol.* **52,** 467–472.
2. Baldwin, K. M., and Winder, W. W. (1977). Adaptive response in different types of muscle to endurance exercise. *Ann. N. Y. Acad. Sci.* **301,** 411–423.
3. Burke, R. E., and Edgerton, V. R. (1975). Motor unit properties and selective involvement in movement. *In* "Exercise and Sport Sciences Reviews" (J. H. Wilmore, ed.), Vol. 3, pp. 31–81. Academic Press, New York.
4. Edgerton, V. R. (1978). Mammalian muscle fiber-types and their adaptability. *Am. Zool.* **18:** 113–125.

5. Gollnick, P. D., Armstrong, R. B., Saubert, C. W., IV, Piehl, K., and Saltin, B. (1972). Enzyme activity and fiber composition in skeletal muscle of untrained and trained men. *J. Appl. Physiol.* **33:** 312–319.

6. Gollnick, P. D., Timson, B. F., Moore, R. L., and Riedy, M. (1981). Muscular enlargement and number of fibers in skeletal muscle of rats. *J. Appl. Physiol.: Respir. Environ. Exercise Physiol.* **50:** 936–943.

7. Gollnick, P. D., and Saltin, B. (1982). Significance of skeletal muscle oxidative enzyme enhancement with endurance training. *Clinical Physiol.* **2:** 1–12.

8. Katz, A. M. (1977). "Physiology of the Heart." Raven Press, New York.

9. Macdougall, J. D., Sale, D. G., Moroz, J. R., Elder, G. G. B., Sutton, J. R., and Howard, H. (1979). Mitochondrial volume density in human skeletal muscle following heavy resistance training. *Med. Sci. Sports* **11:** 164–166.

10. Rifenberick, D. H. and Max, S. R. (1974). Substrate utilization by disused rat skeletal muscle. *Am. J. Physiol.* **226:** 295–297.

11. Roy, R. R., Meadows, I. D., Baldwin, K. M., and Edgerton, V. R. (1982). Functional significance of compensatory overloaded skeletal muscle. *J. Appl. Physiol.: Respir. Environ. Exercise Physiol.* **52:** 473–478.

12. Saltin, B., and Rowell, L. B. (1980). Functional adaptation to physical activity and inactivity. *Fed. Proc., Fed. Am. Soc. Exp. Biol.* **39,** 1506–1513.

13. Spector, S. A., Gardiner, P. F., Zernicke, R. F., Roy, R. R., and Edgerton, V. R. (1980). Muscle architecture and force-velocity characteristics of cat soleus and medial gastrocnemius: Implications for motor control. *J. Neurophysiol.* **44:** 951–960.

14. Walmsley, B., Hodgson, M. A., and Burke, R. E. (1978). Forces produced by medial gastrocnemius and soleus during locomotion in freely moving cats. *J. Neurophysiol.* **41:** 1203–1216.

CHAPTER 2

Cardiovascular Physiology of Exercise

RUSSELL T. DOWELL

Department of Physiology
University of Kansas
Medical Center
Kansas City, Kansas

I. OVERVIEW AND LIMITATIONS

In order to perform physical work of durations in excess of a few seconds, man is obligated to undergo a series of complex cardiovascular adjustments. The nature and magnitude of the required cardiovascular adjustments are determined by the overall work intensity, which, in turn, dictates the oxygen requirements for the skeletal muscles performing the work. Contracting skeletal muscles may utilize both aerobic and anaerobic energy-producing reactions, but the energy required for muscle contraction ultimately involves aerobic oxidation of fuel substrates and tissues eventually receive adequate amounts of oxygen. The by-products of metabolism must also be removed. Among metabolic by-products, considerable quantities of heat need to be dissipated to maintain "normal" environmental conditions within the organism. Thus, the cardiovascular system should be regulated such that the metabolic demands of working skeletal muscles are met. A full appreciation of the circulatory controls associated with muscular

19

Exercise Medicine: Physiological Principles
and Clinical Applications

exercise requires recognition of the unique and complex physiological integration that occurs. However, the potential complexity of exercise responses necessitates certain limitations in the present discussion. First, we will consider exercise responses which occur in normal, moderately fit, male individuals. We will not attempt to examine changes in circulatory control systems that may occur as the result of repetitive, regular bouts of exercise, i.e., exercise training. Finally, our attention will be confined to those exercise responses expected during light to moderate work intensities. Exhaustive exercise, or work performed in extreme conditions of heat, cold, or humidity are not considered.

II. MECHANISMS SUPPORTING SUBSTRATE OXIDATION DURING EXERCISE

Increased oxygen requirements of working muscles are met by (1) increasing the amount of blood flowing through the muscles, and (2) extracting more of the available oxygen in blood delivered to the tissues. Overall mechanisms that serve to increase the amount of blood pumped by the heart (cardiac output) will be addressed below. We now will focus our attention on the two factors regulating oxygen availability to muscle.

Under resting conditions, the amount of blood flowing through each gram of muscle is very low. Low flow rates are due to the high level of intrinsic tone of vascular smooth muscle in skeletal muscle blood vessels (18). During exercise, increased blood flow occurs as the result of factors that overcome normal vasoconstriction to yield blood vessel dilation. The autonomic nervous system is, undoubtedly, involved in this response, particularly in the first few seconds of exercise; however, local factors acting directly on vascular smooth muscle are much more important as work continues and a "steady state" is achieved (10,17,20). Among the factors contributing to local control of muscle blood flow are: (1) reduced tissue oxygen tension, (2) increased levels of carbon dioxide, (3) accumulation of lactic acid, and (4) release of intracellular potassium, histamine, and/or adenine compounds (adenosine) resulting from ATP hydrolysis. No single local factor can totally account for the degree of vasodilation that occurs during exercise (11), but reduced tissue oxygen tension and increased carbon dioxide levels appear to be most rapid and effective.

Because the volume capacity of the muscle vascular system when fully dilated exceeds total blood volume, profound vasodilation of the large vascular bed contained within skeletal muscle requires compensatory vasoconstriction in other vasculature so that blood may be diverted from organs that are either metabolically less active or whose function can be held in abeyance. In normal, resting humans, the visceral organs (heart, liver, kidney, spleen, and gastrointestinal tract) receive about 3.0 liters of blood per minute, the skin about 0.25

liters, and skeletal muscle about 1.0 liter (Fig. 1). During exercise, both the percentage of cardiac output and the actual blood flow volume are decreased below resting levels in the visceral organs (14), with the heart being the single obvious exception. Blood vessels in the skin initially constrict, but upon continued exertion, vascular dilation occurs as locally mediated mechanism divert blood to the skin, thus dissipating heat produced by repetitive muscular contractions. The simplest and most comprehensive mechanistic explanation for this exercise response would be a generalized activation of sympathetic nervous system discharge in all vascular beds, including working skeletal muscle vascular beds. Such activation would effectively divert blood flow via α-adrenergic receptor stimulation of vascular smooth muscle in resistance vessels (6); however, production and accumulation of local vasodilator metabolites would override the prevailing neural signals in the exact vascular beds and to the precise amount necessary to match blood flow volume with metabolic requirements. As an overall final result, the summation of local vasodilation in muscle together with vasoconstrictive diverting mechanisms in other organs increases blood flow through working muscles to a degree that allows muscle oxygen consumption to achieve a value 50–75 times that observed during resting conditions.

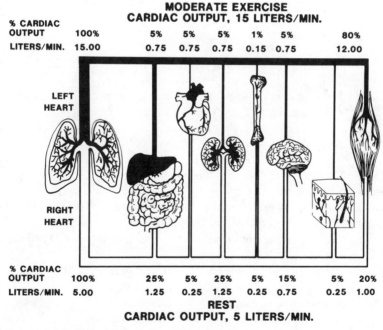

Fig. 1. Schematic drawing showing the relative distribution of blood flow to various organs during exercise. Modified from Astrand and Rodahl (1).

In addition to the delivery of greater volumes of blood to muscle, metabolic conditions within the working tissue facilitate delivery of oxygen to individual skeletal muscle cells. Increased rates of oxygen consumption in the active muscles lower tissue oxygen tension and elevate the oxygen gradient between blood and tissue. Increased carbon dioxide and lactic acid levels shift the hemoglobin–oxygen dissociation curve to the right so that more oxygen is available for diffusion into muscle cells at any given tissue oxygen tension. The cumulative result is to increase the amount of oxygen extracted from arterial blood, thereby widening the arteriovenous (A−V) oxygen difference. During exercise, skeletal muscle oxygen extraction may be increased to three times resting value. Combined influences of (1) a threefold increase in cardiac output, (2) a 10-fold increase in blood flow volume through muscle, and (3) a threefold increase in oxygen extraction permit oxygen delivery to working skeletal muscles that may be 90–100 times ($3 \times 10 \times 3 = 90$) as great as during rest. Thus, physiological mechanisms support the increased oxygen demanded by the metabolic reactions necessary to sustain muscle contraction during exercise (2).

III. CIRCULATORY REGULATION DURING EXERCISE

A. Cardiac Output

In order to deliver the additional oxygen required by contracting muscles, a coordinated response of the heart, resistance vessels, and capacitance vessels is necessary. From an overall functional viewpoint, the most important aspect of circulatory regulation during exercise is the attainment of an appropriate cardiac output. This cardiac output requirement is necessary, not only to increase blood flow to working skeletal muscles, but to adequately increase pulmonary blood flow and respiratory functions as well. At rest in the supine position, adult human cardiac output is 4–5 liters/minute. Cardiac output is slightly reduced when the individual assumes an upright posture due to hydrostatic effects and venous pooling. During exercise, cardiac output increases to a magnitude dependent on work intensity; however, cardiac output does not increase to the same extent as does metabolic rate or pulmonary minute ventilation. For example, with strenuous exercise, whole body oxygen consumption and alveolar ventilation may be increased approximately 24-fold with only an eightfold increase in cardiac output. Therefore, the fundamental circulatory response to exercise would be inadequate to sustain substrate oxidation in working muscles were it not for (1) selective increase in blood flow through the muscles, and (2) greater tissue extraction of available oxygen from the blood that is delivered.

B. Heart Rate and Stroke Volume

Increased cardiac output can be achieved by augmenting heart rate, stroke volume, or both constituents of cardiac output. Heart rate responses during light to moderate exercise accurately reflect the circulatory adjustments required for a given work intensity (Fig. 2). In light work, heart rate may increase to 100 beats/minute, to about 150 beats/minute during moderate work, and to 200 beats/minute or more in very strenuous work. The direct, linear relationship between heart rate and level of work intensity (Fig. 2) converts this simple physiological measurement into an extremely useful clinical tool for evaluating or monitoring patient exercise intensity. Heart rate acceleration begins immediately after exercise is initiated and may, in fact, precede the start of exercise (16). Heart rate is regulated by a complex mechanism involving both neural and humoral factors. Withdrawing inhibitory action of the parasympathetic nervous system (vagus nerve) could allow heart rate acceleration, but complete abolition of vagal influences by atropine produces a heart rate increase of only 30–40 beats/minute, whereas heart rate during exercise may increase by more than 100 beats/minute. Therefore, withdrawal of vagal inhibition cannot be the sole mechanism for elevating heart rate during exercise (6). Heart rate stimulation via the sympathetic nervous system is of equal, or perhaps even greater, importance. Circulating catecholamines emanating from the adrenal medulla and elevated body temperature also serve to increase heart rate (5).

Because enhanced cardiac output is the primary circulatory adjustment required during exercise, stroke volume regulation, as well as heart rate control, must be considered. Major factors influencing stroke volume are (1) the force of

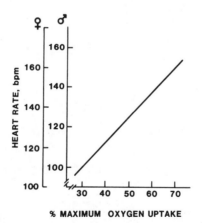

Fig. 2. Relationship between heart rate and work intensity during exercise. Modified from Astrand and Rodahl (1).

ventricular contraction, (2) the resistance in cardiac outflow vessels, and (3) venous return to the heart. Many of the same mechanisms that serve to increase heart rate concurrently increase the force of ventricular contraction. Sympathetic neural stimulation and circulating catecholamines effect marked enhancement of ventricular contractile force by stimulating the enzymatic activity [adenosine trophosphatase (ATPase)] of myocardial contractile proteins. Tachycardia itself may increase contractile element shortening velocity via the "treppe" or Bowditch effect. Sympathetic neural stimulation, circulating catecholamines, and the Bowditch effect all influence stroke volume via positive inotropy or increased ventricular contractility (12, 13). Enhanced contractility is an important cardiac compensatory mechanism during exercise when the physiological components of stroke volume are taken into consideration (3). Left ventricular stroke volume is defined as the difference between end-diastolic volume (LVEDV) and end-systolic volume (LVESV) (Fig. 3). LVEDV is a function of (1) venous return, (2) ventricular outflow resistance, and (3) ventricular filling time. Because ventricular filling occurs during the diastolic period and because diastole is attenuated during exercise due to tachycardia, stroke volume would decrease during exercise (Fig. 3B) were it not for a compensatory reduction in LVESV mediated by increased ventricular contractility (Fig. 3C). Reduced LVESV can either maintain or enhance stroke volume depending on the magnitude of the inotropic effect. It is clear, however, that the Frank–Starling mechanism can contribute little or nothing to stroke volume regulation during exercise under the conditions outlined above (15). In order to apply Starling's law to heart function, two basic conditions must be fulfilled. The first condition is that diastolic heart volume (LVEDV) must be increased with respect to resting LVEDV. The second conditions requires that the magnitude of heart emptying (LVESV) is maximal at rest and remains constant. Some early textbooks state

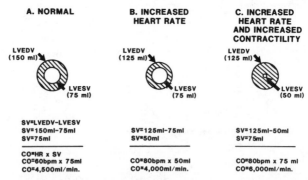

Fig. 3. Schematic illustration of heart rate effects on stroke volume and cardiac output in the presence or absence of increased contractility. LVEDV, left ventricular end-diastolic volume; LVESV, left ventricular end-systolic volume; SV, stroke volume; CO, cardiac output; HR, heart rate.

that LVEDV increases with exercise while LVESV is maintained constant via the increased force of ventricular contraction. The net result would be, of course, a substantial increase in stroke volume. However, modern measurement techniques have shown that diastolic heart volume does *not* increase, but actually decreases during exercise. Therefore, Starling's law cannot explain the increased force of ventricular contraction during exercise.

The final answer to the stroke volume response during exercise requires a distinction between sedentary and exercise trained individuals. The well conditioned (exercise trained) person has a lower resting heart rate as well as an attenuated increase in heart rate during comparable intensities of exercise. Despite slower heart rates, cardiac output is equivalently augmented due to an increase in stroke volume resulting from enhanced reduction in LVESV. In contrast, a sedentary individual's stroke volume does not increase from the value measured at rest in the *supine* position and cardiac output increases during exercise due to an increase in heart rate with little or no increase in stroke volume.

C. Blood Pressure, Systemic Resistance, and Venous Return

Systemic blood pressure is the product of cardiac output and total peripheral vascular resistance. Enhanced cardiac output during exercise would be expected to proportionately elevate blood pressure due to the systemic resistance encountered; however, total peripheral resistance is significantly reduced due to the vasodilation of skeletal muscle vascular beds (21). Thus, the greater oxygen delivery to working muscles can be achieved by elevating cardiac output without imposing a severe pressure load on the heart. Systolic blood pressure does increase, particularly during severe exercise (8), but seldom exceeds 180 mm Hg in normotensive individuals. Diastolic pressure is only slightly elevated (4), yielding a small elevation in mean arterial blood pressure. It should be noted that the exercise blood pressure response described above is that typically observed for dynamic, endurance-type work involving large muscles, e.g., running or cycling (22). Intensities of physical work eliciting significant increases in cardiac output may be achieved during either anaerobic, isometric-type work, or exercise involving relatively small muscle mass (19), e.g., work using only the arms. Under these circumstances, (1) local vasodilatory mechanisms are less effective, (2) total peripheral resistance is *not* reduced to the same extent, and (3) dramatic elevations in mean arterial blood pressure occur. Increased ventricular afterloading and attendant myocardial effects can be anticipated under these circumstances.

During exercise, the extreme vasodilation in skeletal muscle beds coupled with increased blood delivery to these vascular beds would result in significant blood pooling and compromised venous return if appropriate compensatory mechanisms were not engaged. Because veins are thin walled, easily collapsible structures possessing valves to permit flow of blood *only* toward the heart, when muscles surrounding veins contract, blood contained in the veins is compressed. The "backward" flow of blood, i.e., flow toward the capillaries, is prevented by the venous valves, and resulting muscular contraction forces blood flow toward the right atrium. Subsequent muscle relaxation allows the veins to refill with blood, thus creating a "massaging action" of rhythmically contracting muscles that assists venous return to the heart. Naturally occurring ventilatory movements during exercise also promote blood flow from the dependent portions of the body. Large abdominal and thoracic veins constitute a reservoir containing 400–500 ml blood. Valves of the femoral veins and valves of the jugular and subclavian veins create a closed system. During forced inspiration, the thoracic cavity is expanded, resulting in a fall in intrathoracic pressure. Diaphragmatic contraction simultaneously increases intra-abdominal pressure. Because the right atrium is the outlet path of least resistance in this case, venous return to the heart is enhanced by the resulting increase in driving pressure. Alternating inspiration and expiration establishes a "pumping" effect functionally analogous to that seen with skeletal muscle contraction. Massaging actions of skeletal muscles and pressure changes associated with ventilatory movements serve as "booster pumps" to promote venous return during exercise. In addition, sympathetic nervous system mediated stimulation of capacitance vessels occurs (7). This "tightening" of the venous system reduces vascular capacitance, thus aiding venous return by improving venous flow conductance to assure efficient blood transport to the right atrium.

IV. SUMMARY

Performance of muscular exercise requires the activation of coordinated circulatory controls. Enhanced oxygen requirements of working skeletal muscles are met by (1) increasing cardiac output, (2) preferential diversion of blood to working muscles, and (3) extracting greater quantities of oxygen from arterial blood. Appropriate cardiac output levels are attained by elevating heart rate while maintaining stroke volume despite compromised diastolic filling time. Constant stroke volume occurs by facilitating ventricular contractility to reduce end-systolic volume. Peripheral vascular mechanisms of exercise involve (1) reduced total peripheral resistance via local metabolic factors to prevent severe elevations in mean arterial blood pressure, and (2) sympathetic nervous system mediated reduction in venous capacitance in concert with muscle and respiratory "pump" mechanisms promote venous return to the heart. In short, circulatory adjustments during exercise are qualitatively and quantitatively appropriate to meet the metabolic demands imposed on the organism.

REFERENCES

1. Åstrand, P.-O., and Rodahl, K. (1977). "Textbook of Work Physiology, Physiological Bases of Exercise," 2nd ed. McGraw-Hill, New York.
2. Bevegard, B. S., and Shepherd, J. T. (1967). *Physiol. Rev.* **47,** 178–213.
3. Braunwald, E., Sonnenblick, E. H., Ross, J., Jr., Glick, G., and Epstein, S. E. (1967). *Circ. Res.* **20,** Suppl. 1, 44–58.
4. Clausen, J. P., Klausen, K., Rasmussen, B., and Trap-Jensen, J. (1973). *Am. J. Physiol.* **225,** 675–682.
5. Donald, D. E., Ferguson, D. A., and Milburn, S. E. (1968). *Circ. Res.* **22,** 127–134.
6. Donald, D. E., and Shepherd, J. T. (1964). *Am. J. Physiol.* **207,** 1325–1329.
7. Duggan, J. J., Love, V. L., and Lyons, R. H. (1953). *Circulation.* **7,** 869–873.
8. Ekelund, L. G., and Holmgren, A. (1967). *Circ. Res.* **20,** Suppl. 1, 33–43.
9. Folkow, B., Haglund, U., Jodal, M., and Lundgren, O. (1971). *Acta Physiol. Scand.* **81,** 157–163.
10. Guyton, A. C., Jones, C. E., and Coleman, T. G. (1973). "Circulatory Physiology: Cardiac Output and its Regulation," 2nd ed., Saunders, Philadelphia, Pennsylvania.
11. Haddy, F. J., and Scott, J. B. (1968). *Physiol. Rev.* **48,** 688–707.
12. Keul, J., Dickhuth, H. H., Simon, G., and Lehmann, M. (1981). *Circ. Res.* **48,** Suppl. 1, 162–170.
13. Newman, G. F., Rerych, S. K., Upton, M. T., Sabiston, D. C., Jr., and Jones, R. H. (1980). *Circulation* **62,** 1204–1211.
14. Rowell, L. B. (1974). *Physiol. Rev.* **54,** 75–159.
15. Rushmer, R. F. (1959). *Am. J. Physiol.* **196,** 745–750.
16. Rushmer, R. F., and Smith, O. A. (1959). *Physiol. Rev.* **39,** 41–68.
17. Rushmer, R. F., Smith, O., and Franklin, D. (1959). *Circ. Res.* **7,** 602–627.
18. Shepherd, J. T. (1967). *Circ. Res.* **20,** Suppl. 1, 70–81.
19. Shepherd, J. T., Blomqvist, C. G., Lind, A. R., Mitchell, J. H., and Saltin, B. (1981). *Circ. Res.* **48,** Suppl. 1, 179–188.
20. Skinner, N. S., Jr., and Powell, W. J. (1967). *Circ. Res.* **20,** Suppl. 1, 59–67.
21. Smulyan, H., Cuddy, R. P., Vincent, W. A., Kashemsant, U., and Eich, R. J. (1965). *J. Appl. Physiol.* **20,** 437–442.
22. Wolthius, R. A., Froelicher, V. F., Fischer, J., and Triebwasser, J. H. (1977). *Circulation* **55,** 153–157.

CHAPTER 3

Pulmonary Physiology
of Exercise

DANIEL C. DUPONT AND ALLAN P. FREEDMAN
Division of Pulmonary Diseases
Hahnemann University School of Medicine
Philadelphia, Pennsylvania

I. INTRODUCTION

The pulmonary system is a vital part of the body's integrated physiological response to exercise. The lungs serve as the site of oxygen uptake and carbon dioxide excretion. Oxygen is then transported to the peripheral tissues by the cardiovascular system and carbon dioxide is similarly transported back from the tissues to the lung (Fig. 1). Finally, skeletal muscle utilizes the increased supply of oxygen to generate ATP for energy production at the mitochondrial level. Carbon dioxide is produced as a by-product of substrate metabolism. After

29

Exercise Medicine: Physiological Principles
and Clinical Applications

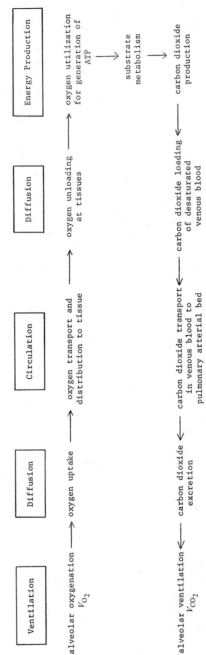

Fig. 1. The consumption of oxygen and excretion of carbon dioxide links several physiological systems.

briefly reviewing pertinent resting pulmonary physiology, we will describe the response of the lung to the demands of exercise.

II. RESTING PULMONARY PHYSIOLOGY

Although the lung has many physiological and metabolic functions, its role in energy output for physical performance centers on oxygen uptake and carbon dioxide removal. Mindful that there is more to pulmonary physiology than gas exchange, we can focus on this area.

A. Ventilation

Total movement of gas by the lung is usually expressed as the expired minute ventilation ($\dot{V}_E$). $\dot{V}_E$ is the product of tidal volume (V_T) and respiratory frequency (f). Tidal volume can be divided into that portion of gas that reaches the alveoli for respiratory exchange and that which occupies the anatomic dead space and nonperfused alveoli. The former is referred to as the alveolar ventilation (V_A) and the latter as dead space ventilation (V_D). Dead space ventilation does not participate in gas exchange with the circulation. V_D/V_T, the ratio of the dead space ventilation to tidal volume, is an expression of the efficiency of alveolar ventilation. Normally, V_D/V_T is close to 0.3, but this ratio increases as ventilation and perfusion become less well matched. The tension of carbon dioxide in arterial blood or expired gas is a rather pure indicator of the ventilatory function of the lungs. This is because carbon dioxide is so readily diffusable across the alveolar–capillary membrane that ventilation rather than membrane transfer is the limiting factor in its excretion.

B. Oxygen Uptake

At any given fraction of inspired oxygen (F_IO_2), there is a pressure gradient for oxygen from the atmosphere to the alveolus to the pulmonary capillary. A gradient in the opposite direction exists for carbon dioxide. It is important to realize that carbon dioxide tension affects alveolar oxygen tension in a reciprocal fashion and may be thought of as diluting the oxygen partial pressure. That is, the higher the partial pressure of CO_2 in the alveolus (P_ACO_2), the lower the partial pressure of alveolar O_2 (P_AO_2). The normal alveolar– arterial (or alveolar–capillary) gradient for oxygen is due both to the membrane diffusion barrier that oxygen must traverse and the fact that a small fraction of blood bypasses the alveolus and is therefore not well oxygenated. This bypass or shunt normally consists of the small quantity of blood in the bronchial circulation and blood traversing the zone of relatively underventilated alveoli. As we shall see, altera-

tion of both ventilation/perfusion relationships and diffusion effect the alveolar–arterial gradient for oxygen.

C. Carbon Dioxide Excretion

The amount of carbon dioxide produced and the amount of oxygen consumed
are frequently expressed relative to one another. The respiratory quotient (RQ) is
the ratio of CO_2 production divided by O_2 consumption. At rest, there are
approximately 200 ml of carbon dioxide produced and 250 ml of oxygen consumed per minute when a diet with normal carbohydrate content is utilized,
giving an RQ of 0.8. If the metabolic fuel is altered (i.e., high carbohydrate diet)
or anaerobic metabolism is necessary, more carbon dioxide is produced per
quantity of oxygen consumed. Thus the respiratory quotient increases, approaching or exceeding unity.

D. Distribution of Ventilation and Perfusion

The entire cardiac output flows through the lungs. This is pumped from the
right ventricle through the low resistance, high compliance pulmonary vascular
bed. However, blood flow is distributed in a regional fashion. The bases of the
lung are preferentially perfused in an upright person due to the influence of
gravity. There is a reactive smooth muscle population in both the pulmonary
vessels and air sacs. This smooth muscle dilates and constricts to alter blood flow
and ventilation on a regional basis. In health, the body attempts to match perfusion and ventilation for the most efficient gas exchange. The concept of ventila-
tion/perfusion matching as well as the abnormalities of shunt and wasted ventilation are depicted in Fig. 2.

E. Control of Ventilation

Control of overall pulmonary ventilation may be even more complex than
regulation of local ventilation. It involves integration of physical, chemical, and
neural stimuli on both a voluntary and involuntary basis. The control of breathing
incorporates central automatic respiratory centers, peripheral chemoreceptors for
oxygen, and both central and peripheral receptors for CO_2 and hydrogen ion
concentration. This multifactorial system closely matches oxygen consumption
and carbon dioxide excretion to body metabolism.

The brainstem contains several regions for involuntary automatic control of
breathing. The upper pons contains a pneumotaxic center that integrates neural
impulses to encourage rhythmic respiration. In the lower pons, the apneustic
center stimulates an inspiratory reflex based on vagal, sensory, and chemical
stimuli. The upper and lateral regions of the medulla contain chemoreceptors that

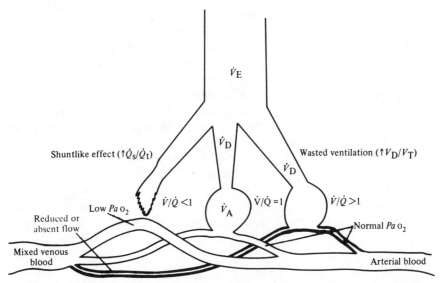

Fig. 2. Ventilation–perfusion relationships: Shuntlike effect and wasted ventilation represent imbalances between ventilation and perfusion. "Ideally" there is precise matching of alveolar ventilation and arterial perfusion ($\dot{V}/\dot{Q} = 1$). The dead space ventilation ($\dot{V}_D$) is the small quantity of air in the proximal tracheobronchial tree. When regions are well ventilated but poorly perfused as shown on the right, there is wasted ventilation with alveolar air adding to the dead space; gas exchange is inefficient. When regions are well perfused but poorly ventilated, there is impaired gas exchange with blood traversing the pulmonary system without being oxygenated (shunt).

respond to hydrogen ion concentration in the surrounding cerebrospinal fluid. The lower medulla harbors a respiratory center specialized in coordinating rhythmic inspiration and expiration. Finally, the brainstem output is modulated by the cerebral hemispheres on a voluntary basis. These respiratory centers are networks of neurons and synaptic relays that evaluate and precisely respond to the body's metabolic status with proportionate gas exchange.

Several systems are present peripherally that supply sensory input to the brainstem respiratory centers. The carotid and aortic bodies are chemoreceptors located in the arterial circulation that respond to decreased oxygen tension and increased carbon dioxide tension in the arterial blood that bathes these nests of cells. Whereas hypoxemia and hypercarbia individually cause the carotid and aortic bodies to increase ventilation, both in combination result in an even greater ventilatory response. Hydrogen ion concentration also affects respiration. Besides the brainstem response to alteration in CSF hydrogen ion concentration, there is believed to be a peripheral response to pH alterations mediated by the carotid and aortic bodies that is independent of the CO_2 tension.

In addition to these peripheral chemoreceptors there are various respiratory stimuli that originate directly from the lungs. Although multiple bronchopulmonary reflexes affecting respiration exist, only several are important in ventilatory control. The inflation reflex, initially described by Herring and Breuer, is an inhibitory reflex generated by distension of the lung. This may be important in regulating the depth and frequency of ventilation so as to minimize the energy used by respiratory muscles for any given minute ventilation. The receptors are located in the smooth muscle of the tracheobronchial tree and a vagal pathway to the brain stem has been demonstrated. A second reflex involving the lung utilizes the J (or juxtapulmonary capillary) receptor located in the interstitium. It elicits an increase in the depth and rate of breathing in response to pulmonary congestion and so-called "capillary hypertension."

This brief discussion of normal physiology and control of breathing is meant to serve only as an introduction to the response of the pulmonary system to exercise. Table I lists many of the variables discussed and gives average values for an

TABLE I

Some Important Terms in Resting Pulmonary Physiology

Term	Definition
Ventilation	
Respiratory frequency (f)	Breaths per minute
Tidal volume (V_T)	Volume of gas per breath
Minute ventilation ($\dot{V}_E$)	Volume of gas expired in 1 minute
Distribution of ventilation and perfusion	
Alveolar volume (V_A)	Volume of each breath that reaches perfused alveoli
Dead space volume (V_D)	Volume of each breath not involved in gas exchange (distributed in airways and nonperfused alveoli)
Dead space tidal volume ratio (V_D/V_T)	Fraction of each breath that occupies dead space
Pulmonary blood flow ($\dot{Q}$)	Cardiac output from right heart
"Shunt" ($\dot{Q}_s/\dot{Q}_T$)	The ratio of shunt blood flow to total blood flow; the fraction of blood that passes from right side of heart to left without being oxygenated
Ventilation–perfusion ratio ($\dot{V}/\dot{Q}$)	The matching of alveolar and capillary units (high $\dot{V}/\dot{Q}$ = wasted ventilation; low $\dot{V}/\dot{Q}$ = shunt effect)
Respiratory gas exchange	
Oxygen consumption ($\dot{V}_{O_2}$)	Volume of oxygen transferred to circulation per minute
Carbon dioxide production ($\dot{V}_{CO_2}$)	Volume of carbon dioxide excreted from circulation per minute
Respiratory quotient (RQ)	Ratio of oxygen utilized to carbon dioxide produced

adult male at rest. Selected texts and monographs are referenced for the interested reader (1–6).

III. EXERCISE PULMONARY PHYSIOLOGY

With increasing muscular work, there is a parallel increase in oxygen demand and carbon dioxide production. The normal pulmonary response to muscular exercise is a precise integration of changes necessary to satisfy these increased demands.

A. Progressive Exercise

What happens as workload is gradually increased? The consequent increase in oxygen demand is met by an increase in minute ventilation. The slope of the curve in Fig. 3 relating minute ventilation to oxygen consumption is the ventilatory equivalent, a measure of ventilatory efficiency. This is expressed as $\dot{V}_E/\dot{V}O_2$; at

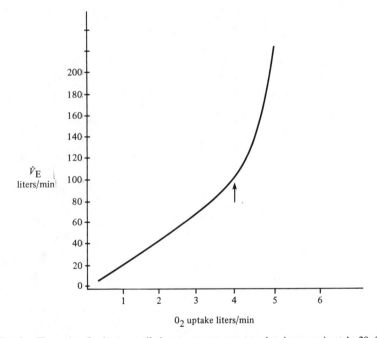

Fig. 3. The ratio of minute ventilation to oxygen consumption is approximately 20–25 liters/liter/minute at rest and low work rates. This ratio approaches 35 liters/liter/minute at maximal work rates. The point (arrow) where the slope of the curve increases approximates the onset of anaerobic metabolism, when ventilatory demand is increased by CO_2 requirements.

rest it is approximately 20–25 liters of minute ventilation per liter of oxygen consumed (7). The point at which the slope of the curve changes represents the anaerobic threshold. At work loads requiring oxygen consumption greater than this level, anaerobic metabolism is relied on for some of the energy production. Pyruvate, the end product of anaerobic glycogenolysis, accumulates and is converted to lactate. The attendant acidemia is mostly buffered by serum bicarbonate and CO_2 is generated. A further increase in ventilation becomes necessary to excrete this additional carbon dioxide and $\dot{V}_E/\dot{V}_{O_2}$ increases. The anaerobic threshold normally occurs at approximately 60% of the maximal oxygen consumption ($\dot{V}_{O_2}$ max).

B. Steady-State Exercise

What happens if a constant level of exercise is maintained? Changes in oxygen consumption during light and heavy exertion are described in Fig. 4. There is an immediate increase in oxygen consumption in response to muscular work. After an increase to steady-state levels, it is maintained throughout the period of exertion. After exercise is terminated, oxygen consumption does not immediately return to resting levels. The initial rise in oxygen consumption lags behind the tissue requirements and thus an oxygen deficit is created. Oxygen stores are limited. As the oxygen bound to hemoglobin, dissolved in plasma, and contained in myoglobin is depleted, tissue oxygen delivery falls. Metabolism then becomes anaerobic and lactate production from glycogenolysis becomes significant. After exercise has ceased, the pulmonary system must still maintain above normal gas

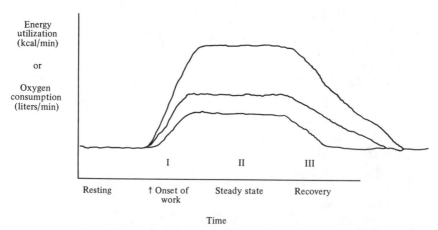

Fig. 4.   Oxygen consumption and energy utilization during exercise. There is a rapid increase in oxygen consumption with the onset of muscular work (I). This is followed by attainment of a steady-state oxygen consumption (II). With termination of exercise there is a variable period of increased oxygen consumption and energy utilization to repay the oxygen debt and replenish oxygen stores (III). The three curves demonstrate increasing work levels.

exchange not only to replete the body's oxygen stores and substrates required for synthesis of high energy phosphate bonds (ATP, ADP, phosphocreatine, etc.), but also to excrete the additional carbon dioxide generated from lactate production. The recovery period during which oxygen debt is repaid is demonstrated in Fig. 4. It is apparent that alterations in resting pulmonary physiology may persist after the actual period of muscular work, depending on its duration and severity (8).

The rapid initial response to exercise is of variable duration, as shown in Fig. 4. In light work, such as walking, this phase is less than 1 minute while in demanding physical exertion it may be up to 10 minutes. Acceleration in oxygen uptake lags behind peripheral oxygen utilization due to the time required for circulating hemoglobin to unload its oxygen and return to the pulmonary system. During this period, aerobic stores are exhausted and glycogen is utilized anaerobically. Oxygen consumption plateaus when equilibrium between uptake and utilization of oxygen is at a steady state. The oxygen deficit initially created is not repleted during this steady-state period (8). The final "recovery phase" is characterized by delayed return of oxygen uptake to resting levels. This variable period of apparently excessive oxygen uptake is necessary to restock the depleted oxygen stores. The time required for recovery of basal oxygen stores can be as long as the actual period of increased work. The aerobic cost of exercise is the amount of oxygen required to perform a task. It can be measured as the total increase in oxygen utilization over resting levels during both exercise and recovery.

C. Mechanics of Increased Ventilation

Increases in minute ventilation are accomplished by alterations in both the respiratory frequency and tidal volume. At low levels of work, the increase in tidal volume is the major component. With progressive increase in work level, the tidal volume plateaus at approximately half the vital capacity (the maximal amount of gas that can be exhaled in a single breath) while respiratory rate continues to increase up to 50 breaths/minute (9). At rest, the expiratory phase of respiration is greater than the inspiratory phase. With increasing respiratory frequency, there is a reduction in the expiratory phase such that the ratio of inspiration to expiration approaches one. This pattern of minute ventilation has been shown to be the most efficient balance of volume and rate for least energy expenditure. Respiratory muscle oxygen consumption usually remains less than 1 ml oxygen/liter minute ventilation, even at maximal work (10).

D. Increase in Efficiency of Gas Exchange

During exercise there are also alterations in alveolar O_2 tension, alveolar–capillary diffusion, and matching of ventilation and perfusion. These adaptations optimize gas transport. The partial pressure of oxygen in the alveolus rises when ventilation exceeds requirements for O_2 supply at higher exercise levels (i.e., above anaerobic threshold). As ventilation rises to levels necessary for elimination of excess CO_2, there is hyperventilation with respect to oxygen requirements (11).

Diffusing capacity is also increased. The transfer of gas from capillary to alveolus is achieved entirely by this passive diffusion. Carbon dioxide is readily diffusable across the alveolar-capillary membrane and its excretion is usually assured by appropriate increases in minute ventilation. Oxygen uptake across this membrane is dependent on more than minute ventilation since the "diffusability" of oxygen is only one-twentieth that of carbon dioxide. During work, the overall diffusion "capacity" of the lung increases for several reasons. There is widening of the partial pressure gradient from alveolus to deoxygenated blood as alveolar P_{O_2} rises and the P_{O_2} in mixed venous blood falls from increased oxygen extraction. Also there is an increase in the surface area available for gas transfer in the lung (12). More alveoli are being ventilated and increased pulmonary blood flow has enlarged the pulmonary capillary bed.

In addition to alterations in alveolar oxygen tension and diffusing capacity, there is less wasted ventilation. Vascular pressures in the pulmonary system increase only slightly during exercise, even at high work rates. The small increase in pulmonary vascular pressure that occurs from increased cardiac output does result in a greater portion of blood flow being distributed to the normally underperfused apical regions of the lung. These upper lobe regions now approach a more normal ventilation perfusion ratio (13). Despite the more rapid transit through the pulmonary capillary bed as heart rate increases, capillary flow and alveolar ventilation are still in "contact" for an adequate period (0.5 seconds) for alveolar and capillary P_{O_2} to equilibrate (14).

Another mechanism for reduction in the amount of wasted ventilation (V_D/V_T) during exercise is the increase in tidal volume (15). A healthy male at rest has a tidal volume of approximately 500 ml, of which dead space comprises 150 ml (giving a V_D/V_T ratio of 0.3). With increasing tidal volumes during muscular work, dead space also increases but at a slower rate. At a relatively large tidal volume of 1500 ml, the total dead space may be only 300 ml (giving a V_D/V_T ratio of 0.2). Table II compares resting and maximal exercise values in a typical healthy adult male.

E.   Control of Breathing during Exercise

The importance of appropriate ventilation for oxygen demand and CO_2 production in exercise is clear. If ventilation is insufficient for the level of muscular work, carbon dioxide accumulates and acidemia occurs. This results in altered cellular function, especially in the heart and central nervous system. Of equal

TABLE II

Pulmonary Response to Exercise in a Healthy Adult Male[a]

Parameter	Rest		Maximal work
Respiratory rate (f)	10	per minute	50 per minute
Tidal volume (V_T)	0.6	liters	3.2 liters
Minute ventilation ($\dot{V}_E$)	6	liters per minute	160 liters per minute
Oxygen consumption ($\dot{V}_{O_2}$)	0.25	liters per minute	4.57 liters per minute
Carbon dioxide production ($\dot{V}_{CO_2}$)	0.20	liters per minute	.52 liters per minute
Respiratory exchange quotient (RQ)	0.79		1.21
Ventilatory oxygen consumption	6	ml per liter per minute	120 ml per liter per minute
Wasted ventilation (V_D/V_T)	0.30		0.12
Pulmonary blood flow ($\dot{Q}$)	4	liters per minute	26 liters per minute
Pulmonary artery mean pressure ($\overline{PA}$)	14	mm Hg	27 mm Hg
Alveolar-arterial oxygen gradient	10	mm Hg	30 mm Hg

[a] Values shown are the results of a maximal work effort by a healthy adult male. The maximal values are frequently expressed with the designation max, e.g., $\dot{V}_{O_2}$ max, $\dot{V}_{CO_2}$ max, $\dot{V}_E$ max.

importance is the avoidance of hyperventilation with consequent hypocapnia and alkalemia that also alter cellular function. It is therefore not surprising that in submaximal exercise, the P_{CO_2} and, therefore, the pH are maintained in the normal range. Even above anaerobic threshold, lactate production causes a component of metabolic acidosis, but compensatory respiratory alkalosis maintains pH in the normal range. Alkalemia is uncommon in exercise, and acidemia, while occurring at maximal work levels, is relatively mild. Significant acidemia may, however, occur in altered respiratory or neurological states; these will be considered in future chapters.

The mechanisms of respiratory control during exercise have been the subject of intensive investigation. Controversy still remains about several issues, particularly the feedback mechanism for preservation of near normal blood gases during submaximal work (16). As shown in Fig. 5, the relationship between minute ventilation and CO_2 production is linear throughout its entire range. Not only is the increase in minute ventilation directly proportional to CO_2 production, but it appears to be almost immediate. Several reflexes have been found that contribute to such precise coordination of minute ventilation with CO_2 production. These include the carotid body chemoreceptors, peripheral muscular and

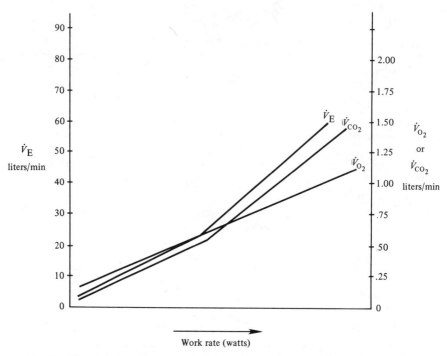

Fig. 5. The relationship of minute ventilation ($\dot{V}_E$), oxygen consumption ($\dot{V}_{O_2}$), and carbon dioxide production ($\dot{V}_{CO_2}$) to work. Note that whereas oxygen consumption increases linearly, CO_2 production and minute ventilation increase more rapidly relative to work when anaerobic metabolism occurs.

thoracic mechanoreceptors, the medullary respiratory center, and a "missing link" (17).

It is instructive to examine the steady-state response to exercise, described by DeJours and others as having two phases (18). At the onset of any given level of increased muscular activity there is an immediate ventilatory adjustment. Although the mechanism for this acute ventilatory response remains controversial several explanations appear plausible. The first is that proprioceptive stimulation from the muscles of exercise (especially the extremities) travels through a neural reflex leading to "exercise hyperpnea" (19). A second explanation for this fast ventilatory response proposes an as yet undiscovered "missing" mechanism that rapidly matches rate of ventilation with carbon dioxide delivery to the lung (17). Wasserman suggests that specific receptors may exist in the arterial circulation that rapidly respond to CO_2 tension and pH changes.

The second, latent phase of respiratory response described by DeJours appears to occur mainly at high work rates. This component is responsive to carbon dioxide tension and is felt to be mediated through the carotid body chemoreceptors. In subjects exercising at work levels above anaerobic threshold, elevation in P_{CO_2} appears to drive the ventilatory response (20). The role of the carotid bodies in mediating this has been demonstrated by the limited ventilatory response to exercise in subjects with surgically removed carotid bodies (21). In addition to the well known insensitivity to hypoxemia that occurs after carotid body resection, response to CO_2 elevation is blunted.

To summarize, the control of respiration appears to be multifactorial and dependent on both peripheral and central stimuli. The regulation of CO_2 tension and pH is rapid and precise throughout the range of exercise. Receptors in the carotid body, peripheral muscles, and arterial circulation appear to modulate this response.

F. The Pulmonary System and Maximal Oxygen Uptake

To conclude this review of the pulmonary aspects of exercise, it is appropriate to compare the role of the lung with that of the cardiovascular and muscular systems. When considering muscular exercise for any significant duration (greater than 10–15 minutes), the limiting factor is the maximal oxygen uptake (22). This "aerobic capacity" for work depends on the individual's age, sex, and body habitus, as well as his physical condition. Limitation to aerobic capacity may be a function of the oxygen transport system (the heart and lungs) or the oxygen utilizing system (the muscles). In examining the oxygen transport system and its limitations three phases can be considered: ventilatory capacity of the lungs, the diffusion of oxygen into blood, and the cardiovascular transport of oxygen. The role of the pulmonary system in oxygenation and ventilation has been presented. When viewed in relation to the cardiovascular aspects of oxygen transport and the muscular phase of exercise, the lungs do not normally limit work capacity. Rather the circulation, both systemic and local, appears to set the limit in the healthy individual. Exercise limitation caused by problems with ventilation or oxygen delivery to the red blood cell constitutes perturbed physiology. These problems will be the topic of Chapter 12.

REFERENCES

1. Cherniack, R. M., Cherniack, L., and Naimark, A. (1972). "Respiration in Health and Disease," 2nd ed. Saunders, Philadelphia, Pennsylvania.
2. Comroe, J. H., Jr. *et al.* (1962). "The Lung: Clinical Physiology and Pulmonary Function Tests." 2nd ed. Year Book Med. Publ. Chicago, Illinois.
3. Comroe, J. H., Jr. (1974). "Physiology of Respiration," 2nd ed. Year Book Med. Publ., Chicago, Illinois.
4. West, J. B. (1974). "Respiratory Physiology-The Essentials," 2nd ed. Williams & Wilkins, Baltimore, Maryland.

5. Bouhuys, A. (1974). "Breathing: Physiology, Environment and Lung Disease." Grune & Stratton, New York.

6. Jones, N. L., and Campbell, E. J. M. (1982). "Clinical Exercise Testing," 2nd ed. Saunders, Philadelphia, Pennsylvania.

7. Åstrand, P. O., and Rodahl, K. (1977). "Textbook of Work Physiology," 2nd ed., p. 228. McGraw-Hill, New York.

8. Asmussen, E. (1965). Muscular exercise. *In* "Handbook of Physiology" (W. D. Fenn and H. Rahn, eds.), Sect. 3, Vol. 2, pp. 939–978. Am. Physiol. Soc., Washington, D.C.

9. Åstrand, P. O., and Rodahl, K. (1977). "Textbook of Work Physiology," 2nd ed., p. 233. McGraw-Hill, New York.

10. Demsey, J. A., and Rankin, J. (1967). Physiologic adaptations of gas transport systems to muscular work in health and disease. *Am. J. Phys. Med.* **46,** 582–647.

11. Asmussen, E., and Nielsen, M. (1960). Alveolo-arterial gas exchange at rest and during work at different 02-tensions. *Acta Physiol. Scand.* **50,** 153–166.

12. Gledhill, N., Froese, A. B., and Dempsey, J. A. (1977). Ventilation to perfusion distribution during health and disease. *In* "Muscular Exercise and the Lung" (J. A. Dempsey and C. E. Reed, eds.), pp. 325–342. Univ. of Wisconsin Press, Madison.

13. West, J. (1962). Regional differences in gas exchange in the lung of erect man. *J. Appl. Physiol.* **17,** 893–898.

14. Johnson, R. L., Spicer, W. S., Bishop, J. M., and Forster, R. E. (1960). Pulmonary capillary blood volume, flow and diffusing capacity on exercise. *J. Appl. Physiol.* **15,** 893–902.

15. Wasserman, K., Van Kessel, A. L., and Burton, G. G. (1967). Interaction of physiological mechanisms during exercise. *J. Appl. Physiol.* **22,** 71–85.

16. Berger, A. J., Mitchell, R. A., and Severinghaus, J. W. (1977). Regulation of respiration. *N. Engl. J. Med.* **297,** 194–201.

17. Wasserman, K. (1978). Breathing during exercise. *N. Engl. J. Med.* **298,** 780–785.

18. Dejours, P. (1965). Control of respiration in muscular exercise. *In* "Handbook of Physiology" (W. O. Fenn and H. Rahn, eds.), Sect. 3, Vol. 1, pp. 631–648. Am. Physiol. Soc., Washington, D.C.

19. Farber, J. P., and Bedell, G. N. (1973). Responsiveness of breathing control centers to CO2 and neurogenic stimuli. *Respir. Physiol.* **19,** 88–95.

20. Kozlowski, S., Rasmussen, B., and Wilkoff, W. G. (1971). The effect of high oxygen tensions on ventilation during severe exercise. *Acta Physiol. Scand.* **81,** 385–395.

21. Wasserman, K., Whipp, B. J., Koyal, J. N., and Cleary, M. G. (1975). Effect of carotid body resection on ventilatory and acid-base control during exercise. *J. Appl. Physiol.* **39,** 354–358.

22. Mitchell, J. H., and Blomquist, G. (1971). Maximal oxygen uptake. *N. Engl. J. Med.* **284,** 1018–1022.

CHAPTER 4

Exercise Metabolism

PAUL A. MOLÉ
*Department of
Physical Education
Human Performance
Laboratory
University of
California
Davis, California*

This chapter summarizes the principal elements of exercise metabolism in man and provides a critical analysis of the major features of (1) phosphocreatine, carbohydrate, and fat metabolism during exercise; (2) the chronic effects of endurance exercise training on carbohydrate and fat metabolism during exercise; and (3) some dietary–exercise interactive effects on metabolism of body proteins, fats, and carbohydrates.

I. ENERGY METABOLISM DURING AND FOLLOWING EXERCISE

A. The Fuel for Muscle Contraction

The energy for muscle contraction arises from the hydrolysis of adenosine triphosphate (ATP) to adenosine diphosphate (ADP) and inorganic phosphate

43

Exercise Medicine: Physiological Principles
and Clinical Applications

(P_i), that is,

$$ATP^{4-} \rightarrow ADP^{3-} + HPO_4^{2-} + H^+ \qquad (1)$$

As shown, the process is entirely anaerobic in that the utilization of oxygen is not involved. The ATP store in muscle is relatively small amounting to about 6 μmoles/g wet weight of muscle (14). This small quantity of ATP can sustain only a few muscle contractions. So a tight coupling between ATP utilization and production must occur to sustain work for more than a few seconds. Both anaerobic and aerobic metabolic processes of ATP production are involved.

1. ANAEROBIC METABOLISM

Anaerobic ATP can occur via coupling the end product of contraction ADP to (a) adenylate kinase reaction

$$2 \, ADP^{3-} \rightarrow ATP^{4-} + AMP^{2-} \qquad (2)$$

in which both ATP and adenosine monophosphate (AMP) are formed; (b) creatine kinase reaction

$$ADP^{3-} + PC^{2-} + n \, H^+ \rightarrow ATP^{4-} + Cr \qquad (3)$$

where phosphocreatine (PC) is another high-energy phosphate store which can be split to form ATP and creatine (Cr); (c) anaerobic glycolysis, which is another pathway in which muscle glycogen is degraded to lactic acid by a number of enzymatic steps with ATP synthesized in the process by substrate-level phosphorylation of ADP.

The adenylate kinase and creatine kinase enzymes are located in the immediate vicinity of the contractile proteins and both can respond very rapidly to any change in muscle [ADP]. Therefore, activities of both enzymes can readily change to increase ATP production at the onset of muscular contractions when ATP is split to ADP. The PC store in muscle is limited, however, amounting to 15–20 μmoles/g muscle. So the capacity for maintaining anaerobic ATP production by PC splitting alone is limited too. The capacity for anaerobic metabolism is greatly extended by the slower process of anaerobic glycolysis. In muscle, glycolysis can be coupled to the resynthesis of PC via its ATP formation and the creatine kinase reaction as

$$0.5 \text{ glycogen unit} + 1.5 \, Cr + 1.5 \, P_i^{2-} \rightarrow \text{lactate}^- + H^+ + 1.5 \, PC^{2-} (4)$$

The net effect of this coupling is to maintain the ATP supply, with some fall in muscle PC and some increase in muscle lactate. If no other mechanism for ATP production were available, then lactacidosis would continue to develop and muscle would stop contracting when its acid maximum is reached. However, ATP also can be produced by aerobic metabolism.

2. OXIDATIVE METABOLISM

Aerobic ATP production occurs via oxidative phosphorylation in mitochondria of muscle involving the consumption of oxygen and the production of carbon dioxide and water as varying proportions of long-chain fatty acids, glycogen, glucose, ketones, and amino acids are oxidized.

3. PARTITION OF ENERGY TRANSFER KINETICS

A schematic for the partition of the energy transfer rate kinetics is presented in Fig. 1 for moderately intense exercise such as cycling or running. Curve 1 illustrates the net rate of utilization of phosphagen, that is, the high-energy phosphate stores comprising the sum of muscle ATP and PC. As shown, phosphagen utilization begins at the onset of exercise at a rate equal to the energy transfer rate required, and then rapidly falls exponentially to a net rate of zero shortly after about 1 minute into exercise. This means any additional phosphagen utilization is balanced by its resynthesis via coupling the creatine kinase reaction with anaerobic glycolysis [Eq. (4)] and oxidative ATP production. Anaerobiosis attributed to lactate production is illustrated by curve 2. It shows net lactate production begins at zero, rises quickly to a peak rate at about 15 seconds into the exercise, and then falls toward zero again. This pattern of response for anaerobic glycolysis can be quite different than shown here, depending on circumstances to be considered later. Curve 3 represents the kinetic response of aerobic fuel utilization. In this regard, it reflects the net rate of O_2 consumption due to the oxidation of various fuels. The curve shows net oxidative metabolism begins at zero and then rises toward an apparent asymptote or steady value that can be equal to or less than the energy requirement, depending on several factors to be described below.

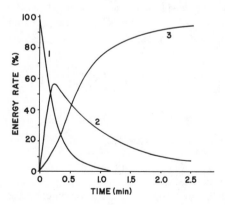

Fig. 1. Schematic of energy transfer kinetics. Net energy equivalents arising from phosphagen (curve 1), anaerobic glycolysis (curve 2), and aerobic fuel utilization (curve 3).

B. Phosphagen Metabolism

Our knowledge of the chemical changes occurring in various muscles of exercising man has been greatly expanded since Bergström (13) introduced the needle biopsy technique. We consider here the essential findings on phosphagen utilization during exercise and its resynthesis during recovery from exercise.

1. PHOSPHAGEN UTILIZATION DURING EXERCISE

After about 2 minutes of exercise, the phosphagen concentration in quadriceps muscle has been shown to be reduced to a constant value relative to rest, with the change proportional to the work rate for bicycle ergometer exercise (14,92). Most of the phosphagen used is phosphocreatine, but there are some ATP stores also used during the early phase of exercise. As implied by curve 1 of Fig. 1, net consumption of phosphagen stores occurs immediately at the onset of exercise and is terminated once other sources of ATP production attain a level that satisfy the contemporary ATP requirement. Regardless of the intensity or duration of exercise, the net phosphagen stores used in the early part are not resynthesized later in the exercise (14,91,92). This finding suggests that when ATP production and utilization attain a new steady state during exercise, new equilibria for the creatine kinase [Eq. (3)] and adenylate kinase [Eq. (2)] reactions are attained. However, the study of this problem by Sahlin et al. (129) showed only the apparent equilibrium constant for creatine kinase (K'_{ck}) increases; that for adenylate kinase was not changed. Because of cellular compartmentalization and the difficulty of identifying the free species of the reactants, it is impossible to explicitly evaluate the mechanism for the increase in K'_{ck}. Of the several possibilities, the alteration of intracellular pH and change in that portion of ADP and ATP which is available to creatine kinase enzyme likely are most important for affecting K'_{ck}. Sahlin et al. (129) found the changes in intracellular pH of muscle is highly related ($r = 0.92$, $n = 34$) to K'_{ck}, that is, the theoretical expression for the equilibrium constant of creatine kinase, when transformed to solve for pH, is

$$pH = -\log \frac{[Cr]\,[ATP]}{[PC]\,[ADP]} + \log K$$

$$pH = -\log(K'_{ck}) + \log K \tag{5}$$

and the relationship actually found was

$$pH = -0.42 \log[K'_{ck}] + 7.38 \tag{6}$$

This finding and the fact that K'_{ck} for adenylate kinase was not observed to change suggested to them the new equilibrium established for creatine kinase during exercise is determined mainly by the change in intracellular pH. That is, H^+ ion activity increases in muscle soon after the onset of exercise, due primarily to lactate production (80), and helps to drive the creatine kinase reaction [Eq. (3)] to the right. The result is a new steady state, achieved with muscle PC maintained at a lower level throughout the remainder of exercise. The net amount of PC used during exercise is proportional to the work rate (14). PC is resynthesized back to its preexercise level only during the recovery period.

2. PHOSPHAGEN RESYNTHESIS DURING RECOVERY FROM EXERCISE

The rate of PC resynthesis appears to be slower at the offset than PC splitting at the onset of exercise (14,58), although it should be noted that data are rather limited. In a study by Saltin *et al.* (131), repeated biopsies taken over short intervals of bicycle exercise at 275 W were obtained for one subject. Based on these data, the calculated half-time for PC splitting is about 10 seconds. In contrast, Harris *et al.* (58) found PC resynthesis could be described by a double exponential, with the half-time for the fast recovery component of 21 seconds and for the slow component of 173 seconds, for 4 men during recovery from bicycle exercise at a mean work of 301 ± 23 W. The slow component appears to be related to the slow return of muscle H^+ to the rest level (58).

There is some uncertainty as to the metabolic processes coupled to PC resynthesis during recovery from exercise. As shown by Eq. (4), PC resynthesis is primarily coupled to anaerobic glycolysis immediately after the onset of exercise where anaerobiosis is the predominant energy-yielding process. At present, it is not known to what extent this coupling diminishes and is replaced by PC resynthesis via the mitochondrial creatine kinase reaction coupled to ATP production via oxidative phosphorylation. It is likely that PC turnover is increased during exercise. Since lactate production, after a transient peaking, diminishes as oxidative metabolism attains a steady level in mild to moderate exercise, it is also likely that the coupling of PC resynthesis shifts from the anaerobic to aerobic mechanism. If this holds true, it means PC resynthesis during recovery from exercise is primarily coupled to oxidative metabolism. Evidence to support this view has been obtained by Harris *et al.* (58), in that they found muscle PC did not change if blood flow to the leg was occluded following exercise; only when circulation was intact was PC resynthesis complete, thereby implying primary dependence on oxidative resynthesis of PC. Thus, additional anaerobic glycolysis during recovery would not be required for restoring muscle PC to the rest level.

C. Lactate Metabolism

1. INTRODUCTION

Three recent publications on this subject are Hultman and Sahlin (80), Moret *et al.* (107), and DiPrampero (35).

Lactate as a product of muscle contraction was first identified by Berzelius in 1807 (110). Lactic acid is the end product of anaerobic glycolysis in which the final enzymatic step catalyzed by lactic dehydrogenase (LDH) is

$$\text{Pyruvate}^- + \text{NADH} + \text{H}^+ \rightleftharpoons \text{lactate}^- + \text{NAD} + \text{H}^+ \tag{7}$$

Lactate production is important in energy metabolism of exercising man in three ways. First, as indicated earlier, it provides a means for anaerobic ATP production. Second, lactate production is an important mechanism in regulating the redox potential of the muscle sarcoplasm through changes in the NAD/ NADH ratio [Eq. (7)]. Third, lactate is an important substrate for oxidative metabolism and for glucose production via gluconeogenesis in other tissues during exercise. We will consider these aspects of lactate metabolism in the following discourse. In addition, the impact of lactate metabolism on acid–base will be considered.

2. LACTATE PRODUCTION IN MUSCLE

Lactate production in muscle provides a means for anaerobic ATP production, with a net formation of 2 ATP per glucose or 3 ATP per glycosyl unit used. In this way, it helps to maintain the supply of ATP and CP in active muscle during the initial transient period (Fig. 1) when anaerobic energy transformations are the predominant processes. It greatly extends the ATP producing power of the performer's muscles beyond that of aerobic metabolism so that much higher exercise intensities can be attained for a longer period of time (35).

Exercise physiologists agree that lactate production increases with the intensity of exercise and all agree that some lactate is formed during the initial, non-steady-state phase of exercise. Moreover, there is a consensus that for severe exercise, where the energy requirement exceeds the aerobic capacity for ATP production (maximum $\dot{V}_{O_2}$), lactate production quickly attains a rate that is virtually proportional to work rate (35). But there is disagreement as to whether net lactate production is sustained in some active muscle fibers once steady state $\dot{V}_{O_2}$ below the subject's maximum is attained. There are two views on this problem which are based on blood lactate concentration. One view, originating with Hill and Lupton (69) and currently championed by Margaria (104) and co-workers (20,35), is that net lactate formation is not sustained at submaximal exercise intensities, that is, for exercise requiring a rate of energy transfer less than that equivalent to max $\dot{V}_{O_2}$, sustained net lactate production is zero. This occurs when blood lactate is constant or falling as exercise continues. The most recent summary of the evidence and arguments for this point of view has been published by DiPrampero (35). The second view is that there exists an "anaerobic threshold" (AT), unique for each performer, at some submaximal work intensity below max $\dot{V}_{O_2}$, which represents the onset of the imbalance between lactate production and removal (146,147). This AT is represented by the onset of a change in blood lactate which can be sustained eventually at some constant level.

Our views on this problem will become apparent in the course of the following discussion.

Controversy exists even after 150 years of study because (1) the problem of lactate metabolism in exercising man is complex; (2) it is not readily possible to measure the rate of lactate production in specific muscle fibers; and (3) we do not really know how the various factors influencing lactate metabolism actually operate *in vivo* during exercise in man. Therefore, it is difficult to ascertain the real meaning of blood lactate changes during exercise.

There are several lines of evidence supporting the view that lactate production exists at all levels of exercise. Studies on the metabolism of radioactively labeled lactate in dogs by Eldridge (36) and Issekutz *et al.* (85), and in man by Jorfeldt (88), reveal that lactate turnover exists both at rest and during exercise. Even at rest, the tissue concentrations of lactate are maintained above zero by a balance between production and removal. Major contributors of blood lactate at rest are erythrocytes, muscle, brain, and leukocytes, with muscle providing about 35% of the amount of lactate entering the blood each minute (80). Thus, at least some skeletal muscles produce lactate when man is at rest.

In the resting state, the rate of lactate removal is proportional to moderate increases in blood lactate concentration brought about by constant infusion (36,85). During prolonged moderate exercise, the same relationship holds, but the removal is about three times greater per unit change in lactate concentration (36, 85), that is, lactate clearance from the blood is enhanced with exercise. Also, clearance is enhanced for exercise even if the concentration of blood lactate is not increased above the rest level. Jorfeldt (88) found a large fraction (52%) of lactate taken up was oxidized at the same time that lactate was produced and released from exercising forearm muscles. Similarly, Issekutz *et al.* (85) and Depocas *et al.* (33) observed oxidation of lactate accounted for about 56 and 75%, respectively, of the lactate turnover. As did Jorfeldt, Issekutz was led to conclude that during mild exercise active muscle produces and releases lactate to the blood at the same time it is taking up and oxidizing lactate from blood. Further, Jorfeldt (88) observed the rate of lactate release from working forearm muscles was time dependent, with release greater at 10 minutes than that at 40 minutes of exercise. This complexity of lactate metabolism of active muscle can be explained in the following way. Skeletal muscles in man are composed of various types of motor units, each with fibers having unique enzymatic, metabolic, and local circulatory characteristics (see Chapter 1). At the onset of exercise, there is a great dependence on anaerobic glycolysis, as revealed by curve 2 of Fig. 1, for the muscle fibers recruited. In addition, there is likely recruitment primarily of fast-glycolytic (FG) motor units initially (57). These two factors combine to give a high lactate production and release from mixed muscle early in exercise. As work continues, there is a decreased demand for anaerobiosis as oxidative metabolism rises toward its steady value (Fig. 1). Also, the recruitment of FG units decreases with time as they are replaced by fast-oxidative-glycolytic (FOG) and slow-oxidative (SO) units (57). The latter units have a greater capacity to take up and oxidize lactate. The combined effect is that lactate production decreases with time and the amount released from mixed muscle not only decreases for this reason, but also because now more of the active units can take up and oxidize the lactate produced and released from other units. In this way, it is possible to have lactate being produced and released in some fibers while others are taking up and oxidizing lactate in an active mixed muscle, with perhaps no change in blood lactate concentration.

Obviously, anaerobic glycolysis is contributing to the energetics of some of the fibers but not others in active mixed muscle, even in mild exercise. Conceivably, differences in motor unit composition, recruitment pattern, and intensity of activity of different active muscles could mean some muscles are in lactate balance, whereas others have a net production and release, and still others have a net uptake and oxidation of lactate during even mild to moderate exercise. To my knowledge, data are not available to quantitatively assess these possibilities. In the following discourse, lactate metabolism is considered in which only the average net responses of mixed muscle are revealed.

3. LACTATE ACCUMULATION IN AND RELEASE FROM ACTIVE MUSCLES

Mixed muscle, sampled with a needle biopsy, contains about 1.0 mmole/kg wet weight of lactate or about 1.3 mmoles/liter muscle H_2O in the resting state. With severe exercise, lactate can attain a concentration of 25–30 mmoles/kg. Although such a change in muscle lactate is taken to represent a dramatic rise in lactate production, it represents in reality an imbalance between production and release from muscle. Both of these processes are functions of time as well as intensity of exercise. These complications and the fact that a means is not available for measuring the active muscle mass associated with a concentration change make it difficult to ascertain the contribution of anaerobic glycolysis to energetics of exercise in man as a whole.

At low work rates, muscle lactate rises to a peak and then falls and returns to the rest level or attains an elevated level, depending on the intensity of exercise and the fraction of aerobic capacity (% maximum $\dot{V}_{O_2}$) elicited by the exercise. For example, Karlsson et al. (93) showed that lactate starts to accumulate in muscle at a relative work load of about 50–55% maximum $\dot{V}_{O_2}$ in untrained subjects. Presumably, below this intensity any transient net lactate production at the onset of exercise leads to oxidative lactate removal in the muscle so that the energetics of lactate metabolism in muscle and the body as a whole can be considered as representing complete oxidation of carbohydrate (CHO). This supposition is consistent with the findings that exercise below this relative intensity does not result in significant release of lactate from muscle (95) and accumulation in blood (93).

Exercise eliciting a $\dot{V}_{O_2}$ greater than 50–55% maximum $\dot{V}_{O_2}$ results in the accumulation of lactate in muscle and blood as shown by Karlsson *et al.* (93). In general, the accumulation of lactate in these tissues is a power function of work rate or percentage maximum $\dot{V}_{O_2}$; that is, lactate accumulation increases approximately as a quadratic function of work rate or percentage maximum $\dot{V}_{O_2}$ (91,95), but the relationship is not constant because there is a time dependency as well. The intensity–time relations have not been fully evaluated mathematically. There is some evidence (11,91,132,145) that between about 50 and 75% maximum $\dot{V}_{O_2}$, lactate accumulation rises to a peak and then falls to an elevated level above rest as exercise continues, with the decline from the peak diminishing as the intensity approaches about 75% maximum $\dot{V}_{O_2}$. Supposedly, in this range of work levels, a new steady state is attained between the rate of production and removal of lactate in the various tissues of the body. In active muscle, there is an increase in the release of lactate with an increase in work intensity in this range, and the lactate release appears to be related to lactate concentration in muscle (80,89). Up to about a fourfold increase in muscle lactate concentration, there is a linear increase in lactate efflux rate from muscle to a maximum of 4–5 mmoles/minute per leg (89). So below this limit, production ultimately can be matched to efflux of lactate from working muscle, thereby permitting muscle lactate to attain a new steady state level. As far as muscle energetics is concerned, anaerobic energy production from lactate starts before the capacity for aerobic energy production is fully utilized. In my opinion, an "anaerobic threshold" for muscle metabolism occurs when there exists a sustained lactate efflux which develops perhaps at about 25–50% maximum $\dot{V}_{O_2}$, well below any sustained change in blood lactate (blood lactate threshold).

Exercise requiring a $\dot{V}_{O_2}$ of 70–80% maximum $\dot{V}_{O_2}$, or greater, involves increases in lactate production rates without further changes in lactate efflux rate in muscle. In this case, lactate accumulates in active muscle in a disproportionate fashion with work intensity because production increases without a change or even a decrease in efflux. Further, lactate accumulation is time dependent through the exercise period. Clearly, at any point during such exercise, contemporary changes in muscle lactate are not reflected in proportional changes in blood lactate once the transport limit is achieved, and a steady state between muscle and blood lactate cannot be achieved.

The blood is an open system with respect to lactate so the amount of this metabolite accumulating in this tissue is determined by the balance between influx and efflux processes. Translocation in both directions appears to involve passive mediated transport of lactate in that the process reveals saturation kinetics (80). Moreover, lactate efflux from muscle is complicated by its apparent dependency on intracellular and extracellular pH and bicarbonate concentrations (70,102,137). Essén *et al.* (40) have shown lactate is released from muscle during work when glycogen content is "normal," but is taken up by muscle when its glycogen content is low. Further, the concentration gradient for lactate alters the efflux of lactate from working muscle (88); the higher the blood lactate level the lower the efflux rate. In addition to the enzymatic profiles of the muscle cells, it is also likely that local blood flow and the rate of oxidation of the fibers also influence the amount of lactate released from the mixed muscle to the blood. These complexities for muscle lactate efflux clearly illustrate the difficulty of using blood lactate as an index for the existence or nonexistence of anaerobic glycolysis in working muscles. The problem is compounded further when processes for lactate removal from blood are considered.

4. LACTATE ACCUMULATION IN AND EFFLUX FROM BLOOD

The removal of lactate from the blood during exercise involves oxidation, glyconeogenesis and excretion. Below about 75% maximum $\dot{V}_{O_2}$, the rate of lactate removal is roughly proportional to the relative work rate (percentage maximum $\dot{V}_{O_2}$); therefore, it is approximately linearly related to steady-state cardiac output and oxygen consumption of the exercise. So in addition to the blood lactate concentration dependency already mentioned earlier, lactate removal is also influenced by the amount of lactate delivered to tissues (flow times concentration) and perhaps the metabolic rate of the tissues. More than half of the lactate eliminated from blood is oxidized during submaximal exercise (33,85,88). By far skeletal muscles, both active and inactive, are the major tissues involved in oxidative removal of blood lactate. Heart also uses lactate as a substrate for oxidation (95), as can liver and kidney, during exercise in man, but their quantitative contributions to whole body oxidative removal of lactate are considered minor relative to that of skeletal muscle at least over the first 40 minutes of exercise (80).

Studies on splanchnic removal of lactate in man at rest and during exercise suggest very little is oxidized and most is used to form glucose via gluconeogenesis. At rest about 14–15% of hepatic glucose output arises from lactate (78,113,144). For exercise lasting up to about 40 minutes, most of the three- to fourfold increase in hepatic glucose output arises from glycogen degradation, with a 2.5- to threefold increase in lactate uptake relative to that at rest (144). Although hepatic glucose output is related to submaximal work intensity, hepatic lactate uptake is not, and is probably related to the progressive reduction in blood flow to the liver which occurs as exercise intensity increases (142). This finding and the likelihood that flow to the kidneys also decreases in a similar fashion to that of the liver support the contention that oxidative lactate removal is the predominant process during the first 40 minutes of exercise and it occurs primarily in active and nonactive skeletal muscles. With prolonged, submaximal exercise up to 240 minutes, gluconeogenesis becomes progressively more important in contributing to hepatic glucose production as glycogen stores and glycogenolysis diminishes (5). Hepatic lactate uptake increases with a greater fractional extraction, particularly at 240 minutes of exercise. This finding and the observation (76) that lactate uptake and gluconeogenesis from lactate is markedly enhanced during exercise when the subjects have been on a CHO-poor diet illustrate the point that blood lactate removal due to splanchnic metabolism is strongly influenced by the dietary state of the individual and metabolic state of the liver with respect to its glycogen store and ability for glycogenolysis.

Lactate is removed from circulation by the kidney and could involve oxidation, gluconeogenesis, and urinary excretion. To my knowledge, there are no measurements of lactate uptake by the kidney during exercise in man. Only small amounts of lactate are excreted in urine at resting arterial lactate levels (31, 37,86,98) and most of the loss appears to arise from "new" production by the kidney itself (37). There is tubular reabsorption of filtered lactate so little lactate is lost to the urine at blood concentrations below 5–6 mmoles/liter (34). Only above this blood level is there increasing quantities of filtered lactate lost in urine. Thus, tubular transport of lactate has a maximum just as found for lactate efflux from muscle (89). This transport maximum and the fact that renal blood flow becomes markedly reduced as exercise intensity is increased (148), just as occurs for hepatic flow, could help to limit the clearance of lactate from blood. Thus, blood lactate could increase not only because there is enhanced influx, but also because there is a decreased efflux.

5. THE MEANING OF THE BLOOD LACTATE THRESHOLD

The blood lactate threshold is determined by the onset of a sustained rise in blood lactate concentration above the rest value. This threshold usually develops at about 55–60% maximum $\dot{V}_{O_2}$ for exercise lasting 20 minutes or longer. Shorter exercise bouts, where steady-state lactate production and fluxes between compartments are not achieved, could elicit a rise in blood lactate below this threshold. It should be realized, therefore, that the threshold is not necessarily an invariant property of the performer, since it is dependent on the intensity–time profile of the exercise test used, as well as the dietary and acid–base status of the individual, among others.

Obviously, the onset of blood lactate accumulation means there develops at this point an imbalance between influx and efflux rates in blood. From the foregoing evidence presented, it is clear the threshold does not mark the onset of muscle lactate production; lactate production exists at rest in a variety of tissues, including muscle, and it increases in active muscles for all mild to moderate exercise intensities studied. A threshold for lactate production, therefore, does not exist. The older view of the failure of blood lactate concentration to increase during mild to moderate exercise below the threshold as meaning the nonexistence of lactate production in the body is incorrect. ATP production arising from anaerobic glycolysis exists for some working muscle fibers under all exercise loads. Whether there is net ATP production from anaerobic glycolysis for the whole mixed muscle during exercise depends on whether there is net efflux of lactate from that muscle. This likely occurs well below the 55–60% maximum $\dot{V}_{O_2}$ work level before muscle and blood lactate begin to accumulate, because the efficiency of lactate removal from these tissues is markedly enhanced by the increase in perfusion within and between various organ systems and by their increased metabolism (33,36,85). Thus, increased lactate efflux from active muscle and blood occurs without a change in lactate concentration. In this case, the onset of change in muscle and blood lactate concentrations signifies the initiation of neither net lactate production nor net ATP production from anaerobic glycolysis in working muscle.

The law of conservation of mass and energy dictates net anaerobic glycolysis contributes to energy metabolism of exercise for the body as a whole when there is sustained lactate accumulation in the body which usually occurs above the blood lactate threshold of 55–60% maximum $\dot{V}_{O_2}$. Whether the lactate accumulated accounts for all of the anaerobic glycolytic contribution to the energetics depends on the energy balance between production and removal of lactate. As mentioned earlier, more than 50% of blood lactate removed during exercise involves oxidation. So this portion of lactate production can be considered as part of whole body carbohydrate oxidation. That is, although a portion of muscle energetics involves ATP production from anaerobic glycolysis, this part of the energetics of exercise for the whole body represents carbohydrate oxidation. A large part of the remaining lactate, which is metabolically removed, involves gluconeogenesis. This process requires energy which ultimately is derived from oxidative metabolism. Although there is uncertainty regarding the quantification of various aspects of gluconeogenesis relevant to the problem considered here (121), it is reasonable to assume as a first approximation that no significant gain in ATP occurs for the fraction of lactate production involved in gluconeogenesis in the body as a whole. In this case, any net loss of lactate carbon would be accounted for by net glucose oxidation. Thus, below the lactate threshold any net carbohydrate used by the body can be assumed to be accounted for by carbohydrate oxidation, since any small amount of lactate removed not included with oxidation and gluconeogenic fractions can be neglected. To the extent that these simplifications are reasonable, the lactate threshold in blood could signify when net anaerobic glycolysis begins to contribute significantly to the energetics of exercise in the body as a whole. Under no circumstances, however, does it represent the onset of net lactate production in working muscle.

Although it is not possible to adequately quantify the contribution that lactate production and removal processes make to the disproportionate rise in muscle and blood lactate that develop above the threshold as work intensity is increased, it does appear that both aspects of lactate metabolism are involved. It would appear that lactate production dramatically increases at work loads above the threshold. This could develop because of a disproportionate recruitment of the fast-glycolytic motor units combined with an intensification of firing frequency of the motor units involved as increased amounts of force are needed with increasing power output of exercise (108). Also, as exercise increases above the performer's lactate threshold the efficiency of lactate removal becomes progressively impaired. In working muscle, the efflux rate reaches its limit and H^+ ion activity and lactate concentrations rise, thereby enhancing the accumulation of lactate in working muscle. Further, progressively more circulation is diverted from inactive muscles and splanchnic tissues and in this way delivery of lactate to these tissues is not increased in proportion to the rise in blood lactate. This coupled with a decrease in fractional extraction by removal sites such as the liver (at least for the first 40 minutes of exercise) likely contribute to the impairment in the efficiency of lactate removal by the performer at work intensities above his threshold. Thus, blood lactate accumulates dramatically.

6. H^+ ION ACTIVITY AND ANAEROBIC FUEL UTILIZATION

H^+ ion activity and anaerobic fuel utilization have recently been considered (107). Therefore, the following discourse will focus on elements essential to understanding the extent to which pulmonary CO_2 production ($\dot{V}O_2$) is a measure of oxidative fuel utilization.

As illustrated in Eq. (3), the creatine kinase reaction for ATP production involves the removal of n H^+ ions/PC used, with the number of ions, n, actually consumed depending on the pH (107). Relatively more H^+ ions are taken up by the CK reaction as the pH falls. The CK reaction produces a relative alkalinization at the onset of exercise as it is the predominant ATP-producing process. Then, as anaerobic glycolysis comes into play shortly after the beginning of exercise, it becomes functionally coupled to the CK reaction as shown by Eq. (4). This effectively reverses the alkalinization process to one of net H^+ ion formation which then leads to a relative acidification of working muscle.

A theoretical presentation of these events in working muscle is shown by the schematic for the kinetics of H^+ ion change in Fig. 2 for two cases. Curve A represents the H^+ ion response for exercise above the lactate threshold, say at 80% maximum $\dot{V}O_2$, where there is a sustained net lactate production and release from working muscle and a sustained accumulation of lactate in muscle and blood once $\dot{V}O_2$ attains a steady value. Curve B is for milder exercise below the lactate threshold at say 30% maximum $\dot{V}O_2$, where muscle and blood lactate concentration changes are not sustained at steady-state $\dot{V}O_2$. The CK reaction and anaerobic glycolysis interact as described above to produce the kinetic changes in H^+ ion.

That this schematic is a reasonable presentation of the H^+ ion response is suggested by the research of Steinhagen et al. (137), where they showed the equivalent pattern of change for interstitial pH of working gastrocnemius muscle of the dog. As they pointed out, the change of interstitial pH could be caused by rapid permeation of H^+, OH^-, CO_2, and HCO_3^- across the muscle cell mem-

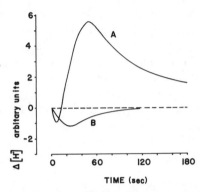

Fig. 2. Schematic of net hydrogen ion activity in active muscle. Curve A is theoretical response at 80% maximum $\dot{V}o_2$; curve B is for exercise at 30% maximum $\dot{V}o_2$.

brane. The most likely candidate, however, is CO_2 because it can rapidly move across membranes (1). In this case, CO_2 exchange across the working muscle cell membranes becomes a complex process involving oxidative CO_2 production and bicarbonate-derived CO_2 production arising from changes in intracellular and extracellular H^+ ions. As yet, we cannot distinguish quantitatively between these processes for CO_2 production. I suppose the onset of mild exercise involves a rapid influx of CO_2 into working muscle such that there occurs a relative retention of CO_2 in the body; that is, there is relatively less CO_2 loss from the lungs than expected from oxidative CO_2 production at the onset of mild exercise because the H^+ consumed by PC splitting causes the bicarbonate buffer system to be driven to the right of Eq. (8).

$$H_2O + CO_2 \rightleftharpoons H_2CO_3 \rightleftharpoons H^+ + HCO_3^- \qquad (8)$$

This relative retention of CO_2 is rapidly reversed as lactic acid production comes into play; with the magnitude of the reversal and the time course of change in CO_2 reflected by the kinetics of H^+ ion response shown in Fig. 2. Thus, the reversal would mean relatively more CO_2 is produced and lost from the body than predicted from oxidative fuel utilization in the later stages of exercise where there is CK coupling with anaerobic glycolysis. To the extent that this coupling is continued during exercise, there would be bicarbonate-derived CO_2 production contributing to pulmonary CO_2 exchange. This becomes particularly evident at exercise intensities above the blood lactate threshold in that pulmonary CO_2 excretion becomes increasingly inadequate to compensate for H^+ ion production and release from working muscle to blood; blood pH drops even though there is bicarbonate-derived CO_2 excreted by the lungs because the ventilatory mechanism is not capable of completely compensating for H^+ accumulation. There must be an increasing proportion of pulmonary CO_2 production arising from bicarbonate-derived CO_2 formation in this situation. These considerations raise the question as to the extent that working muscle gas exchange ratio and ventilatory gas exchange ratio at the lungs ($R = \dot{V}_{CO_2}/\dot{V}_{O_2}$) accurately reflect only the oxidative fuel mixture.

D. Oxidative Fuel Utilization

1. INTRODUCTION

It is a dictum in bioenergetics that the energy transformed in the body in response to physical exercise ultimately arises from the combustion of the three major foodstuffs, including mixtures of fats, carbohydrates, and proteins, when the exercise as well as the recovery period is considered. Some of the energy transformed by combustion is contemporary to the exercise and represents the oxidation of primarily fat and carbohydrate stores, with a minor fraction due to catabolism of body proteins and subsequent oxidation of the derived amino acids. The remainder of the energy derived from combustion occurs during complete recovery from the exercise and represents the energy required to re-synthesize fuel stores used during exercise and the ill-defined alterations in metabolic processes involved in the adaptive responses induced by the exercise. The latter, for example, include the prolonged changes in metabolic rate (12). Complete recovery requires consumption of food.

The simultaneous assessment of whole body net oxidation of fats, carbohydrates, and proteins from body stores requires measurements of O_2 consumption, CO_2 production, and nitrogen (N) production under steady-state conditions. This means the stores of O_2, CO_2, and urea N are not changing so that O_2 uptake by and losses of CO_2 and N from the body represent only the dynamics of oxidative metabolism. Although this steady-state condition can be readily satisfied over relatively long periods of measurement in the resting state, the case for an equivalent steady state for the exercise condition apparently has never been verified, except on a 24-hour basis for prolonged mild exercise in which both exercise and recovery over this period were assessed (8a,9). The fundamental question remains as to whether moment to moment measures of CO_2 and N excretion from the body represent the contemporary oxidative CO_2 production and N production, respectively. This question is particularly relevant for exercise intensities above the blood lactate threshold because (1) there are dynamic changes in acidification of body compartments, thereby altering the CO_2 stores in the body, and (2) there are dramatic shifts in the distribution of blood flow away from skin and the splanchnic bed which alters sweat gland N excretion and modifies liver and kidney functions related to N metabolism and excretion. These problems of CO_2 and N excretion not representing contemporary combustion are markedly exaggerated in the transition from rest to exercise where it is obvious the required steady-state condition cannot be satisfied. We raise these issues here because indirect calorimetry has been and continues to be the fundamental method of assessing oxidative fuel utilization of exercise in the body as a whole and it is the reference for which data on oxidation and substrate exchange within and between organ systems are interpreted. Yet, the concerns raised about the potential non-steady-state nature of CO_2 and N excretion have not been universally recognized and/or have not been adequately considered. Because of this unfortunate development, we will attempt to show some of the important interpretations concerning oxidative metabolism of exercise based on R ($\dot{V}_{CO_2}/\dot{V}_{O_2}$) have not been entirely justified. We begin by considering R data since it is one of the fundamental measurements most often used to assess the oxidative fuel mixture of exercise metabolism.

2. CRITIQUE OF SOME FUNDAMENTAL CONCEPTS

Current theory states the primary fuels sustaining oxidative metabolism of working muscles are long-chain fatty acids mobilized from lipolysis of triglycerides in adipocytes, muscle glycogen, and blood glucose. Amino acid and ketone oxidation can and do contribute to muscle energetics, but it is thought their involvement is minor. The specific contribution of these fuels, however, is determined by (1) the immediate and long-term intake of mixtures of carbohydrates (CHO), proteins (PRO), and fats (FAT); (2) the time during exercise when measurements are made; (3) the intensity of the exercise relative to the aerobic capacity of the performer; and (4) the endurance trained state of the performer. There are important effects of ambient temperature and altitude on exercise metabolism, but these are not considered here. We will first describe the general character of each of these relations as can be found in standard texts on exercise physiology (8).

For calorically adequate diets, the composition of the foodstuffs establishes the metabolic mixture (the oxidative fuel mix of metabolism) at rest and for mild exercise. Here we consider only CHO and FAT mix in the diet using the ventilatory exchange ratio ($R = \dot{V}_{CO_2}/\dot{V}_{O_2}$) as a measure of the metabolic mixture. When all the oxidation arises from FAT, the R is 0.707 and conversely when only CHO is oxidized the $R = 1.00$. A R of 0.854 would represent an equal mix of FAT and CHO oxidation. The classical studies of Benedict and Cathcart (12), Krogh and Lindhard (96), and Christensen and Hansen (25) clearly illustrate the relationship between FAT and CHO composition in the diet and R. They showed the higher the dietary CHO composition, the higher the R at rest and during prolonged mild exercise on the bicycle ergometer. Conversely, the higher the FAT content in the diet, the lower the R for rest and exercise. So, as reflected by average R, the apparent oxidative fuel mix of both rest and mild exercise was shown to be established by dietary intake of FAT and CHO; high dietary CHO intake produced a larger fractional CHO oxidation for both rest and exercise conditions. It is also significant to note that the metabolic mixture was found to be virtually the same for rest and mild exercise. So although diet changes the fuel mix, mild to moderate intensities of exercise do not, at least over the first 20–40 minutes of exercise.

What is the time course for R during prolonged, mild exercise? For the dietary effects considered above, the average R changes were used. Disregarding the initial transient period of exercise for the moment, the study of Krogh and Lindhard (96) showed that after about 40 minutes of exercise R tended to rise from its low value when their subjects were on a high fat diet, but R decreased progressively from its high value when the subjects were on a high CHO diet. Christensen and Hansen (25) also have shown R to fall during prolonged exercise for both normal mixed and high CHO diets. These findings have been interpreted to mean that oxidative fuel mixture changes with time of mild to moderately intense exercise. According to this concept, at the onset of exercise CHO, mainly in the form of muscle glycogen, is the predominant fuel supporting muscle oxidation, but as the exercise is continued, there is a gradual shift so that combustion is sustained more by FAT oxidation. What CHO is oxidized during the latter stages of exercise is thought to arise progressively more from blood glucose derived from liver gluconeogenesis.

The kinetics of R have been effectively evaluated by Linnarsson (99) using a breath-by-breath technique and averaging three trials for eight male subjects while exercising on a bicycle ergometer at various intensities. Two of the average R responses at about 31 and 78% maximum $\dot{V}O_2$ relative work loads are idealized and presented in Fig. 3A to show the essential features of the kinetic response. For both intensities after a short delay, R falls from the "zero-load" exercise reference value, reaches a minimum, and then rises, with the R for mild exercise returning approximately to the reference value of about 0.78, while the R for the more intense exercise rises well above this level to a value slightly above unity after which it gradually falls. In neither case, below or above the expected blood lactate threshold, does the R initially rise above the reference value as would be expected if there were a rapid increase in CHO oxidation as the aforementioned concept proposes. To what extent do these R kinetics reflect the metabolic events occurring in the body? If so, how much of the change is due to alterations in oxidative fuel mixture? How much is the result of change in acid–base balance due to PC splitting and anaerobic glycolysis (Fig. 2)? As yet, we cannot answer these essential questions.

A second feature to notice for the R kinetics of Fig. 3A is that the reference and mild exercise R values (curve 1) are essentially the same after the initial transient period. This finding confirms the results of the aforementioned studies in which the resting and average exercise R values were found to be virtually the same. In the postabsorptive condition, R at rest and during mild exercise is determined by the CHO and FAT mix of the diet consumed over several days prior to exercise.

A third feature illustrated in Fig. 3A is that, after the initial transition, R for

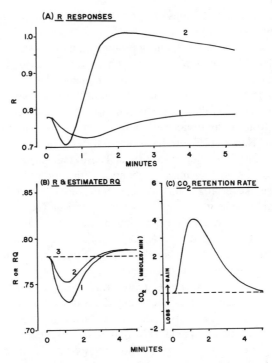

Fig. 3. Experimental and theoretical kinetics of the ventilatory exchange ratio (R) and respiratory quotient (RQ) during exercise. (A) Scheme of measured R for 31 and 78% maximum $\dot{V}O_2$ from Linnarsson (1974). (B) Measured R (curve 1, Linnarsson, 1974) at 31% maximum $\dot{V}O_2$ and possible RQ responses (curves 2 and 3). (C) Net CO_2 retention rate estimated as difference between measured CO_2 production and estimation oxidative CO_2 production during exercise at 31% maximum $\dot{V}O_2$.

intense exercise above the expected blood lactate threshold attains a higher value than the reference R. One finds R to increase in a disproportionate fashion with exercise intensity, particularly above the blood lactate threshold (84,109). So below the threshold, R attains a level virtually equal to the rest or reference R, but above the threshold intensity R attains progressively higher values as exercise intensity is increased. Exercise eliciting maximum $\dot{V}O_2$ results in R values ranging from about 1.0 and 1.4 with an average of about 1.15. These observations have led to the notion that CHO utilization dramatically increases with the intensity of exercise, particularly above the blood lactate threshold. Muscle biopsy studies have supported this conclusion with findings showing muscle glycogen depletion and lactate accumulation occurs during exercise and that these measures of glycogen utilization dramatically increase with exercise intensity (15,55,56,65,72). In this regard, the increasing contribution of CHO to exercise energetics is thought to involve both increases in lactate production and

CHO oxidation from muscle glycogen, at least during the early phase (first 20–40 minutes) of exercise, as considered here. The concept generally accepted for the relation between oxidative fuel mixture and exercise intensity is that the fractional contribution of CHO oxidation increases and that of FAT oxidation decreases as the exercise intensity increases above the lactate threshold so that at a work load that elicits maximum $\dot{V}o_2$, the performer is oxidizing virtually all CHO (132). But it should be noted that the rise in R with exercise intensity above the blood lactate threshold has never been shown to be due only to an increase in the fractional oxidation of CHO. As a matter of fact, the change in R has been shown to be proportional to the increase in blood lactate (84), and to decreases in blood bicarbonate (109). Further, Wasserman et al. (145) have shown the arterial bicarbonate changes inversely to lactate. These findings show there remains the question as to the actual partition of the increased CHO utilization that occurs with exercise intensity. Just how much of the rise in R is due to an increase in the fractional CHO oxidation and how much is due to increases in HCO_3^--derived CO_2 production arising from lactic acid accumulation in body compartments? In fact, one can seriously ask where is the hard evidence that oxidative fuel mixture changes with work intensity? Could it be that most, if not all, of the R increase above the reference value is due to HCO_3^--derived CO_2 production from neutralization of accumulated lactic acid? If so, it would mean the unchanging oxidative fuel mix observed with increases in intensity below the lactate threshold either changes very little or not at all, as the intensity increases above the threshold. Thus, whatever the oxidative fuel mix, it would be established for both rest and exercise by dietary intake of CHO and FAT, with the exercise respiratory exchange ratio (RQ = oxidative CO_2 production/O_2 consumption) invariant with respect to exercise intensity. In this case the increase in CHO utilization with exercise intensity would represent primarily a greater net anaerobic glycolysis.

Repeated daily exercise of large muscle groups, such as with cycling, walking, jogging, or running, at intensities of about 60% maximum $\dot{V}o_2$, or above, for 20 minutes or longer is referred to as endurance exercise training. This form of training produces cardiorespiratory and muscular adaptations which operate synergistically to increase maximum aerobic power (maximum $\dot{V}o_2$) of the performer elicited during exercise (26,71,130,133). The adaptations in maximum $\dot{V}o_2$ can be characterized as involving increases (1) in the capacity for systemic nutrient flow needed to support metabolite exchange between organ systems and blood and their oxidative metabolism; (2) in the capacity for perfusion of working muscles leading to better delivery of nutrients and exchange of metabolites at the individual fibers; and (3) in the capacity of active muscle fibers to take up and use the nutrients needed to sustain oxidative metabolism.

In regard to adaptations in oxidative fuel mixture of submaximal exercise, the intial peak or plateau of R is found to be lower in the trained compared to the untrained state of the individual when exercise time and intensity as well as diet are all held constant (65,72,132). Not only is R lower at all submaximal exercise intensities in the trained compared to the untrained state, but it changes less with intensity and the rise in R, when it does occur, develops at a high intensity for the blood lactate threshold. These adaptations in R have been interpreted to mean there is a decrease in CHO utilization accompanied by an increase in FAT oxidation. Qualitatively, this conclusion is supported by muscle biopsy studies (65,72,132), in which glycogen concentration decreases less and muscle and blood lactate concentrations increase less for the trained individual during exercise at the same absolute intensity ($\dot{V}o_2$). On the surface, these data would appear to indicate that CHO oxidation is reduced as FAT oxidation is increased during submaximal exercise. But this interpretation may not be entirely correct because the decrease in R and carbohydrate utilization may also include adaptive changes in lactate metabolism. There is about 19 times more ATP per glucose used when CHO is oxidized as compared to its degradation to lactate. So for the same ATP requirement for exercise, less muscle glygogen would be used if more of it was oxidized and less ended up as lactic acid. A decrease in CHO oxidation would decrease the R and the reduction in lactate accumulation and CO_2 formation from bicarbonate neutralization of lactic acid would also decrease R. In addition to some reduction in lactate production being responsible for the lower lactate accumulated in muscle and blood, this reduction in lactate also could be due to an increased lactate anion removal from blood for glucose production via gluco-neogenesis and lactate oxidation. For both cases of lactate removal, there would be one OH^- formed/lactate ion metabolized (27,28). This relative alkalinization would effectively drive the bicarbonate buffer reaction [Eq. (8)] to the right, thereby leading to a relative retention of CO_2 and ulimately to a decrease in the CO_2 excreted by the lungs. In this case, the R would appear lower, not only because less CHO was oxidized but also because more lactate was removed via oxidation and gluconeogenesis. So dramatic adaptive changes in lactate metabolism could significantly contribute to the lowering of exercise R so that the R change produced by training is not simply a shift from CHO oxidation to greater FAT oxidation.

II. CARBOHYDRATE AND FAT METABOLISM DURING EXERCISE

A. Muscle Glycogen Utilization

1. INTRODUCTION

The first comprehensive report on variations of muscle glycogen in man with diet and exercise was published by Hultman (73). It summarized his research

(72) and several other studies (15,65). Muscle glycogen utilization was assessed by measuring changes in its concentration in small muscle samples taken serially with the needle biopsy technique of Bergström (13), as described by Hultman (74).

Muscle glycogen is an essential fuel for exercise. Its utilization always occurs during exercise. Only the extent of its utilization varies with exercise mode (38,39), exercise intensity and time (65,77,91,132), dietary conditions (15,56, 65,72,73), state of training (65,77,132), and ambient conditions of temperature (44) and altitude (132).

2. EXERCISE INTENSITY, TIME, AND MODE

For a given work load, muscle glycogen degradation is most rapid at the onset of exercise and its rate decreases thereafter in a curvilinear fashion with time of exercise (38,65,73,77,132). Nevertheless, at any moment during exercise the rate of glycogen utilization is greater the higher the exercise intensity (77,132). Essén (38) has summarized data from the literature showing both the initial degradation rate and the rate of decline in muscle glycogen with time are affected by the mode of exercise. In this regard, it appears that at the same relative exercise intensity (% maximum $\dot{V}_{O_2}$), the rate of utilization follows the order: bicycle exercise greater than treadmill running uphill greater than treadmill running on the level. Essén (38) and Gollnick et al. (54,55) have discussed this phenomenon.

3. GLUCOSE INGESTION AND GLYCOGEN UTILIZATION

Exercise at 70–80% maximum $\dot{V}_{O_2}$ leads to exhaustion, in which the work load can no longer be maintained, in approximately 1–2 hours and coincides with nearly complete depletion of muscle glycogen (65). The initial glycogen content in muscle prior to exercise has been shown to be highly correlated with maximum time exercise at 70–80% maximum $\dot{V}_{O_2}$ can be sustained before exhaustion occurs (15,94). This finding demonstrates the strict dependence on muscle glycogen for sustaining exercise at this intensity. Such an interpretation is supported by the finding that glucose infusion throughout the exercise bout elevates blood glucose to between 200 and 600 mg/200 ml, yet the amount of glycogen lost in muscle is identical to that for the same exercise performed without glucose infusion (73,75). Glucose uptake by exercising muscle is enhanced with glucose ingestion (2,3), but this extra CHO does not conserve muscle glycogen (75). Only at exercise intensities below about 50% maximum $\dot{V}_{O_2}$ is there evidence suggesting blood glucose utilization can replace that of glycogen in active muscle (75). Thus, it seems that above about 70% maximum $\dot{V}_{O_2}$, glycogen utilization is an essential fuel for sustaining muscular work at least for the first 40–60 minutes of exercise. As muscle glycogenolysis diminishes, muscle glucose uptake and utilization from liver glycogenolysis and gluconeogenesis become progressively more prominent as the CHO fuel for muscle (2,4).

It is unknown if glucose ingestion or infusion can substitute for muscle glycogen utilization in the later stage of hard prolonged exercise, thereby helping to sustain the same intensity of exercise. It is possible that progressive enhancement of glucose uptake not only involves a greater glycolysis, but also a proportionately greater glycogen synthesis. Hultman (75) has shown the percentage of the I (active) form of glycogen synthetase during exercise is dependent upon the glycogen content of muscle; the lower the glycogen concentration, the greater percentage I form found. Moreover, he showed that the expected glycogenolysis occurs in the previously unworked leg muscles, containing normal glycogen levels, whereas net glycogen resynthesis occurred in working muscles of the opposite leg which had been previously worked to markedly reduce its glycogen content. Further, Essén et al. (40) have shown lactate release from muscle during work when glycogen content is intact, but is taken up by muscle when its glycogen content is low, as occurs during prolonged hard exercise. The fate of this muscle lactate uptake is not established, but it is reasonable to assume some of it is oxidized and some is used to synthesize glycogen, particularly in the latter stages of exhaustive exercise, just as considered here. All these considerations suggest some muscle becomes progressively geared toward glycogen synthesis and not glycogenolysis; the uptake of glucose and lactate probably is shunted more toward glycogen resynthesis in those fibers with low glycogen content. This would severely diminish their capacity to sustain glycolysis, thereby requiring the recruitment of other "fresh" fibers to maintain the power output required for the exercise (54–56). In these newly activated fibers, glycogenolysis, not glycogen resynthesis, would be expected to predominate. It is unknown whether glucose ingestion would help to maintain glycolysis in these presumably fast-twitch fibers (54), but probably would help to enhance glycogen resynthesis in the glycogen-depleted fibers. Nevertheless, it should be kept in mind that glucose utilization increases as glycogenolysis decreases, thereby helping to maintain CHO utilization during prolonged hard exercise. The fat and CHO oxidative fuel mix of muscle may not change as much as is thought during prololonged severe exercise.

4. DIET AND GLYCOGEN RESTITUTION

Muscle glycogen does not vary significantly over the course of normal daily activity as long as usual meal patterns are followed (73). But with starvation, its concentration gradually falls over a 5- to 6-day period. On calorically adequate but virtually CHO-free diet, glycogen falls in muscle but more slowly than during starvation (73). Glucose or fructose infusion increases muscle glycogen content only modestly in a 6-hour period of rest (73). However, this is not the case in the recovery of muscle previously exercised and glycogen depleted. Even without food intake in the immediate recovery period, muscle glycogen is re-synthesized, both in rest and during active recovery at a reduced exercise intensity, presumably using blood glucose from accelerated glyconeogenesis (4), and using enhanced lactate uptake by muscle (67). There remains, however, a controversy as to the extent lactate disappearance during recovery represents oxidation and glycogen resynthesis (17,18,49,67). Nevertheless, complete restitution of muscle glycogen requires food intake, since it has been shown that endogenous substrates do not lead to full recovery, at least over 4–5 (101) to 20 hours (73). A mixed diet does replenish glycogen by between 24 hours (101) to 46 hours (118). Presumably this difference in rate of restitution depends on the intensity and duration of the preceding exercise and the extent the exercise has depleted muscle glycogen. Also, some of the differences in the glycogen restitution rate of the last two studies, which used different exercise protocols, could be related to differences in blood glucose and insulin levels produced by each exercise. For the prolonged hard exercise of Piehl, blood glucose and insulin levels fell (2–4) and remained low for some time during recovery, whereas in the short intermittent severe exercise of MacDougall, blood glucose and insulin were elevated at the end and following exercise. So presumably, there is accelerated resynthesis of glycogen in the latter case thereby promoting significant glycogen accumulation within 2 hours even without food, and complete recovery occurs in 24 hours with consumption of a 3100-kcal mixed diet.

For muscle glycogen depletion produced by prolonged exercise, it appears the composition of food intake is important in determining both the rate and extent of glycogen repletion. With a calorically adequate diet of fat and protein, glycogen resynthesis is slow and incomplete even after 4 days (73). In contrast, a day of fasting after exhaustive exercise, followed by CHO ingestion, nearly restores glycogen in the next 24 hours and produces ''supercompensation'' of glycogen stores in 2 days (73). Supercompensation means the glycogen stores increase to a level markedly above the predepletion content. It can amount to three to four times control over a 3-day period of CHO feeding (16). This supercomposition of glycogen repletion produced by exhausting exercise and CHO feeding is specific to the muscles exercised; nonexercised muscles increase their glycogen content only slightly (16).

5. AVAILABILITY OF FAT AND MUSCLE GLYCOGEN

Unlike glucose ingestion or infusion, which increases glucose utilization without substantially affecting muscle glycogen depletion, ingesting fat not only diminishes glucose, but also muscle glycogen utilization during prolonged hard exercise (30,68,124,125); energy transfer by fat oxidation replaces that derived from muscle glycogen and blood glucose utilization in working muscle. This decreases in CHO utilization apparently involves both a decrease in CHO oxidation (as assessed by $\dot{V}_{O_2}$ and R) as well as in CHO degradation to lactate, in that less lactate accumulates in muscle and blood (30). Both the uptake of glucose into muscle and lactate production have been shown to be decreased when oleate is perfused in the exercising rat hind quarter preparation that is well oxygenated (124). The increased availability of fatty acids in blood enhances fatty acid uptake and oxidation in working muscle and leads to inhibition of CHO utilization by increasing glucose 6-phosphate (G6P) and citrate levels in muscle (124,125). Elevated citrate inhibits glycolysis by reducing the activity of phosphofructokinase, the key regulatory enzyme of the glycolytic pathway. G6P accumulates and inhibits hexokinase activity, which regulates glucose uptake and phosphorylation. In this way, both glycogen and glucose utilization decrease in working muscle as more fatty acids are made available to them.

6. TRAINING AND MUSCLE GLYCOGEN

Adaptation to endurance exercise training involves a number of changes in the metabolism of prolonged submaximal exercise which can be generally characterized as an acceleration of fat oxidation and sparing of body stores of CHO. Glycogen utilization during exercise at a given work load and time is reduced after training. Hermansen et al. (65) studied glycogen depletion during exercise at 77% maximum $\dot{V}_{O_2}$, and later Saltin and Karlsson (132) investigated the response at the same $\dot{V}_{O_2}$ and percentage maximum $\dot{V}_{O_2}$ in trained and untrained subjects. They showed the rate of glycogen depletion during such exercise was reduced in the trained, as compared to the untrained state. Not only is there relatively less CHO utilized because FAT oxidation replaces CHO oxidation, but also because less lactate accumulates in muscle and blood (65,132). The latter could mean less CHO is used because there is a reduced lactate production and/or more of the lactate formed is removed by oxidation and gluconeogenesis.

It is of interest to highlight findings of Henriksson (63) because they illustrate the difficulty in identifying what are the specific adaptations in exercise metabolism produced by endurance training. Only one leg was endurance trained by bicycle exercise for 2 months; the untrained leg served as the control for the six subjects studied. As expected, maximum $\dot{V}_{O_2}$ increased for the trained leg but not for the untrained leg. During 50 minutes of two-leg bicycle exercise at about 67% maximum $\dot{V}_{O_2}$, whole body oxidative fuel utilization ($\dot{V}_{O_2}$ and R) and metabolic exchange across both legs were studied after the training period. The trained leg (TL) R was significantly lower than that of the untrained leg (UL) even though TL O_2 uptake and force development was greater, indicating the TL was producing a greater power output than UL. From these data, it was estimated the average combustion of fat was 29 and 16% of caloric expenditure for the TL and UL, respectively. This greater relative fat oxidation also was found to be accompanied by relatively greater plasma free fatty acid (FFA) uptake in the TL, thereby supporting Henriksson's contention that training induced a shift in oxidative fuel utilization to greater fat combustion. This conclusion is disconcerting, in that other findings suggest a more comprehensive interpretation of the local adaptive response. For example, no difference was found for the amount of glycogen degraded or of lactate accumulated in working muscle in TL and UL over the 50 minutes of exercise, yet the pattern for the rate of lactate released for the two legs was markedly different over the period. More specifically, lactate release was significantly greater for the UL than TL throughout exercise; the TL actually revealed net uptake of lactate at 50 minutes. Moreover, glucose uptake was slightly, but not significantly, greater and the free glucose concentration was higher in the TL, compared to the UL. Since CO_2 and lactate are released from muscle together (45), the higher R for the UL may not only be due to a greater CHO oxidation but also to a greater bicarbonate-derived CO_2 production. On the other hand, the lower R for TL, in addition to reflecting a relatively greater fat oxidation, could be due to a greater intramuscular oxidation and gluconeogenesis from lactate, thereby stoichiometrically producing OH^- and requiring the retention of relatively more CO_2 arising from oxidative metabolism. Thus, it is possible the relative CHO oxidation is overestimated for the UL but underestimated for the TL. It should be clear that measurements of net exchange across mixed muscles, with heterogeneous fiber types and metabolic patterns, do not provide sufficient information to fully (1) elucidate the partition of aerobic and anaerobic components, (2) define the contribution of CHO and fat to combustion, or (3) evaluate the extent of CHO utilization involves oxidation and lactate production. All these elements of muscle metabolism must be adequately assessed before the essential features of the exercise-induced adaptations of muscle metabolism can be identified. All we can say with assurance about the metabolic adaptations is that relatively more fat is oxidized and correspondingly less glycogen is utilized by working muscle in the endurance trained state.

7.   AMBIENT TEMPERATURE AND MUSCLE GLYCOGEN

Extremes of ambient temperature alter metabolism. Rest and exercise metabolic rate increase either when the ambient temperature is low enough to cool the body, or when it is high enough to heat the body (29). Extremes of temperature also affect the oxidative fuel mixture; cold exposure increases the mobilization and oxidation of fatty acids, whereas a hot environment shifts metabolism toward greater CHO utilization relative to the thermal neutral environment. For example, Fink et al. (44) reported severe exercise (70–85% maximum $\dot{V}o_2$) in the heat (41°C) produced a greater rate of muscle glycogen depletion, smaller reduction in muscle triglyceride content, and greater blood lactate level than exercise in the cold (9°C). The elevated blood lactate during exercise in the heat has been corroborated by the study of Irondelle and Freund (81). This finding and the research of Rowell and others (see ref. 126, for details and references) have led to the notion that the greater CHO utilization and lactate accumulation in the heat develops primarily because of the relative ischemia induced in muscle and splanchnic beds as a result of shunting of blood to the skin for heat dissipation. In this way, more CHO is utilized because there is more lactate produced with relatively less ATP yield/glucose and also perhaps because less lactate can be removed via oxidation and gluconeogenesis. The metabolic response to the cold presumably is affected by changes in circulatory as well as neurohumeral functions. The cold stimulus leads to shunting of blood from the skin to the core, thereby increasing the effective volume flow of blood to working muscle and splanchnic regions, thus enhancing lactate oxidation and gluconeogenesis. In addition, sympathetic stimulation of fat cells, coupled with cold-induced catecholamine discharge into blood, enhances lipolysis of triglycerides, thereby mobilizing more fatty acids. This effectively enhances delivery, uptake, and oxidation of FFA by working muscle. The result is CHO is more readily conserved during exercise in the cold.

8. ALTITUDE AND MUSCLE GLYCOGEN

In acute exposure to altitude (reduced inspired Po_2), the rate of CHO utilization is markedly accelerated during the first 4–5 minutes of exercise, as evidenced by increased muscle glycogen depletion and lactate accumulated in muscle and blood (132). Presumably these responses reflect a greater anaerobic contribution to energy transfer due to reduced arterial Po_2 (87), at least during the early part of exercise. The results of the study of Jones et al. (87) suggest that there is an enhanced mobilization, uptake, and oxidation of FFA in the hypoxic relative to the normoxic condition. It could be that exercise in hypoxia dramatically shifts CHO to fat oxidation as more CHO is degraded to lactate. We must await further quantification of these processes before this proposal can be further evaluated.

B. Glucose Metabolism

1. INTRODUCTION

Glucose metabolism during exercise has been reviewed by Wahren (142) and Felig and Wahren (43). Hultman (76) and Hultman and Nilsson (78,79) have discussed liver glycogen. It is now recognized that blood glucose is an important fuel for working muscle. The source of endogenous glucose is derived from liver glycogenolysis and gluconeogenesis and, perhaps, from kidney gluconeogenesis. The availability of glucose is an important factor affecting the rate of glucose utilization, and this, in turn, is dependent on the amount of CHO and FAT eaten, as well as the amount of glucose and FFA mobilized from the liver and adipose tissue, respectively. Thus, it is to be expected that glucose utilization during exercise is affected by the intensity and duration of the exercise, and both the immediate and more long-term dietary status of the performer. These relations will be developed in the following discourse.

2. HEPATIC GLUCOSE PRODUCTION

Unlike skeletal muscle, liver glycogen is rapidly degraded during starvation so that by 24 hours it is nearly depleted, and stores can be rapidly repleted by a CHO diet (78,79). Thus, liver glycogen stores represent a dynamic balance between synthesis and degradation. Blood glucose also turns over rapidly and its constancy represents a dynamic steady state between production and influx of glucose from primarily the liver and utilization by peripheral tissues. Forces affecting glucose homeostasis are dramatically altered with exercise. Arterial glucose levels change very little during the first 40 minutes of mild to moderate exercise intensities, but increase with time, particularly with continuous hard (143) to severe intermittent exercise intensities (66,101). As mild to moderate exercise is continued beyond 40 minutes, there is a progressive decline in blood glucose which eventually leads to hypoglycemia (glucose < 60 mg/100 ml) at exhaustion when the work intensity can no longer be maintained (2–5).

Glucose production by the liver increases with exercise (4,79,127,128,144). For exercise lasting up to about 40 minutes, the rate of glucose production increases with both time and intensity of exercise (4,143,144). Since blood glucose levels change little during the early phase (< 40 minutes) of prolonged exercise, the rate of glucose utilization must increase in proportion to liver glucose production during this period in order to sustain blood glucose homeostasis. The glucose produced by liver for this exercise arises almost entirely from accelerated glycogenolysis since gluconeogenesis does not increase significantly above the rest level over the first 40 minutes of exercise (144). Consequently, as the exercise intensity is increased, the rate of glycogenolysis increases out of proportion to that of gluconeogenesis to increase liver production of glucose, thereby affecting a progressive reduction in the fractional production of glucose from gluconeogenesis (144). Liver glycogen falls during exercise (78,79), thereby limiting the ability of the liver to sustain the rate of glycogenolysis. Nevertheless, liver glucose production is maintained between 40–180 minutes and 40–120 minutes by progressive increases in the rate of gluconeogenesis during exercise at 30% (5) and 58% maximum $\dot{V}_{O_2}$ (4), respectively. However, beyond these times liver glycogen presumably diminishes further and glycogenolysis drops to the extent that even further increases in gluconeogenesis cannot sustain glucose production by the liver (2–5). Consequently, blood glucose falls to hypoglycemic levels.

As already mentioned, gluconeogenesis in liver increases after about 40 minutes of exercise and also increases with exercise intensity when the response at 30% maximum $\dot{V}_{O_2}$ (143) is compared to that at 58% maximum $\dot{V}_{O_2}$ (4). The principal substrates for gluconeogenesis are lactate, glucogenic amino acids, glycerol, and pyruvate (42,144), with the contribution of each given in descending order. The glucogenic amino acids contributing most to glucose production at

40 minutes of exercise are alanine, glycine, serine, threonine, tyrosine, and phenylalanine (42). However, it should be noted glutamate and glutamine also are important substrates, but were not measured in this study. Alanine is the main amino acid for glucose production by the liver. Its rate of release from working muscle increases with work rate out of proportion to its uptake by liver, thereby arterial alanine concentration increases progressively to higher levels as submaximal exercise intensity is increased. The fractional extraction of alanine by liver also increases, thereby increasing the contribution it makes to glucose production.

By far lactate makes the greatest contribution to glucose production from gluconeogenesis. This occurs primarily by increases in its fractional extraction, just as occurs with alanine uptake, since splanchnic blood flow decreases with exercise. Until recently, the source of lactate was thought to arise solely from that released from working muscle. However, Alhborg and Felig (4) have shown this holds true only during the first 90 minutes of exercise at 58% maximum $\dot{V}_{O_2}$. Thereafter, lactate release from working leg muscle became insignificant, whereas release from relatively inactive forearm muscle was found now to be an important site contributing to lactate delivery to the splanchnic bed. They estimated from simultaneous measurements of glucose uptake that if all glucose were to be degraded to lactate, then glucose uptake would account for at most 20–67% of forearm lactate release after 2–3.5 hours of exercise. So some of the lactate release from forearm muscle would have to arise from muscle glycogenolysis. This unusual pattern of inactive muscle transferring its CHO store in the form of lactate to other tissues for oxidation and gluconeogenesis apparently occurs only late in prolonged exercise where blood lactate levels are maintained within the normal resting range. For more intense exercise lasting between 20 and 40 minutes, either one leg (6,46) or arm exercise (6) elevated arterial lactate to 3.8–4.4 mmoles/liter, and lactate was taken up by the inactive leg for both modes of exercise. So the duration of exercise and the arterial lactate level may be important factors determining if inactive muscle is the site for release or uptake of lactate.

The glycerol precursor for liver glucose production arises from lipolysis of adipose tissue triglycerides in which one glycerol molecule and three long-chain fatty acids are produced and released to blood. Glycerol release is faster than its utilization so glycerol accumulates in the blood with time during exercise. Its rate of accumulation is greater the higher the exercise intensity suggesting the lipolysis rate is a function of work load. In general splanchnic uptake of glycerol increases with time of exercise (2–4), but there are only small, perhaps insignificant increases in rate of uptake as exercise intensity is increased (4,5,144). Nevertheless, splanchnic gluconeogenesis is enhanced for exercise, relative to rest, and relative glucose production from glycerol increases as exercise progresses.

To put the relative contribution from gluconeogenesis to hepatic glucose production in perspective, it should be mentioned glucose output from this process increases from about 25% in the postabsorptive resting state to 45% during prolonged (3.5–4 hours) exercise (5). This represents about a threefold increase in the absolute rate of gluconeogenesis. There is a doubling of hepatic uptake of alanine, pyruvate, and lactate, with an approximate 10-fold increase in glycerol uptake. The changes occur in spite of the reduction in splanchnic blood flow because the fractional extraction of these glucose precursors is dramatically enhanced during exercise. However, this accelerated gluconeogenesis is not sufficient to sustain hepatic glucose production as glycogenolysis diminishes, particularly after 120 minutes or more depending on intensity of exercise. Since glucose becomes the primary CHO fuel for muscle as exercise progresses and muscle glycogenolysis decreases, hypoglycemia develops and exercise must be terminated. Exhaustion from such prolonged exercise is characterized by low levels of blood glucose and of glycogen in muscle and liver.

Glucose feeding has been found to diminish splanchnic uptake of glucogenic precursors (lactate, glycerol, alanine, and pyruvate), thereby decreasing gluconeogenesis (2,3).

The factor responsible for enhancing hepatic glucose production during prolonged exercise have not been fully identified. Plasma insulin levels generally fall during mild to moderately intense prolonged exercise (119, 144) and would be expected to stimulate hepatic glycogenolysis and gluconeogenesis. Also, glucose production could be increased by the increase in plasma glucogen that occurs as mild hypoglycemia develops (5). Increases in catecholamine (4, 50,140) and growth hormone (134) also could contribute. But as Wahren (142) has pointed out, these factors may not be the sole determinants of hepatic glucose production in exercise. Exercise-induced glucose production occurs even when glucose, insulin, and glucagon in plasma are made to be constant or when hyperinsulemia is induced and maintained.

3. GLUCOSE UPTAKE AND UTILIZATION

Glucose uptake and utilization by muscle occurs at rest (7) and increases in active muscle with both time (2–5,144) and intensity of exercise (142,144). The partition of glucose uptake by active mixed muscle could involve glycogenesis, oxidation, and lactate formation and accumulation, as well as lactate transport from one to another fiber for oxidation and gluconeogenesis. Moreover, *in situ* studies of glucose exchange in forearm and leg preparations using the Fick technique of arteriovenous (A−V) differences and plasma flow do not simply represent exchange in homogenous muscle, but include changes produced by metabolism of adipocytes, skin, blood cells, and active and inactive muscle fibers of different types. These complexities are beyond the Fick technique for elucidating specific progresses of glucose utilization as they typically have been applied. We introduce this issue here to suggest that we cannot fully quantify how muscle uses the glucose it takes up from blood. Therefore, there exists considerable flexibility in how one can further analyze data on glucose uptake. So it should not be too surprising if there is controversy as to interpretation of the data. Yet it is not the case in the above cited studies, most likely because the same paradigm is used by essentially the same group of excellent scientists.

For subjects who have been on an uncontrolled mixed diet but now in a postabsorptive state, the R across the forearm is quite variable, ranging from 0.64 to 1.02, perhaps reflecting the accumulative errors associated with the measurements of arteriovenous O_2 and CO_2 differences and the derived ratio of $\dot{Q}_{CO_2}/\dot{Q}_{O_2}$, as well as individual differences and uncontrolled food intakes for the subjects. As reported in Table 7 by Andres $et\ al.$ (7), the mean $\pm$ SEM for the measured R is 0.797 ± 0.030 for 14 subjects. In their Table III, the $(A-V)$ O_2 is 3.24 ± 0.32 and $(V-A)\ CO_2$ is 2.50 ± 0.20 mmoles/liter with the average $R = (V-A)\ CO_2/(A-V)\ O_2 = 0.772$. It is not clear why there is this difference in R for the same subjects. The R values would mean that about 30.7% in the former case and 22.2% in the latter of forearm O_2 consumption at rest is due to CHO oxidation. In the same subjects, they found glucose to be taken up and lactate to be released. They calculated, by assuming no net glycogenolysis and all of the lactate released is derived from glucose taken up, that 61% of the glucose was degraded to lactate and the other 39% was oxidized amounting to 7% of the O_2 used. As calculated, this means glucose oxidation accounts for all CHO combusted. So the R calculated from this assessment is 0.728, which is quite different than those of 0.797 and 0.772, given above. Why is the measured CO_2 release greater than that predicted from the glucose and lactate estimate? For example, with $(A-V)\ O_2$ of 3.24, the R values of 0.797, 0.772, and 0.728 would give $(V-A)\ CO_2$ values of 2.58, 2.50, and 2.36 mmoles/liter. The differences in measured and estimated CO_2 released are $(2.58-2.36) = 0.22$ and $(2.50-2.36) = 0.14$ mmole/liter. Obviously, some glycogenolysis could occur, thereby invalidating the calculation of R using glucose and lactate. This would mean the R is higher and CO_2 released is closer to the measured value. But measurements of glycogen degradation in the resting condition have been shown to be slow (72), as estimated by the needle biopsy technique. It is conceded this technique is likely too gross to adequately assess small changes in net glycogen utilization. Therefore, some of the discrepancy in R and CO_2 release is suggested to be due to neglecting the glycogen contribution. Is there any other process involved that has not been considered? Recall that lactate is released, and as described recently by Hultman and Sahlin (80), lactate released from working muscle appears to occur with H^+ ion release too. Fletcher and Hopkins (45) and Needham (110) have reviewed evidence showing lactate release is accompanied by CO_2 release in muscle. Thus, some of the extra CO_2 estimated in the above calculations may be derived from lactate metabolism. In this regard, it is interesting to note that Andres *et al.* (7) found the $(V-A)$ lactate difference to be 0.11 mmole/liter. If there is a stoichiometric CO_2 release, then something like $0.11/0.22 = 0.5$ to $0.11/0.14 = 0.8$ of the extra CO_2 could be accounted for by the lactate (or CO_2) released. Therefore, CO_2 from bicarbonate buffering of lactic acid could make a significant contribution to the measured CO_2 production across the muscles in the forearm even in the resting state. Obviously, this would lead one to overestimate the contribution of CHO oxidation when using O_2 uptake and R. As shown in the study of Andres *et al.* (7), 22–31% of O_2 uptake was estimated to be due to CHO oxidation with R and O_2 data. On the other hand, the estimate of 7% due to glucose oxidation derived from glucose and lactate exchange is likely too low for total CHO oxidation. Taking the average to be 65% for extra CO_2 released, presumably derived from buffering lactic acid, then the estimated true RQ would be about 0.74 and the estimated oxidative fuel mixture of inactive muscle would be about 11% CHO and 89% FAT. In this case, the total O_2 exchange of 3.24 mmoles/liter would mean a total of 0.343 mmole/liter is used for CHO oxidation, of which 0.227 mmole/liter (66%), presumably is consumed by glucose oxidation and 0.1166 mmole/liter (34%) is used for oxidation of other carbohydrates (glycogen and lactate).

In a more extensive series of experiments, Baltzan *et al.* (10) found measured R across the resting forearm to be 0.76 ± 0.02 in 42 young men. The estimation of R using glucose and lactate exchange data on 70 subjects was 0.75. Glucose oxidation accounted for 17.5% of O_2 uptake, whereas the estimate based on R indicated 18.4% of O_2 uptake could be due to CHO oxidation. The discrepancy between CO_2 release of 0.11 μmole CO_2/minute/100 ml forearm for the R values of 0.76 and 0.75 certainly is not significant and is much less than the measured lactate release of 0.47 μmole/minute/100 ml. Thus, unlike the more limited case given above, glucose appears to be the primary (if not only) net CHO utilized in the forearm and it contributes about 18% to total O_2 used. The other 82% of $\dot{Q}O_2$ apparently involves FAT oxidation. The fraction of glucose uptake accounted for by lactate release was 0.412.

During 20 minutes of mild exercise, where the forearm O_2 uptake increased about threefold above the rest value, the average R decreased slightly from 0.72 to 0.70 in the four men studied (152). Glucose oxidation increased from the rest level but its relative contribution to O_2 uptake did not change relative to that at rest. It is interesting to note that the estimation of glucose oxidation from the glucose uptake and lactate release data indicated that 16% of the O_2 uptake should be due to glucose combustion at rest and during exercise. So the R should be 0.75 but measured R was 0.72 and 0.70 in rest and exercise, respectively. This means CO_2 production and release from the forearm muscles, as measured, is less than that expected from estimated glucose oxidation. The apparent CO_2 retention would probably be even more exaggerated if net glycogen utilization, which increases during exercise, is also considered alone with CO_2 release from lactic acid neutralization. Does this discrepancy mean glucose uptake is directed more to glycogen synthesis for such mild exercise and less CHO is oxidized than estimated? Is there lactate anion removal with OH^- production? Probably some of the CO_2 retention could come about from PC splitting and H^+ ion removal (Fig. 2), as well as other alkalinizing reactions. Unlike the examples considered above for rest, where measured forearm R overestimates or equals the apparent true RQ, this example of mild exercise, which admittedly is only on four men, illustrates that R across the muscle bed may be underestimated. This raises the question asked earlier: How much does the oxidative fuel mixture of muscle during exercise change from that at rest which is established by the immediate and more long-term dietary condition? Figure 3B is a schematic showing the R response for mild exercise and two possibilities for the true RQ response, one independent of time (curve 3), and the other a more attenuated response (curve 2) relative to the R pattern shown (curve 1). We cannot say which model is correct. Curve 2 is probably closer to the true RQ response in mild exercise.

More intense forearm exercise than considered above, markedly diminishes the arterial−deep vein (A−DV) glucose difference; that is, it falls to a minimum by about 1.5 minutes where there is a small net release of glucose, then it rises to that of the rest level by 5 minutes and thereafter continues to increase to give a greater glucose uptake than that of rest (141,143). It is not known whether this pattern is typical for less intense exercise. Nevertheless, it clearly indicates that glucose uptake from blood by muscle, which is the major source of net CHO utilization of inactive muscle, must suddenly become less important at the onset of severe exercise. Net glycogen degradation (132) and lactate accumulation and release (90) are maximum over the first several minutes of exercise. So glycogen must be the predominant CHO fuel used early on. But as already discussed, the rate of glycogen utilization falls. The rate of glucose uptake by the forearm gradually increases with time during exercise (90,143). Even at 60 minutes, the rate of uptake is increasing. Thus, blood glucose utilization by muscle becomes progressively more prominent as the CHO fuel used. This places an increasing demand on the liver for glucose production. This demand can be met by accelerating liver glycogenolysis, but as liver glycogen becomes limiting, the acceleration of gluconeogenesis apparently cannot sustain liver production; consequently, blood glucose gradually falls to hypoglycemic levels at exhaustion.

The question is how is this increasing glucose uptake by working muscle utilized. As suggested above, glucose utilization appears to replace glycogen in a progressive fashion as the degradation rate of the latter diminishes during prolonged mild to hard exercise. Muscle lactate concentration and release diminish with time. Presumably, lactate production decreases from some peak value in the early phase of exercise to some constant level that is in steady state with net removal via oxidation and gluconeogenesis within the muscle plus net release from the whole muscle. Since the oxidative fuel mixture is shifting from CHO to

FAT (based on O_2 uptake and R) only moderately in mild to moderate exercise or not at all in more intense exercise, the progressive increase in glucose uptake and decrease in lactate release have been taken to mean more glucose is oxidized and less net lactate is produced. For mild exercise at 30% maximum $\dot{V}o_2$, Ahlborg *et al.* (5) have shown, using the difference between glucose uptake and lactate release as representing maximum glucose oxidation, that leg glucose oxidation could account for 27% of leg O_2 uptake at 40 minutes, 41% at 90 minutes, 36% at 180 minutes, and 30% at 240 minutes of bicycle exercise. In another series of experiments (2), estimations of glucose oxidation in the same way gave values of 28% at 40 minutes and 35% of leg O_2 uptake at 90 minutes of exercise at 30% maximum $\dot{V}o_2$. Then 200 g of glucose was ingested at 95 minutes into the exercise and the percentage O_2 uptake attributed to glucose oxidation, comparing glucose with the nonglucose control, was 60% versus 36% at 180 minutes and 63% versus 30% at 240 minutes of exercise. Thus, exogenous glucose markedly enhanced glucose uptake and apparently the greater glucose utilization by muscle involved enhanced oxidation. Liver glucose production also was enhanced, but gluconeogenesis by this organ was found to be inhibited (2,3). But is some of this glucose taken up by muscle used for glycogen synthesis directly or indirectly from lactate? Studies of this problem have not been reported in the literature.

C. Fat Metabolism

1. INTRODUCTION

Zierler (151), Gollnick (53), Keul *et al.* (95), Paul (116), and Felig and Wahren (43) have reviewed various aspects of fat metabolism during exercise. It is now well established that long-chain fatty acid oxidation is essential for aerobic production of ATP in working muscle, and utilization arises from lipolysis of intramuscular and extramuscular stores of triglycerides in which one glycerol and three fatty acids are formed. What is still unresolved include (1) the quantitative partition of fatty acid and CHO contribution to aerobic metabolism of working muscle as affected by exercise intensity and time; (2) the contribution of the intramuscular and extramuscular triglyceride stores to fatty acid oxidation; and (3) the mechanisms regulating these features of mobilization and utilization of fatty acids as well as the CHO and FAT contribution to oxidation of working muscle.

2. SOURCES AND TYPES OF LIPIDS

Sources and types of lipids metabolized during exercise are being actively researched. Long-chain fatty acids are the principal fuels for fat oxidation. The possible sources of fatty acids supplied to muscle are (1) the plasma lipids, including chylomicrons, lipoproteins and free fatty acids (FFA); (2) intracellular lipid pools of triglycerides and phospholipids; and (3) extracellular lipid pools of triglycerides in adipose tissue between muscle fibers (19). Although it was known since the research of Pettenkofer and Voit in 1866 [see description by Lusk (100)] that fat oxidation could support energy transfer of exercising animals, it was nearly 92 years later when muscle was shown to oxidize fatty acids. Fritz *et al*. (47) by measuring $^{14}CO_2$ evolved from ^{14}C-labeled acetate, octanoate and palmitate showed *in vitro* latissimus dorsi and diaphragm muscles of the rat oxidized these substrates at rest and in increased amounts during activity. Prior to this finding, neither the total lipid content of muscle could be shown to change consistently with activity (151) nor could lipid uptake, as measured by the $(A-V)$ difference in total serum lipids, be demonstrated at rest or during activity of the forearm (7). Zierler (151) has outlined the technical difficulties responsible for these findings. Nevertheless, the research of Andres *et al*. (7), as considered above, showed that glucose uptake could only account for at most 7–30% (mean 18%) of forearm O_2 uptake at rest. This finding and the fact that forearm R averaged 0.76 clearly suggested fat oxidation was the major fuel for muscle oxidation both for rest and activity.

It was not until methods to quantify the FFA fraction in plasma were developed, contamination by interfiber adipose tissue in muscle was identified, and radioisotope studies were performed that definitive evidence was obtained showing fatty acids are the major lipid fuel for muscular work and that fatty acid oxidation is the primary process for aerobic ATP production in resting and mild to moderately active muscle.

Relative to other lipids, fatty acids turn over rapidly. As muscle fibers take up fatty acids from arterial blood, adipocytes between fibers also release fatty acids to venous blood leaving muscle, thereby making it impossible to identify muscle uptake of fatty acids by the $(A-V)$ difference technique. Recognizing this possibility, Rabinowitz and Zierler (120) inhibited adipose fatty acid release by infusing insulin, and with the improved method of FFA analysis, they were able to consistently show FFA uptake. Calculations indicated that, if all FFA taken up were oxidized, it would account for only 60% of forearm O_2 uptake. But the R data indicated a larger fraction of O_2 consumption should have been derived from fat oxidation. This discrepancy was also verified by [^{14}C]oleate and [^{14}C]palmitate oxidation experiments in that the contribution to forearm O_2 uptake of 41, 26, and 17% for oleate, palmitate and glucose, respectively, amounted to a total of 84%. Thus, 16% of the unaccounted O_2 consumption presumably represented oxidation of other fatty acids. To what extent is this unaccounted for fatty acid oxidation due to lipolysis of muscle triglyceride (TG) stores?

Neptune *et al*. (111) reported labile fatty acids of rat diaphragm muscle decreased *in vivo* in rats fasting for 24–48 hours and *in vitro* in the same tissue over a 4-hour incubation. But there was conflicting evidence as to the source of this lipid utilization. George and Naik (51) showed histochemically a decrease in lipid content of muscle fibers from pigeon breast, thereby identifying the red fibers as a site for lipid utilization. In contrast, Masoro *et al.* (105) found neither the composition nor content of lipid esters changed with exercise in muscles of monkeys. George and Vallyathan (52) found blood, liver, and adipose FFA to decrease, but muscle FFA to increase, when pigeon breast muscle was exercised for 30 minutes. Carlson (19) showed the triglyceride content decreased, but not that of cholesterol and phospholipids, in both heart and the red portion of gastrocnemius muscle of exercised rats. Moreover, when mobilization of plasma FFA was blocked with administration of nicotinic acid, Carlson was able to show TG content of this muscle to decrease even at rest. These last two studies provided data suggesting (1) intramuscular triglycerides likely turn over; (2) this lipid pool may be the immediate source of fatty acids for oxidation; and (3) whether the local TG content changes depends on an imbalance between uptake of FFA from blood to support local TG synthesis and lipolysis of TG from this pool and oxidation of the derived fatty acids. Subsequent studies have confirmed that muscle TG decreases with prolonged exercise in man (44,48) and in the rat (123).

These findings are qualitatively consistent with ^{14}C-labeled fatty acid turnover studies by Issekutz *et al.* (82,83), Paul (116), Paul and Issekutz (117), Spitzer and Gold (135), Spitzer and Hori (136), and Havel *et al.* (59–62). These studies showed plasma FFA turnover increases with exercise in both dog and man, but the increase in muscle uptake and oxidation of plasma FFA cannot account for all of the fat oxidized. Local TG stores, therefore, must be oxidized in working muscle. Nevertheless, considerable debate over the quantitative contribution of intracellular and extracellular TG stores continues to this day. This is an extremely important problem because it is linked to understanding (1) the specific mechanism of fatty acid oxidation; (2) whether the kinetics of FFA oxidation depends on the kinetics for delivery of exogenous FFA to muscle; and (3) the partition of CHO and fatty acid oxidation of muscle during the transition from rest to the apparent steady-state $\dot{V}_{O_2}$ of exercise.

3. DIRECT OR INDIRECT PATHWAY

Are exogenous fatty acids oxidized directly or are they incorporated into the muscle TG pool before oxidation? This question developed as it became clear that muscle TG is a source of fatty acids and as it became apparent ^{14}C-labeled fatty acid uptake during rest and exercise was greater than could be accounted for by $^{14}CO_2$ production from plasma FFA. For example, although all the FFA taken up could be accounted for by its immediate and complete oxidation during exercise of the hind limb in dogs, Spitzer and Gold (135) could not detect any $^{14}CO_2$ evolution of [^{14}C]FFA taken up at rest. This suggested that none of the [^{14}C]FFA extracted from blood by muscle is oxidized directly in the resting state. Spitzer and Hori (136) showed only 36 and 60% of FFA uptake by hind limbs of the dog was accounted for by $^{14}CO_2$ evolution during rest and exercise, respectively. Havel *et al.* (59,60,62) showed only about 25% $^{14}CO_2$ appeared at rest in fasting men and less than 50% of [^{14}C]FFA disappearance was due to $^{14}CO_2$ during exercise. Issekutz *et al.* (83) and Paul and Issekutz (117) likewise showed in dogs, during rest and exercise on the treadmill, that FFA oxidation as a fraction of uptake varied with arterial FFA concentration as well as exercise intensity expressed as $\dot{V}O_2$. More fatty acids are taken up than oxidized. For a given workload, the arterial [FFA] increases with time. They found the higher the arterial [FFA], the higher the uptake and oxidation of plasma FFA, but the slope of uptake versus [FFA] was greater than that for the relation of FFA oxidation versus [FFA] (117). So only a fraction of the FFA uptake is oxidized at a given arterial [FFA]. But these relations vary also with rate of aerobic metabolism in a way that the fractional oxidation relative to uptake increases with exercise intensity. Does this mean that as FFA turnover increases with metabolic rate more of the FFA uptake is oxidized directly? Could it indicate the intramuscular TG pool turns over faster as the metabolic rate increases such that the faster [^{14}C] uptake also labels the TG pool faster, thereby providing a proportionately greater $^{14}CO_2$ production from the oxidation of [^{14}C]FFA derived from lipolysis of the [^{14}C]TG pool? We cannot identify which of these two processes is correct or whether both are contributing to FFA oxidation of muscle. Unfortunately, most studies of [^{14}C]FFA utilization are based on steady-state techniques, and therefore are not useful in resolving this issue.

Time course data and kinetic analysis would be helpful in distinguishing between the direct and indirect route for FFA oxidation. Both Havel *et al.* (60) and Malmendier *et al.* (103) evaluated the kinetics of FFA oxidation, the former during prolonged hard exercise and the latter at rest. Their data led both to postulate a direct route for FFA oxidation and a route to lipid ester storage with return to oxidation. It would appear the muscle TG turnover rate is important in determining the time course of the partition. At rest when metabolic turnover is minimal most of the [^{14}C]FFA uptake is not rapidly released as $^{14}CO_2$ (62,117). As Zierler (151) has reported, his group found [^{14}C]oleic acid uptake attained a steady level in about 10 minutes, but $^{14}CO_2$ evolution was not even detected until 30 minutes after the start of constant infusion in the forearm of subjects at rest. This delay and the finding of a huge discrepancy between plasma FFA uptake and oxidation at rest (the latter about 20% of the former) argue that the major, and perhaps the sole, pathway of FFA oxidation in resting muscle arises directly from lipolysis of intramuscular lipid esters, primarily the TG stores. The delay in the evolution of $^{14}CO_2$ from [^{14}C]FFA taken up from plasma, therefore, could mean no plasma FFA is oxidized directly when TG stores are intact and local TG lipolysis can function at a rate in steady state with FFA oxidation. Thus, according to this hypothesis of Zierler (151), plasma FFA are taken up by muscle in proportion to the arterial [FFA], esterified to TG, and incorporated into lipid granules. Hydrolysis of these TG stores releases FFA and become the major immediate fat fuel for oxidation by muscle at rest and during exercise. But is there a delay in $^{14}CO_2$ evolution during exercise as found for rest?

We are unaware of any study showing a delayed $^{14}CO_2$ production from plasma [^{14}C]FFA at the transition from rest to exercise, but there certainly is a lag in $^{14}CO_2$ evolution. For example, after 1 hour of [^{14}C]FFA perfusion at rest, and then 30 minutes of exercise with the perfusion continued, FFA uptake continues to increase with time because arterial [FFA] is increasing (117). In this non-steady-state condition, $^{14}CO_2$ production lags behind [^{14}C]FFA uptake kinetics (117), as if the [^{14}C]TG pool specific activity is progressively increasing. This view is supported by the following observations: (1) Lactate levels are changing very little after the first 20 minutes of exercise and NaH$^{14}CO_3$ studies show steady state for $^{14}CO_2$ evolution after this time (106,117), so little of the $^{14}CO_2$ progression after 20 minutes should be affected by changes in the bicarbonate buffering system, (2) Even though plasma FFA specific activity is constant from 1 to 4 hours of exercise, the fraction of FFA uptake that is oxidized progressively increases with time (117). This could mean that the plasma [^{14}C]FFA uptake and direct oxidation is progressively becoming the dominant pathway, but only if one assumes the specific activity of muscle lipid pools are not changing, (3) Moreover, R is not changing significantly over the short periods where percentage $^{14}CO_2$ of [^{14}C]FFA uptake is changing. Therefore, the increase in fractional oxidation of plasma [^{14}C]FFA uptake would not be due to an increase in contribution of fat oxidation, (4) If muscle TG and FFA pools increase with exercise as they appear to do in some cases (52,139) or the TG pool decreases (44,48) as the FFA pool increases, then it is likely the specific activities of these pools will continue to be functions of time. In this case, the lag in $^{14}CO_2$ production relative to [^{14}C]FFA uptake at the onset of exercise would not reflect a shift in the oxidative FFA partition between the direct plasma FFA and indirect TG pathways. It would mean more unlabeled CO_2 is derived from TG hydrolysis at the beginning of exercise because the [^{14}C]TG specific activity is relatively low. As the unlabeled is used and as the [^{14}C]FFA uptake accelerates, the [^{14}C]TG specific activity increases, and consequently more $^{14}CO_2$ immediately arises from TG hydrolysis in muscle so that [^{14}C]FFA oxidation approach that of [^{14}C]FFA uptake, the fraction depending on the extent plasma FFA uptake equals TG-derived FFA oxidation and [^{14}C]TG specific activity. The higher the metabolic rate, the higher the TG turnover rate, and the sooner and more complete is the [^{14}C]TG specific activity attained during exercise.

This hypothesis is consistent with the findings of Issekutz *et al.* (83) which demonstrated the importance of muscle [^{14}C]TG utilization for supporting fatty acid oxidation in exercising dogs. For example, they showed (after preliminary exercise to partially deplete TG stores followed by [^{14}C]palmitate infusion for 190 minutes to label TG stores), that $^{14}CO_2$ production sharply increased even though plasma [^{14}C]FFA specific activity had fallen to a nominal level 5 minutes into exercise after infusion was stopped. Some 25 minutes after terminating the infusion, $^{14}CO_2$ production remained elevated during exercise. The amount of [^{14}C]FFA uptake was negligible such that between 10 and 40 minutes of exercise $^{14}CO_2$ release relative [^{14}C]FFA uptake was 120 times greater. A similar experiment with $NaH^{14}CO_3{}^-$ infusion instead of [^{14}C]palmitate showed only a fraction of the elevated $^{14}CO_2$ production could be due to a decrease in the $HCO_3{}^-$ pool as lactic acid is neutralized. Thus, when the specific activity of plasma [^{14}C]FFA is low and presumably muscle [^{14}C]TG is high, the major portion of the $^{14}CO_2$ production arises from muscle TG-derived [^{14}C]FFA oxidation during exercise. Even at the onset of exercise $^{14}CO_2$ rose rapidly when muscle [^{14}C]TG was the source of labeled FFA. Thus, any delay at rest or lag during the early phase of exercise in $^{14}CO_2$ evolution from plasma [^{14}C]FFA uptake would appear to reflect not a shift in the pathway between direct plasma FFA oxidation and the TG indirect process, but the non-steady-state nature of muscle [^{14}C]TG specific activity. In this case, $^{14}CO_2$ production does not accurately reflect the rate of FFA oxidation from muscle TG pools, either at rest or during exercise.

The problem of quantification of muscle FAT oxidation is much more complicated than argued here. The preceding analysis suggests muscle TG is the immediate source of FFA oxidation at rest and at the onset of exercise. Thus, intrafiber TG-derived FFA would be oxidized. Presumably, there is a rapid increase in turnover rate for this TG pool as metabolic rate of the fiber increases with contractile activity. Also, the turnover rate of the interfiber TG pool also must increase in the active muscle. Is the fiber uptake of FFA derived from this interfiber TG pool oxidized directly with that rapidly taken up from plasma at the onset of exercise, or must these extrafiber FFA first go to intrafiber TG before they are oxidized, or both? If the latter, what is the partition between the serial intrafiber TG route and the direct route of extrafiber FFA oxidation? We cannot answer these important questions. It is noteworthy that Ahlborg et al. (5) showed with [^{14}C]oleate infusion that the exercising legs progressively increased oleate uptake and release, with the ratio of uptake to release changing from 0.94 at rest to 1.38, 1.90, 1.25, and 1.54 at 40, 90, 180, and 240 minutes, respectively, during bicycle exercise at 30% maximum $\dot{V}_{O_2}$. Clearly, uptake involving lipogenesis and oxidation changed faster than release representing lipolysis. Since changes in $^{14}CO_2$ from FFA oxidation lags uptake, lipogenesis may be increasing in one or both of the muscle TG pools faster than lipolysis so that pool size is increasing during the initial phase of exercise. In muscle fibers this could come about initially by the rapid change in glycolysis with the formation of α-glycerophosphate and acetyl-CoA from leucine oxidation, both of which are required for TG synthesis. However, in interfiber and extra muscular adipose tissue lipolysis would tend to change faster and be predominate over lipogenesis at the onset and even more so thereafter because of rapid increase in sympathetic nervous stimulation of some fat cells, which then would be followed by greater stimulation from the rise in plasma catecholamines and release of inhibition by the fall in insulin. Likewise, muscle lipolysis would be accelerated by catecholamines and insulin in the same way. With α-glycerophosphate and acetyl-CoA levels returning back toward preexercise levels, lipogenesis could then attain a lower rate relative to the initial acceleration so that now lipolysis and lipogensis could be more in balance in the active muscle fibers.

Qualitatively, it would appear that both inter- and intrafiber TG pools contribute significantly to muscle FFA oxidation, particularly at the onset and during the early phase (20 minutes) of exercise when plasma [FFA] is low. As exercise continues, plasma [FFA] rises progressively and thereby promotes the uptake and utilization of FFA. The result is proportionately more of the oxidative fuel arises from oxidation of plasma FFA (either directly or indirectly, or both) in muscle as exercise is continued. Regardless of the specific route, most of the FFA oxidized by muscle arises ultimately from lipolysis of adipose TG, since the amount of intrafiber TG and FFA is small relative to that used during prolonged exercise. So, if muscle fiber TG is the immediate fuel for FFA oxidation, its turnover rate would have to be markedly increased during exercise in order for all of the extrafiber FFA to pass through this small TG pool in active muscle fibers.

III. CONCLUDING REMARKS

We have not considered other important aspects of exercise metabolism. For example, the question of cellular and neuroendocrine mechanisms of metabolic regulation were not considered. The reader should consult the reviews by Terjung (138), Williamson (149,150), and Newsholme (112). Also, the important topics of protein metabolism (97) and amino acid metabolism (22–24,41) during and following exercise should be reviewed by the interested reader. Finally, the exercise-induced changes in body composition (114) and important exercise–nutrition interrelations (115) have not been reviewed.

REFERENCES

1. Adler, S., Roy, A., and Relman, A. S. (1965). Intracellular acid-base regulation. *J. Clin. Invest.* **44,** 8–30.
2. Ahlborg, G., and Felig, P. (1976). Influence of glucose ingestion on fuel-hormone response during prolonged exercise. *J. Appl. Physiol.* **41,** 683–688.
3. Ahlborg, G., and Felig, P. (1977). Substrate utilization during prolonged exercise preceded by ingestion of glucose. *Am. J. Physiol.* **233,** E188–E194.
4. Ahlborg, G., and Felig, P. (1982). Lactate and glucose exchange across the forearm, legs, and splanchnic bed during and after prolonged leg exercise. *J. Clin. Invest.* **69,** 45–54.
5. Ahlborg, G., Felig, P., Hagenfeldt, L., Hendler, R., and Wahren, J. (1974). Substrate turn-

over during prolonged exercise in man. Splanchnic and leg metabolism of glucose, free fatty acids, and amino acids. *J. Clin. Invest.* **53,** 1080–1090.

6. Ahlborg, G., Hagenfeldt, L., and Wahren, J. (1975). Substrate utilization by the inactive leg during one-leg or arm exercise. *J. Appl. Physiol.* **35,** 718–723.

7. Andres, R., Cader, G., and Zierler, K. L. (1956). The quantitatively minor role of carbohydrate in oxidative metabolism by skeletal muscle in intact man in the basal state. Measurements of oxygen and glucose uptake and carbon dioxide and lactate production in the forearm. *J. Clin. Invest.* **35,** 671–682.

8. Åstrand, P.-O., and Rodahl, K. (1977). "Textbook of Work Physiology." McGraw-Hill, New York.

8a. Atwater, W. O., and Benedict, F. G. (1903). Experiments on the metabolism of matter and energy in the human body. *USDA Off. Exp. Stn. Bull.* No. 136.

9. Atwater, W. O., and Rosa, E. B. (1899). Description of new respiration calorimeter and experiments on the conservation of energy in the human being. *USDA Off. Exp. Stn. Bull.* No. 63.

10. Baltzan, M. A., Andres, R., Cader, G., and Zierler, K. L. (1962). Heterogeneity of forearm metabolism with special reference to free fatty acids. *J. Clin. Invest.* **41,** 116–125.

11. Bang, O. (1936). The lactate content of blood during and after muscular exercise in man. *Skand. Arch. Physiol.* **74,** 51–82.

12. Benedict, F. G., and Cathcart, E. P. (1913). "Muscular Work." Carnegie Institute, Washington, D.C.

13. Bergström, J. (1962). Muscule electrolytes in man; determined by neutron activation analysis on needle biopsy specimens. *Scand. J. Clin. Lab. Invest., Suppl.* **68.**

14. Bergström, J. (1967). Local changes of ATP and phosphorylcreatine in human muscle tissue in connection with exercise. *AMA Monogr.* **15,** 91–96.

15. Bergström, J., Hermansen, L., Hultman, E., and Saltin, B. (1967). Diet, muscle glycogen and physical performance. *Acta Physiol. Scand.* **71,** 140–150.

16. Bergström, J., and Hultman, E. (1966). Muscle glycogen synthesis after exercise. An enhancing factor localized to the muscle cells in man. *Nature (London)* **210,** 309–310.

17. Brooks, G. A., Brauer, K. E., and Cassens, R. G. (1973). Glycogen synthesis and the metabolism of lactic acid after exercise. *Am. J. Physiol.* **224,** 1162–1166.

18. Brooks, G. A., and Gaesser, G. A. (1980). End points of lactate and glucose metabolism after exhausting exercise. *J. Appl. Physiol.* **49,** 1057–1069.

19. Carlson, L. A. (1967). Lipid metabolism and muscular work. *Fed. Proc., Fed. Am. Soc. Exp. Biol.* **26,** 1755–1759.

20. Cerretelli, P., and Ambrosoli, G. (1973). Limiting factors of anaerobic performance in man. *In* "Limiting Factors of Physical Performance" (J. Keul, ed.), pp. 157–165. Thieme, Stuttgart.

21. Cerretelli, P., Sikard, R., and Farhi, L. E. (1966). Readjustments in cardiac output and gas exchange during the onset of exercise and recovery. *J. Appl. Physiol.* **21,** 1345–1350.

22. Chang, T. W., and Goldberg, A. L. (1978). The origin of alanine produced in skeletal muscle. *J. Biol. Chem.* **253,** 3677–3684.

23. Chang, T. W., and Goldberg, A. L. (1978). The metabolic fates of amino acids and the formation of glutamine in skeletal muscle. *J. Biol. Chem.* **253,** 3685–3695.

24. Chang, T. W., and Goldberg, A. L. (1978). Leucine inhibits oxidation of glucose and pyruvate in skeletal muscles during fasting. *J. Biol. Chem.* **253,** 3696–3701.

25. Christensen, E. H., and Hansen, O. (1939). Arbeitsfahigkeit und Ehrnahrung. *Skand. Arch. Physiol.* **81,** 150–171.

26. Clausen, J. P. (1977). Effects of physical training on cardiovascular adjustments to exercise in man. *Physiol. Rev.* **57,** 779–815.

27. Cohen, R. D., Barnett, D., Iles, R. A., Howell, M. E. O., and Strunin, J. (1971). The effect of

changes in lactate uptake in the intracellular pH of the perfused rat liver. *Clin. Sci.* **41**, 159–164.

28. Cohen, R. D., Simpson, B. R., Goodwin, F. J., and Strunin, J. (1967). The early effects of infusion of sodium bicarbonate and sodium lactate on intracellular hydrogen ion activity in dogs. *Clin. Sci.* **33**, 233–238.

29. Consolazio, C. F., Johnson, R. E., and Pecora, L. J. (1963). "Physiological Measurements of Metabolic Functions in Man." McGraw-Hill, New York.

30. Costill, D. l., Coyle, E., Dalsky, G., Evans, W., Fink, W., and Hoopes, D. (1977). Effects of elevated plasma FFA and insulin on muscle glycogen usage during exercise. *J. Appl. Physiol.* **43**, 695–699.

31. Crescitelli, F., and Taylor, C. (1944). The lactate response to exercise and its relationship to physical fitness. *Am. J. Physiol.* **141**, 630–640.

32. Davies, C. T. M., DiPrampero, P. E., and Cerretelli, P. (1972). Kinetics of cardiac output and respiratory gas exchange during exercise and recovery. *J. Appl. Physiol.* **32**, 618–625.

33. Depocas, F., Minaire, Y., and Chatonnet, J. (1969). Rates of formation and oxidation of lactic acid in dogs at rest and during moderate exercise. *Can. J. Physiol. Pharmacol.* **47**, 603–610.

34. Dies, F., Ramos, G., Avelar, E., and Lennihoff, M. (1969). Renal excretion of lactic acid in the dog. *Am. J. Physiol.* **216**, 106–111.

35. DiPrampero, P. E. (1981). Energetics of muscular exercise. *Rev. Physiol., Biochem. Pharmacol.* **89**, 143–222.

36. Eldridge, F. L. (1975). Relationship between turnover rate and blood concentration in lactate in exercising dogs. *J. Appl. Physiol.* **39**, 231–234.

37. Eldridge, F. L., T'so, L., and Chang, H. (1974). Relationship between turnover rate and blood concentration of lactate in normal dogs. *J. Appl. Physiol.* **37**, 316–320.

38. Essén, B. (1977). Intramuscular substrate utilization during prolonged exercise. *Ann. N.Y. Acad. Sci.* **301**, 30–44.

39. Essén, B. (1978). Studies on the regulation of metabolism in human skeletal muscle using intermittent exercise as an experimental model. *Acta Physiol. Scand., Suppl.* **454.**

40. Essén, B., Pernow, B., Gollnick, P. D., and Saltin, B. (1975). Muscle glycogen content and lactate uptake in exercising muscles. *Int. Symp. Biochem. Exercise* **2**, 130–134.

41. Felig, P. (1977). Amino acid metabolism in exercise. *Ann. N.Y. Acad. Sci.* **301**, 56–63.

42. Felig, P., and Wahren, J. (1971). Amino acid metabolism in exercising man. *J. Clin. Invest.* **50**, 2703–2714.

43. Felig, P., and Wahren, J. (1975). Fuel homeostasis in exercise. *N. Engl. J. Med.* **29**, 1078–1084.

44. Fink, W. J., Costill, D. l., and Van Handel, P. J. (1975). Leg muscle metabolism during exercise in the heat and cold. *Eur. J. Appl. Physiol.* **34**, 183–190.

45. Fletcher, W. M., and Hopkins, F. G. (1916). Croonian Lecture: The respiratory process in muscle and the nature of muscular motion. *Proc. R. Soc. London, Ser. B* **89**, 444–467.

46. Freyschuss, V., and Strandell, T. (1968). Circulatory adaptation to one and two leg exercise in supine position. *J. Appl. Physiol.* **25**, 511–515.

47. Fritz, I. B., Davis, D. G., Holtrop, R. H., and Dundeee, H. (1958). Fatty acid oxidation by skeletal muscle during rest and activity. *Am. J. Physiol.* **194**, 379–386.

48. Fröberg, S. O., and Mosefeldt, F, (1971). Effect of prolonged strenuous exercise on the concentration of triglycerides, phospholipids and glycogen in muscle of man. *Acta Physiol Scand.* **82**, 167–171.

49. Gaesser, G. A., and Brooks, G. A. (1980). Glycogen repletion following continuous and intermittent exercise to exhaustion. *J. Appl. Physiol.* **49**, 722–728.

50. Galbo, H., Host, J. J., and Christensen, N. J. (1975). Glycogen and plasma catecholamine response to graded and prolonged exercise in man. *J. Appl. Physiol.* **38**, 70–76.

51. George, J. C., and Naik, R. M. (1958). Relative distribution and chemical nature of the two types of fibers in the pectoralis major muscle of the pigeon. *Nature (London)* **181,** 709.
52. George, J. C., and Vallyathan, N. V. (1964). Effects of exercise on fatty acid levels in the pigeon. *J. Appl. Physiol.* **19,** 619–622.
53. Gollnick, P. D. (1977). Free fatty acid turnover and the availability of substrates as a limiting factor in prolonged exercise. *Ann. N.Y. Acad. Sci.* **301,** 64–71.
54. Gollnick, P. D., Armstrong, R. B., Saubert, C. W., IV, Sembrowitch, W. L., Shepherd, R. E., and Saltin, B. (1973). Glycogen depletion patterns in human skeletal muscle fibers during prolonged work. *Pfluegers Arch.* **344,** 1–12.
55. Gollnick, P. D., Piehl, K., and Saltin, B. (1974). Selective glycogen depletion pattern in human muscle fibers after exercise of varying intensities and at varying pedalling rates. *J. Physiol. (London)* **241,** 45–57.
56. Gollnick, P. D., Piehl, K., Saubert, C. W., IV, Armstrong, R. G., and Saltin, B. (1972). Diet, exercise and glycogen changes in human muscle fibers. *J. Appl. Physiol.* **33,** 421–425.
57. Grimby, L., and Hannerz, J. (1968). Recruitment order of motor units on voluntary contraction: Changes induced by proprioceptive different activity. *J. Neurol., Neurosurg. Psychiatry.* **31,** 565–573.
58. Harris, C., Edwards, R. H. T., Hultman, E., Nordejo, L.-O., Nylind, B., and Sahlin, K. (1976). The time course of phosphocreatine resynthesis during recovery of the quadriceps muscle in man. *Pfluegers Arch.* **367,** 137–142.
59. Havel, R. J., Carlson, L. A., Ekelund, L.-G., and Holmgren, A. (1964). Turnover rate and oxidation of different free fatty acids in man during exercise. *J. Appl. Physiol.* **19,** 613–618.
60. Havel, R. J., Ekelund, L.-G., and Holmgren, A. (1967). Kinetic analysis of the oxidation of palmitate-1-^{14}C in man during prolonged heavy exercise. *J. Lipid Res.* **8,** 366–373.
61. Havel, R. J., Naimark, A., and Borchgrevink, C. F. (1963). Turnover rate and oxidation of free fatty acids of blood plasma in man during exercise: Studies during continuous infusion of palmitate-1-^{14}C. *J. Clin. Invest.* **42,** 1054–1062.
62. Havel, R. G., Pernow, B., and Jones, N. L. (1967). Uptake and release of free fatty acids and other metabolites in the legs of exercising men. *J. Appl. Physiol.* **23,** 90–99.
63. Henriksson, J. (1977). Training induced adaptation of skeletal muscle and metabolism during submaximal exercise. *J. Physiol. (London)* **270,** 661–675.
64. Henry, F. M., and DeMoor, J. C. (1956). Lactic and alactic oxygen consumption in moderate exercise of graded intensity. *J. Appl. Physiol.* **8,** 608–614.
65. Hermansen, L., Hultman, E., and Saltin, B. (1967). Muscle glycogen during prolonged severe exercise. *Acta Physiol. Scand.* **71,** 129–139.
66. Hermansen, L., Preutt, E. D. R., Osnes, J. B., and Giere, F. A. (1970). Blood glucose and plasma insulin in response to maximum exercise and glucose infusion. *J. Appl. Physiol.* **29,** 13–16.
67. Hermansen, L., and Vaage, O. (1977). Lactate disappearance and glycogen resynthesis in human muscle after exercise. *Am. J. Physiol.* **233,** E422–E429.
68. Hickson, R. C., Rennie, M. J., Conlee, R. K., Winder, W. W., and Holloszy, J. O. (1977). Effects of increased plasma fatty acids on glycogen utilization and endurance. *J. Appl. Physiol.* **43,** 829–833.
69. Hill, A. V., and Lupton, H. (1923). Muscular exercise, lactic acid, and the supply and utilization of oxygen. *Q. J. Med.* **16,** 135–171.
70. Hirche, H. J., Hombach, V., Langohr, H. D., Wacker, U., and Busse, J. (1975). Lactic acid permeation rate in working gastrocnemii of dogs during metabolic alkalosis and acidosis. *Pfluegers Arch.* **356,** 209–222.
71. Holloszy, J. O., and Booth, F. W. (1976). Biochemical adaptations to endurance exercise in muscle. *Annu. Rev. Physiol.* **38,** 273–291.

72. Hultman, E. (1967). Studies on muscle metabolism of glycogen and active phosphate in man with special reference to exercise and diet. *Scand. J. Clin. Lab. Invest., Suppl.* **94,**

73. Hultman, E. (1967). Physiological role of muscle glycogen in man, with special reference to exercise. *AMA Monogr.* **15,** 99–112.

74. Hultman, E. (1967). Muscle glycogen in man determined in needle biopsy specimens. Methods and normal values. *Scand. J. Clin. Lab. Invest.* **19,** 209–217.

75. Hultman, E. (1971). Muscle glycogen stores and prolonged exercise. *In* "Frontiers of Fitness" (R. J. Shephard, ed.), pp. 37–60. Thomas, Springfield, Illinois.

76. Hultman, E. (1979). Regulation of carbohydrate metabolism in liver during rest and exercise with special reference to diet. *Int. Symp. Biochem. Exercise* **3,** 99–126.

77. Hultman, E., and Bergström, J. (1973) Local energy-supplying substrates as limiting factors of different leg muscle work in normal man. *In* "Limiting Factors of Physical Performance" (J. Keul, ed.), pp. 113–125. Thieme, Stuttgart.

78. Hultman, E., and Nilsson, L. H. (1971). Liver glycogen in man. Effect of different diets and muscular exercise. *In* "Muscle Metabolism during Exercise" (B. Pernow and B. Saltin, eds.), pp. 143–151. Plenum, New York.

79. Hultman, E., and Nilsson, L. H. (1973). Liver glycogen as a glucose-supplying source during exercise. *In* "Limiting Factors of Physical Performance" (J. Keul, ed.), pp. 179–189. Thieme, Stuttgart.

80. Hultman, E., and Sahlin, K. (1980). Acid-base balance during exercise. *Exercise Sport Sci. Rev.* **8,** 41–128.

81. Irondelle, M., and Freund, H. (1977). Carbohydrate and fat metabolism of unacclimatized men during and after submaximal exercise in cool and hot environments. *Eur. J. Appl. Physiol.* **37,** 27–38.

82. Issekutz, B., Issekutz, A. C., and Nash, D. (1970). Mobilization of energy sources in exercising dogs. *J. Appl. Physiol.* **29,** 691–697.

83. Issekutz, B., Miller, H. I., Paul, P., and Rodahl, K. (1964). Source of fat oxidation in exercising dogs. *Am. J. Physiol.* **207,** 583–589.

84. Issekutz, B., and Rodahl, K. (1961). Respiratory quotient during exercise. *J. Appl. Physiol.* **16,** 606–610.

85. Issekutz, B., Shaw, W. A. S., and Issekutz, A. C. (1976). Lactate metabolism in resting and exercising dogs. *J. Appl. Physiol.* **40,** 312–319.

86. Johnson, R. E., and Edwards, H. T. (1937). Lactate and pyruvate in blood and urine after exercise. *J. Biol. Chem.* **118,** 427–432.

87. Jones, N. L., Robertson, D. G., Kane, J. W., and Hart, R. A. (1972). Effects of hypoxia on free fatty acid metabolism during exercise. *J. Appl. Physiol.* **33,** 733–738.

88. Jorfeldt, L. (1970). Metabolism of L(+)-lactate in human skeletal muscle during exercise. *Acta Physiol. Scand., Suppl.* **338.**

89. Jorfeldt, L., Juhlin-Darnfeldt, A., and Karlsson, J. (1978). Lactate release in relation to tissue lactate in human skeletal muscle during exercise. *J. Appl. Physiol.* **44,** 350–352.

90. Jorfeldt, L., and Wahren, J. (1970). Human forearm muscle metabolism during exercise. V. Quantitative aspects of glucose uptake and lactate production during prolonged exercise. *Scand. J. Clin. Lab. Invest.* **26,** 73–81.

91. Karlsson, J. (1971). Lactate and phosphagen concentrations in working muscle of man. *Acta Physiol. Scand., Suppl.* **358.**

92. Karlsson, J., Diamant, B., and Saltin, B. (1970). Muscle metabolites during submaximal and maximal exercise in man. *Scand. J. Clin. Lab. Invest.* **26,** 385–394.

93. Karlsson, J., Nordesjo, L.-O., Jorfeldt, L., and Saltin, B. (1972). Muscle lactate, ATP and CP levels during exercise after physical training in man. *J. Appl. Physiol.* **33,** 199–203.

94. Karlsson, J., and Saltin, B. (1971). Diet, muscle glycogen and endurance performance. *J. Appl. Physiol.* **31,** 203–206.
95. Keul, J., Doll, E., and Keppler, D. (1972). "Energy Metabolism of Human Muscle." Karger, Basel.
96. Krogh, A., and Lindhard, J. (1920). The relative value of fat and carbohydrate as sources of muscular energy. *Biochem. J.* **14,** 290–363.
97. Lemon, P. W. R., and Nagle, F. J. (1981). Effects of exercise on protein and amino acid metabolism. *Med. Sci. Sports Exercise* **13,** 141–149.
98. Liljestrand, S. H., and Wilsson, D. W. (1925). The excretion of lactic acid in the urine after muscular exercise. *J. Biol. Chem.* **65,** 773–782.
99. Linnarsson, D. (1974). Dynamics of pulmonary gas exchange and heart rate changes at start and end of exercise. *Acta Physiol. Scand., Suppl.* **415.**
100. Lusk, G. (1928). "The Elements of the Science of Nutrition." Saunders, Philadelphia, Pennsylvania.
101. MacDougall, J. D., Ward, G. R., Sale, D. G., and Sutton, J. R. (1977). Muscule glycogen repletion after high-intensity intermittent exercise. *J. Appl. Physiol.* **42,** 129–132.
102. Mainwood, G. W., and Worsley-Brown, P. (1975). The effects of extracellular pH and buffer concentration on the efflux of lactate from frog satorius muscle. *J. Physiol. (London)* **250,** 1–22.
103. Malmendier, C. L., Delcroix, C., and Berman, M. (1974). Interrelations in the oxidative metabolism of free fatty acids, glucose, and glycerol in normal and hyperlipemic patients. *J. Clin. Invest.* **54,** 461–476.
104. Margaria, R. (1976). "Biomechanics and Energetics of Muscular Exercise." Oxford Univ. Press (Clarendon), London and New York.
105. Masoro, E. J., Rowell, L. B., McDonald, R. M., and Steiert, B. (1966). Skeletal muscle lipids. II. Nonutilization of intracellular lipid esters as an energy source for contractile activity. *J. Biol. Chem.* **241,** 2626–2634.
106. Miller, H. I., Issekutz, B., and Rodahl, K. (1963). Effects of exercise on the metabolism of fatty acids in dogs. *Am. J. Physiol.* **205,** 167–172.
107. Moret, P. R., Weber, J., Haissly, J.-Cl., and Denolin, H., eds. (1980). "Lactate: Physiologic, Methodologic and Pathologic Approach." Springer-Verlag, Berlin and New York.
108. Moritani, T. (1980). Anaerobic threshold determination by surface electromyography. Ph.D. Dissertations, University of Southern California, Los Angeles.
109. Naimark, A., Wasserman, K., and McIlroy, M. (1964). Continuous measurement of ventilatory exchange ratio during exercise. *J. Appl. Physiol.* **19,** 644–652.
110. Needham, D. M. (1971). "Machine Carnis." Cambridge Univ. Press, London and New York.
111. Neptune, E. M., Sudduth, H. C., and Foreman, D. R. (1959). Labile fatty acids of rat diaphragm muscle and their possible role as a major endogenous substrate for maintenance of respiration. *J. Biol. Chem.* **234,** 1659–1660.
112. Newsholme, E. A. (1977). The regulation of intracellular and extracellular fuel supply during sustained exercise. *Ann. N.Y. Acad. Sci.* **301,** 81–91.
113. Nilsson, L. H., Furst, P., and Hultman, E. (1973). Carbohydrate metabolism of liver in normal man under varying dietary conditions. *Scand. J. Clin. Lab. Invest.* **32,** 331–337.
114. Oscai, L. B. (1973). The role of exercise in weight control. *Exercise Sport Sci. Rev.* **1,** 103–123.
115. Parizkova, J., and Rogozkin, V. A., eds. (1978). "Nutrition, Physical Fitness, and Health." Univ. Park Press, Baltimore, Maryland.
116. Paul, P. (1971). Uptake and oxidation of substrates in the intact animal during exercise. *In* "Muscle Metabolism during Exercise" (B. Pernow and B. Saltin, eds.), pp. 225–247. Plenum, New York.

117. Paul, P., and Issekutz, B. (1967). Role of extra muscular energy sources in the metabolism of exercising dogs. *J. Appl. Physiol.* **22,** 615–622.
118. Piehl, K. (1974). Time course for refilling of glycogen stores in human muscle fibers following exercise-induced glycogen depletion. *Acta Physiol. Scand.* **90,** 297–302.
119. Pruett, E. D. R. (1970). Glucose and insulin during prolonged work stress in men living on different diets. *J. Appl. Physiol.* **28,** 199–209.
120. Rabinowitz, D., and Zierler, K. L. (1962). Role of free fatty acids in forearm metabolism in man, quantitated by use of insulin. *J. Clin. Invest.* **41,** 2191–2197.
121. Radziuk, J. (1982). Developments in the tracer measurements of gluconeogenesis and glycogenesis in vivo: An overview. *Fed. Proc., Fed. Am. Soc. Exp. Biol.* **41,** 88–90.
122. Raynaud, J., Bernal, H., Bourdarias, J. P., David, P., and Durand, J. (1973). Oxygen delivery and oxygen return to the lungs at the onset of exercise in man. *J. Appl. Physiol.* **35,** 259–262.
123. Reitman, J., Baldwin, K. M., and Holloszy, J. O. (1973). Intramuscular triglyceride utilization by red, white, and intermediate skeletal muscle and heart during exhausting exercise. *Proc. Soc. Exp. Biol. Med.* **143,** 628–631.
124. Rennie, M. J., and Holloszy, J. O. (1977). Inhibition of glucose uptake and glycogenolysis by availability of oleate in well-oxygenated perfused skeletal muscle. *Biochem. J.* **168,** 161–170.
125. Rennie, M. J., Winder, W. W., and Holloszy, J. O. (1976). A sparing effect of increased plasma fatty acids on muscle and liver glycogen content in the exercising rat. *Biochem. J.* **156,** 647–655.
126. Rowell, L. B. (1977). Competition between skin and muscle for blood flow during exercise. *In* "Problems with Temperature Regulation during Exercise" (E. R. Nadel, ed.), pp. 49–76. Academic Press, New York.
127. Rowell, L. B., Kraning, K. K., Evans, T. O., Kennedy, J. W., Blackman, J. R., and Kusumi, F. (1966). Splanchnic removal of lactate and pyruvate during prolonged exercise in man. *J. Appl. Physiol.* **21,** 1773–1783.
128. Rowell, L. B., Masoro, E. J., and Spencer, M. J. (1965). Splanchnic metabolism in exercising man. *J. Appl. Physiol.* **20,** 1032–1037.
129. Sahlin, K., Harris, R. C., and Hultman, E. (1975). Creatine kinase equilibrium and lactate content compared with muscle pH in tissue samples obtained after isometric exercise. *Biochem. J.* **152,** 173–180.
130. Saltin, B., Blomquist, G., Mitchell, J. H., Johnson, R. L., Wildethal, K., and Chapman, C. B. (1968). *Circulation, Suppl.* **7,** 1–78.
131. Saltin, B., Gollnick, P. D., Piehl, K., and Eriksson, B. (1971). Metabolic and circulatory adjustments at the onset of exercise. *In* "Onset of Exercise" (A. Gilbert and P. Guille, eds.), pp. 63–67. University of Toulouse, Toulouse.
132. Saltin, B., and Karlsson, J. (1971). Muscle glycogen utilization during work at different intensities. *In* "Muscle Metabolism during Exercise" (B. Pernow and B. Saltin, eds.), pp. 289–300. Plenum, New York.
133. Scheuer, J., and Tipton, C. M. (1977). Cardiovascular adaptations to physical training. *Annu. Rev. Physiol.* **39,** 221–251.
134. Shephard, R. J., and Sidney, K. H. (1975). Effects of physical exercise on plasma growth hormone and cortisol levels in human subjects. *Exercise Sport Sci. Rev.* **3,** 1–30.
135. Spitzer, J. J., and Gold, M. (1964). Free fatty acid metabolism by skeletal muscle. *Am. J. Physiol.* **206,** 159–163.
136. Spitzer, J. J., and Hori, S. (1969). Oxidation of free fatty acids by skeletal muscle during rest and electrical stimulation in control and diabetic dogs. *Proc. Soc. Exp. Biol. Med.* **131,** 555–559.
137. Steinhagen, C., Hirche, H. J., Nestle, H. W., Bovenkamp, U., and Hosselmann, I. (1976).

The interstitial pH of the working gastrocnemius muscle of the dog. *Pfluegers Arch.* **367,** 151–156.

138. Terjung, R. 1. (1979). Endocrine response to exercise. *Exercise Sport Sci. Rev.* **7,** 153–180.

139. Vallyathan, N. V., Grinyer, I., and George, J. C. (1970). Effect of fasting and exercise on lipid levels in muscle. A cytological and biochemical study. *Can. J. Zool.* **48,** 377–383.

140. von Euler, U. S. (1974). Sympatho-adrenal activity in physical exercise. *Med. Sci. Sports* **6,** 165–173.

141. Wahren, J. (1970). Human forearm muscle metabolism. IV. Glucose uptake at different intensities. *Scand. J. Clin. Lab. Invest.* **25,** 129–135.

142. Wahren, J. (1977). Glucose turnover during exercise in man. *Ann. N.Y. Acad. Sci.* **301,** 45–53.

143. Wahren, J., Ahlborg, G., Felig, P., and Jorfeldt, J. (1971). Glucose metabolism during exercise in man. *In* "Muscle Metabolism during Exercise" (B. Pernow and B. Saltin, eds.), pp. 189–203. Plenum, New York.

144. Wahren, J., Felig, P., Ahlborg, G., and Jorfeldt, L. (1971). Glucose metabolism during leg exercise in man. *J. Clin. Invest.* **50,** 2715–2725.

145. Wasserman, K., Van Kessel, A. L., and Burton, G. G. (1967). Interaction of physiological mechanisms during exercise. *J. Appl. Physiol.* **22,** 71–85.

146. Wasserman, K., Whipp, B. J., and Davis, J. A. (1981). Respiratory physiology of exercise: Metabolism, gas exchange, and ventilatory control. *Int. Rev. Physiol. Respir. Physiol.* **23,** 150–211.

147. Wasserman, K., Whipp, B. J., Koyal, S. N., and Beaver, W. L. (1973). Anaerobic threshold and respiratory gas exchange during exercise. *J. Appl. Physiol.* **35,** 236–243.

148. Wesson, L. G. (1960). Kidney function in exercise. *In* "Science and Medicine of Exercise and Sports" (W. R. Johnson, ed.), pp. 270–284. Harper, New York.

149. Williamson, J. R. !1976). Mitochondrial metabolism and cell regulation. *In* "Mitochondria: Bioenergetics, Biogenesis, and Membrane Structure" (L. Packer and A. Gomez-Puyon, eds.), pp. 79–107. Academic Press, New York.

150. Williamson, J. R. (1979). Mitochondrial function in the heart. *Annu. Rev. Physiol.* **41,** 485–506.

151. Zierler, K. L. (1977). Fatty acids as substrate for heart and skeletal muscle. *AMA Monogr.* **54,** 35–39.

152. Zierler, K. L., Maseri, A., Klassen, G., Rabinowitz, D., and Burgess, J. (1968). Muscle metabolism during exercise in man. *Trans. Assoc. Am. Physicians* **81,** 266–272.

CHAPTER **5**

Foods and Nutrition for Exercise

GABE MIRKIN

Department of Physical Education
University of Maryland
College Park, Maryland 20740

Exercise Medicine: Physiological Principles
and Clinical Applications

I. INTRODUCTION TO NUTRIENTS

This chapter provides a brief review of food sources and food metabolism as it relates to exercise and individuals, including athletes, who exercise. Because of the fadism related especially to nutrition and exercise, an attempt is made to provide insight into some commonly held concepts among athletes regarding nutrition and to provide a basis for good nutrition in people who exercise.

Foods contain 44 nutrients that the body needs to maintain health. No specific nutrient will produce a better athlete, but lack of even a single one can impair athletic performance.

The 44 Essential Nutrients

Water
Glucose
Linoleic acid
7 Amino acids
13 Vitamins
21 Minerals

Some manufacturers of food supplements make inaccurate and unfounded claims that their product will result in better athletic performance. It is clear that protein supplements are no better than the protein in foods and in addition cost more. Bee pollen is not better than the pollen derived from plants, and vitamin B_{15} (pangamic acid, calcium pangamate) may not even exist. The Food and Drug Administration found a variety of different chemicals in bottles labeled vitamin B_{15}.

Since the body does not absorb whole foods, all foods must be broken down into single components. Carbohydrates are broken down into (simple) sugars. Protein is broken down into single amino acids, and fat is broken down into monoglycerdies, i.e., glycerol and fatty acids.

Foods contain basic nutrients that are the same as those which make up normal body structure. Glucose, found in fruits, is the same as the glucose in the bloodstream; and the amino acid lysine, found in meats, is the same as the lysine found in the red blood cells.

II. CARBOHYDRATES

Carbohydrates are sugars in various combinations. They can exist as a single sugar molecule, or as two or more sugar molecules bound together. The single sugars are called monosaccharides. Two sugar molecules bound together are called disaccharides. Polysaccharies are found in foods as chains of hundreds, thousands, or even millions of sugar molecules joined together. Disaccharides and polysaccharides must be broken down into monosaccharides before the body can use them. There are many single sugars in foods. But only four, glucose, fructose, galactose, and mannose, can pass from the upper intestine into the bloodstream. All other monosaccharides as well as all disaccharides and all polysaccharides must be broken down chemically in the upper intestine into one of the four acceptable monosaccharides before being absorbed into the circulation. Once they leave the intestines, the four acceptable sugars are taken up by the liver via the portal circulation.

Glucose may pass unchanged through the liver to circulate, but fructose, galactose, and mannose are absorbed by the liver and converted to glucose before reentering the bloodstream.

Therefore, all ingested carbohydrates, from corn to candy bars, end up as glucose before going into the general circulation for use by the body.

A. Why Carbohydrates Are Needed

Carbohydrates are a basic fuel for movement. They are one of the main sources of energy for skeletal muscles during exercise. Muscles will metabolize either sugar or lipid during exercise. Sugar comes from ingested carbohydrates, whereas lipid comes either from ingested fats or from stored body fat, which is mobilized for energy. However, the body can convert sugar to fat for fat storage.

The main advantage of lipid as a fuel is that the body can store vast reserves of it, whereas the main advantage of carbohydrate (glucose) as a fuel is that it is more efficient. Lipid metabolism is always aerobic; carbohydrate metabolism can be either aerobic or anaerobic.

During heavy exercise when oxygen cannot be delivered to the working muscle adequately, muscles utilize sugar (glucose) almost exclusively. At rest when oxygen delivery is adequate muscles utilize nearly only lipid (1). Between extremes, the balance between lipid and sugar varies, depending on the intensity of exercise and level of fitness.

B. Glycogen

Glucose is stored in the muscles for use as fuel in the form of glycogen. Exercise endurance of muscles depends on how much glycogen is stored prior to exercise (2,3). The more sugar stored in muscle, the greater the duration of the exercise.

Patients on a low carbohydrate diet, which limits intake of fruits, sugared foods, and grains, will not be able to sustain long, hard exercise (4). Muscles will have so little glycogen that even minimal activity can produce fatigue.

C. Common Problems in Endurance Athletes

When dealing with problems in long-distance runners, several symptoms and questions arise frequently.

1. HITTING THE WALL

When an exercising muscle runs out of stored glycogen, individual muscle function is impaired. Use and coordination are reduced significantly, and often painful cramps occur.

2. DEPLETION

Marathon runners may develop symptoms of muscles glycogen depletion (the "wall") anywhere from the fifteenth to twenty-sixth mile of a marathon. To improve glycogen stores in muscle, it is necessary to exercise them almost to the point of glycogen depletion about once a week. Following a long run, for example, muscle will take up increased amounts of carbohydrate. Runners training for marathons use this depletion–restoration process to increase muscle glycogen stores prior to long runs. Marathon runners will run more than 15 miles once a week, bicycle racers will ride for 4–6 hours, and the cross-country skiers may spend 10–12 hours on a continuous skiing program.

Because of the increased popularity of marathons, many people are participating in these long (26.2 miles) races before they have achieved enough training to improve muscle glycogen stores. That is why at the finish of many marathons, there are large numbers of runners staggering, limping, and in pain. These people are consuming their own muscle as fuel at the end of the race.

3. CARBOHYDRATE PACKING

The procedure called carbohydrate packing is useful (5) for adapting skeletal muscles to store more glycogen. Four days before a long-distance race, the runner should be advised to exercise intensely to deplete muscle glycogen. To accomplish this, many marathoners run 4–6 miles rapidly. Then for the next 3 days, regular meals are eaten but in addition extra carbohydrates such as bread, spaghetti, macaroni, potatoes, pancakes, and fruits are consumed. The major reason for an increase in sugar (glycogen storage is the combination of initial muscle depletion, increased carbohydrate ingestion, and the period of reduced exercise prior to the race.

Interestingly, most top runners do not gain added benefit from carbohydrate packing. They do so much exercise each day that they are depleting their muscles regularly and they eat so much carbohydrate each night that they are packing each evening. Moreover, there are some limitations to carbohydrate packing:

1. Carbohydrate packing will be a benefit only if the anticipated event involves strenuous continuous exercise lasting longer than 30 minutes.

2. Carbohydrate packing will reduce performance speed in events that requires great speed over shorter distances. Each gram of stored glycogen requires three additional grams of water so that the muscles will be much heavier than usual.
3. Maximum muscle capacity for glycogen is achieved in 3 days. Carbohydrate loading beyond that time will cause ingested sugars to be converted to fat.
4. The precompetition meal has very little to do with carbohydrate loading. Since more than 10 hours are needed to load muscle with glycogen, the most important meal is on the night before the event (6).

4. BONKING

Bonking is an expression used by long-distance bicycle racers to describe a hypoglycemic state that occurs when the liver glycogen stores are depleted. It is common in long-distance bicycle racers who do not eat during a race.

Muscles, brain, and other tissues are contantly consuming glucose from the blood for energy. There is only enough glucose stored in the blood to last about 3 minutes. To keep blood sugar levels from dropping, the liver releases glucose slowly and constantly into the circulation. At rest, there is enough glucose stored in the liver to last 12 hours (7) During exercise, muscles draw sugar from the blood even faster so that the liver must release sugar more rapidly into the bloodstream. Under conditions of prolonged exercise, the liver can run out of its stored sugar supply in much less than 12 hours. During vigorous exercise for an extended period of time, the liver can become depleted of its stored glucose, blood glucose will fall, and cerebral dysfunction (bonking) will occur. Headache, tachycardia, sweating, dizziness, confusion, and motor paralysis may result. Since the brain obtains 98% of its energy from glucose in the bloodstream, low blood sugar levels may result in syncope.

5. EATING BEFORE ATHLETIC EVENTS

Usually about 12 hours elapse from the time of the evening meal until awakening in the morning. This situation results in relatively lower liver stores of glucose in the morning. Beginning morning exercise without eating breakfast is more likely to result in low sugar and early fatigue than if a morning meal is ingested prior to exercising.

6. SUGAR INGESTION PRIOR TO EXERCISE

Sugar intake within 3 hours of exercising can result in fatigue (8). Ingestion of a large amount of sugar will raise blood sugar levels, induce insulin release, and subsequent reduction of blood glucose. If exercise is done during this high insulin period, early fatigue may result.

The combination of high blood insulin levels and the rapid glucose utilization by exercising muscles can cause blood sugar to fall, producing early fatigue even though adequate calories have been stored in the body.

7. SUGAR INGESTION DURING EXERCISE

Individuals participating in events which lasting less than 2 hours probably do not need extra calories during exercise. On the other hand, for prolonged exercise lasting more than 2 hours continuously, it is a good idea to take in extra food during exercise (9). The extra calories will help to preserve muscle and liver sugar stores and prevent fatigue.

8. EATING DURING COMPETITION

Almost any food can be used for energy production. The body can utilize the sugars in carbohydrates directly, it can use the fat directly, and it can convert the protein to sugar and use it for energy.

Bicycle racers often eat chicken, marmalade, peanut butter sandwiches, and bananas during a race. Any of these foods is a good source of nutrition on long hikes or bicycle tours.

Although protein can be broken down into organic acids and ammonia, both of which must be eliminated by the kidneys, there should be little concern about these compounds as long as urine output is maintained during exercise and fluid intake is adequate.

9. FLUID INTAKE DURING EXERCISE

For continuous exercise lasting 2 hours or less, there is no advantage to eating during exercise, but adequate fluid intake must be maintained. The best drink during exercise is water. Sweat is hypotonic and serum sodium and potassium levels usually rise. Serum calcium is unchanged and serum magnesium may fall slightly. Thus, salt tablets are unnecessary and may be frankly dangerous.

Drinks with minerals are absorbed slightly more quickly than pure water, but the difference is not significant (10). In competitive events that last less than 2 hours, one should not drink fluids that contain more than 2.5% sugar (11). At percentages greater than this, absorption of fluid from the gastrointestinal tract is markedly delayed. Orange juice, most other fruit juices, and most soft drinks contain about 10% sugar. Manufacturers commonly add sugar to enhance sweetness. Many of these drinks would have less pleasant taste with sugar levels much below 10%.

Cold drinks are less likely to cause cramps than warm ones. The rate of absorption of fluids depends on how quickly they leave the stomach. Since cold drinks leave the stomach more quickly than warm ones, cold drinks are more desirable during exercise (12).

During warm-weather exercise lasting more than 30 minutes, water should be taken before a thirst sensation occurs. Since sweat contains far more water than salt, the concentration of salt in the blood will rise. Osmoreceptors in the brain will not signal a thirst sensation until blood salt concentration rises considerably. By that time 1–2 liters of water may have been lost, and it will be impossible to catch up on this loss during exercise (13). Thus, before starting exercise on a warm day, a cup of cold water should be taken, and repeated every 15 minutes during exercise.

10. DOES FRUCTOSE IMPROVE ENDURANCE?

Fructose is taken up by the liver and converted to glucose before it is released into the bloodstream. Thus, fructose will cause an insulin response even though it might be delayed and not as high. Fructose does not increase endurance and it costs 15 times as much as glucose. Thus there is no advantage to fructose ingestion, and indeed the cost would indicate that glucose is a better choice.

11. HONEY VERSUS SUGAR

Honey and fruit contain glucose and fructose, respectively. Granulated table sugar contains sucrose (glucose and fructose linked—a disaccharide). When table sugar reaches the intestine, it is converted to glucose and fructose. Thus, there is no difference between table sugar, fruit sugar, and honey. Although it is true that honey contains more calcium and iron than sugar, it would be necessary to ingest 3 cups of honey to meet your daily needs for calcium and iron. However, 3 cups of honey contain 2500 calories so that a significant excess of calories will occur if honey is used to supply these minerals.

12. FRUIT SUGARS VERSUS TABLE SUGAR

Granulated table sugar and fruit sugar provide the same carbohydrates. However, fruits contain vitamins and minerals, and the sugar in fruit is released more slowly. Thus, the rise in blood sugar is slightly delayed when ingesting sugar from fruits.

13. IS THERE A WAY TO EAT SO THAT YOU RECOVER FASTER FROM EXERCISE?

You will recover faster from endurance exercise if you eat a diet that is rich in carbohydrates. The average athlete takes in about 250 grams of carbohydrate per day, which will not help him to completely fill his muscles with glycogen.

If the athlete takes in 600 grams of carbohydrate per day, he can usually completely refill his muscles with glycogen.

III. PROTEINS

Protein is the basic structural material for all plants and animals. Proteins are made up of amino acids, all of which contain the element nitrogen, whereas carbohydrates and fat do not. The liver can remove nitrogen from amino acids and convert what is left to fat or sugar. Since protein can be changed into energy-producing substances, it can be used for energy, but only indirectly. Protein is never a source of immediate energy, as fat and carbohydrates are, because it requires extra processing.

All proteins are made up of various combinations of the 22 amino acids, but only 21 of them are found in humans. Of these 21, nine must come from the diet; the body can manufacture the other 12. Because the nine dietary amino acids cannot be made internally, either *de novo* or in minute amounts, they are called the "essential" amino acids. All individual must be sure to get enough of these essential amino acids in their diet.

The 21 Amino Acids

Glycine	Cystine
Alanine	Cysteine
Valine*	Methionine*
Leucine*	Tyrosine
Isoleucine*	Phenylalanine*
Serine	Tryptophan*
Threonine*	Proline
Aspartic acid	Histidine*
Glutamic acid	Glutamine
Lysine*	Asparagine
Arginine	

*Essential amino acids.

Animal protein (meat, fish, poultry, eggs, and milk products) contains all nine essential amino acids. Vegetable protein usually lacks one or more. However, even vegetarians can get all the essential amino acids by combining vegetables and other plant products in their diet. For instance, individually, neither corn nor beans have all essential amino acids, but the two in combination do.

A. Protein Utilization

The body uses the building blocks of each nutrient group to supply its needs. In carbohydrates, the building blocks are sugars. In protein, they are amino acids.

Just as carbohydrates must be broken down into single sugars, protein must be broken down into single amino acids before the body can absorb and use it.

Protein breakdown takes place in the stomach and upper intestines, and the single amino acids go to the liver.

The liver can recombine them to make new proteins essential for normal function, or it can route the amino acids into the bloodstream to be picked up by other parts of the body to be used as needed, or it can eliminate or convert excess amino acids. The body has no way of storing amino acids so any surplus must be eliminated or converted to fat or sugar. If excess protein is consumed, the liver breaks down the surplus amino acids into two basic components: nitrogen and organic acids. The nitrogen becomes ammonia to be eliminated in the urine. The organic acids may also leave the body via the kidneys; however, if a large protein excess occurs, the liver and kidneys will not eliminate all of the organic acids. In this case, the liver can convert them to sugar or fat to be used for energy or stored. Thus, the converted organic acids can ultimately become body fat, just as can excess carbohydrates and dietary fat.

B. Protein Requirements during Exercise Training

Since so much of the body is made up of protein, these compounds are needed for normal tissue and organ function. Since protein is not a major source of energy for muscles during exercise, it takes almost as much protein to sit in a chair as it does to run a marathon. Protein requirements do not rise significantly with exercise (14–16).

C. Will Protein Supplements Improve Strength?

By consuming extra protein, muscular strength will not increase. Indeed, excess protein intake can result in muscle weakness. Only small amounts of extra protein are needed to increase muscle mass. The most important stimulus to muscle growth is exercise against resistance, such as lifting heavy weights or pushing on special strength machines. The stimulus to muscle growth under a chronic load is so strong that a muscle will enlarge with strength training even if the athlete is fasting and losing weight and all other muscles are getting smaller (17).

Even on an intensive strength training program which results in a gain of one pound of muscle per week, protein needs are not increased. Significantly one pound of muscle is 72% water and contains only about 100 g protein. One hundred grams of protein divided by 7 days in a week equals 15 g/day, equivalent to the amount of protein you will find in a handful of corn or beans. Taking extra protein can be harmful during exercise in hot weather. Since the body cannot store extra protein, excess protein is converted to ammonia and organic acids, which are excreted in the urine. These organic compounds act as diuretics and can cause dehydration and increase the risk for heatstroke (18). Taking extra protein can also cause loss of appetite and diarrhea.

IV. FATS

Fats are made up of fatty acids and glycerol. They are the principal fuel for muscles at all times except during heavy exercise, which requires anaerobic metabolism. Dietary fat, however, is not necessary for the energy supply to muscle. Protein and sugar can both be converted to fat by the liver.

There is one fatty acid, linoleic acid, which is essential i.e., it cannot be made by the body. This fatty acid is used to form cell membranes, hormones, and other things. The fat-soluble vitamins A, D, E, and K require fats in the gastrointestinal tract for proper absorption. The American population obtains almost 50% of their calories from fat. The amount appears excessive compared to other populations. High fat ingestion has been incriminated in increasing the chance of getting certain cancers, e.g., colon, lung, breast, and uterus; it may also increase the incidence of coronary artery disease. To reduce fat intake, individuals should limit red meat intake to not more than three times a week, avoid all skin and organ meats, drink skim milk, and avoid fried foods. Patients with hyperlipidemias should avoid eating nuts and seeds.

Eggs are a common source of calories from fat. Most of the calories in eggs come from the lipid cholesterol, but it appears to be healthful to eat a few eggs a week. More than 80% of the cholesterol is made by the liver; less than 20% comes from food sources. With increased cholesterol ingestion, the liver produces less, and blood cholesterol is maintained nearly constant. The current American diet contains more than 700 mg cholesterol/day and the added 300 mg from one egg is unlikely to affect blood cholesterol levels. In addition, eggs are an excellent source of 11 basic nutrients and they contain high quality protein as well.

Fat Intake prior to Competitive Events

The type of food eaten before participating in a competitive event is not critical as long as the stomach is empty at the time exercise begins.

Fats delay stomach emptying, but as long as the stomach is empty at the start of exercise, they pose no problem. The purpose of the pregame meal is to supply liver and not muscle with stores of sugar. It is not important to ingest an excess of carbohydrates.

V. VITAMINS

Most vitamins are chemical compounds that combine with other chemicals to form enzymes. Extra vitamins are not needed when exercising.

As components of catalytic enzymes, vitamins help process other nutrients, and they facilitate a wide range of other vital chemical reactions.

For example, three B vitamins must be present for breakdown of sugar for energy. Without them sugars would not be metabolized properly and the brain, which obtains more than 98% of its energy from sugar, would be in danger of starvation. Vitamins are present in most foods. They pass directly from the gastrointestinal tract into the bloodstream after they have been dissolved, either in water or fat.

Common and Correct Names of the Vitamins

Original name	Current names
Vitamin A	Vitamin A (retinol)
Vitamin B	Vitamin B_1 (thiamine)
	Vitamin B_2 (riboflavin)
	Niacin (nicotinic acid, niacinamide, nicotinamide)
	Vitamin B_6 (pyridoxine)
	Vitamin B_{12} (cobalamin, cyanocobalamin)
	Folacin (folic acid, pteroylglutamic acid)
	Pantothenic acid
	Biotin
Vitamin C	Vitamin C (ascorbic acid)
Vitamin D	Vitamin D (calciferol)
Vitamin E	Vitamin E (α-tocopherol)
Vitamin K	Vitamin K (menaquinone, phylloquinone)

A. Vitamin Needs

A catalyst provides the environment necessary for a certain chemical reaction to occur. But, though it must be present, the catalyst does not *cause* the reaction. Since it is not a direct participant, hardly any of the catalyst is used up in the reaction. Thus, most of the catalyst's components, including vitamins, are available for recycling. For this reason, most people do not need vitamin supplements. Vitamins last a considerable time in the body, and those that are depleted are easy to replace. The National Academy of Sciences has established a recommended daily allowance, or RDA, for each vitamin (20). The RDAs for most vitamins are readily available in the standard American diet, and vitamins taken above these levels are wasted. Having more vitamins than necessary will not make body chemical reactions take place any better or any faster. The excess vitamins will create another disposal chore. For example, following ingestion of a large dose of vitamin C, more than 80% of the dose is excreted in the urine and feces shortly after ingestion.

B. Do Athletes Need More Vitamins?

With only three exceptions, namely, thiamine, niacin, and riboflavin, requirements for vitamins do not increase with exercise. These three vitamins are consumed in the breakdown of carbohydrates and fats to form energy, and during exercise, muscles utilize both (21). These three vitamins are found in most places where carbohydrates are found: in grains and cereals. So unless an athlete is living mostly on refined sugar which contains no vitamins, he or she need not worry about getting enough of them.

Breads made from white flour, in which these three vitamins have been removed, are supplemented with the vitamins. It is illegal to ship bread in interstate commerce that does not contain the three B vitamins. Virtually all breads have them added.

C. Vitamin Excess

For individuals who feel a vitamin supplement is helpful and who want to assure adequate intake, a daily multivitamin tablet will suffice. The dosages in such pills are not high enough to cause any vitamin toxicity. At worst the vitamins will be unused and excreted in the urine. However, beware of exceeding the RDAs appreciably. Too many vitamins can be dangerous or even fatal (22). Chronic vitamin A overdose can result in skin cracking, hair loss, joint and bone pain, and severe headache. Overdoses of vitamin D can cause extreme muscle weakness and stiffness, calcium deposition in muscles and kidneys, high blood pressure, anemia, and death from kidney failure. Overdoses of vitamin E can cause headaches, blurred vision, diarrhea, muscle weakness, and extreme fatigue. With excess vitamin C, patients can develop diarrhea, kidney stones, and a chemical dependence so that when vitamin C is stopped, symptoms develop of vitamin C deficiency even though current intake would normally have satisfied requirements for that vitamin. Large doses of niacin can cause jaundice, liver disease, stomach ulcers, and joint pain.

The reason for these adverse effects from vitamins stems from their specific functions in the body. In some cases, large overdoses can exaggerate these functions and produce abnormal effects. For example, vitamin D aids in absorption and storage of calcium. With excess vitamin D intake, patients absorb and retain so much calcium that the calcium is deposited in the kidneys to form stones and in soft tissue, causing calcification of muscles, ligaments, and tendons.

Niacin functions as an aid in conversion of sugar to energy and helps the liver in processing sugar. Excess niacin will cause high blood levels of sugar and liver damage. Vitamins can also produce unwanted effects in high doses which are due to other actions of the vitamin which are not their primary action.

D. Vitamin C and Protection from Colds

There are at least eight well-controlled studies on vitamin C and the common cold. Seven of them show no benefit whatever (23–29). The eighth by Anderson *et al.* (29a) did show a slight protective effect on Canadian Army troops on maneuvers in the Arctic. The study was repeated 2 years later and did not demonstrate any protective effect by vitamin C.

E. The Vitamin That Is Not

There is no evidence that vitamin B_{15} improves athletic performance (30). In fact what is vitamin B_{15} (31)? The Food and Drug Administration has tested several different brands, and they appear to contain different things. At the present time, some manufacturers of this compound disagree among themselves each claiming that only they have the real thing. The people who introduced B_{15} into this country claim that it is a methylating agent and sent some of it to Dr. William Darby, then chairman of the Department of Chemistry at Vanderbilt University. He found no such activity. Doctor Darby sent some of the so-called vitamin B_{15} to Dr. Victor Herbert, a vitamin expert, who found that it was the simple sugar lactose, found in milk. It was introduced as a vitamin but a vitamin is a compound needed in the diet, which if missing, causes a deficiency syndrome. Neither need nor deficiency has ever been demonstrated for B_{15}. It is absurd to call it a vitamin. The Food and Drug Administration has obtained legal permission to remove vitamin B_{15} from the drug market, but it is difficult to keep this drug off the market. Since nobody knows what vitamin B_{15} is, when the government gets a court order to take it off the market, the producer can refill the bottle with another chemical compound, like the Greek god Proteus who, when captured in his human form, would change into something such as a snake or a cloud and escape. To make matters even worse, one recent study showed that the material in one of the preparations may cause cancer.

VI. MINERALS

With the exception of the need for iron for some menstruating women, there is no need to take mineral supplements.

A. Iron

Most men get all the iron they need from the food that they eat. And women would too, if they ate better and if they did not menstruate. The extra blood lost through menstruation causes one out of every four women in this country to be iron deficient. The iron in meat, fish, and poultry is absorbed quite well, but the iron from grains is absorbed poorly. So women who eat very little meat, fish, and poultry are most likely to benefit from taking iron supplements.

With exercise, the muscles require large amounts of oxygen, which is carried bound to the iron containing pigment hemoglobin.

With inadequate hemoglobin, oxygen transport by the blood is impaired and early fatigue will occur. Iron deficiency can also impair performance in the absence of frank anemia (32). Iron is stored in red blood cells and other plasma proteins as well as in tissues such as muscle, bone marrow, and liver. Reduced blood hemoglobin does not occur until the body has run out of almost all its reserve iron. Thus, one can be iron deficient and still have a normal red blood cell count.

With inadequate tissue stores of iron, tiredness may occur more quickly. Testing for adequate tissue reserves of iron requires bone marrow examination, and since this test is expensive and painful, it should only be used in refractory cases where iron deficiency is suspected as a cause of established anemia. Serum ferritin levels can serve as a fairly dependable measure of iron reserves.

B. Potassium

Low levels of potassium can cause tiredness, muscle weakness, cardiac arrhythmias, heat stroke, and even sudden death (33). Most healthy exercisers do not need potassium supplements. Their diets contain all the electrolykes that they need. Excess potassium can also cause cardiac rhythm disturbances by interfering with the conduction system. Potassium is present intracellularly in the highest concentration of all cations. It is necessary for normal muscle contraction and normal heartbeat. In contrast, sodium is present primarily in the extracellular fluids.

Muscle contraction is instituted by an action potential, which is activated when sodium moves into the muscle cell. This sodium passage is immediately followed by a flux of potassium from the cells. When potassium stores are low, the blood level is proportionately lower than concentration in muscle cells, the electrical potential across the cell membrane is greater, and muscles do not function properly. Potassium deficiency thus results in chronic fatigue and weakness.

Since the heart is a muscle, the cardiac electrical impulses are altered by low potassium and cardiac arrhythmias may develop. In extreme cases of hypokalemia, severe cardiac arrhythmia and death may occur. Potassium also prevents the body from overheating. Muscles generate large amounts of heat from the sugar and fat metabolized during exercise. More than 70% of the food that is burned is lost in heat.

As muscles begin to overheat, they release potassium into the bloodstream, causing vasodilation and increased blood flow through the muscle (34,35). This increased flow of blood carries large amounts of heat from the muscle to the skin, where it can be dissipated. When total body potassium is low and exercise is attempted, muscles do not regulate temperature as well, body temperature can rise, and heat stroke can occur.

A potassium-rich diet may provide some protection from high blood pressure. Several studies have shown that people who eat a diet rich in potassium and low in sodium are the ones least likely to develop high blood pressure. Since potassium is found within cells, any food that contains cells also contains potassium. A diet that is rich in fresh fruits, vegetables, and whole grain and low in prepared foods and meat, best fits this description. Prepared foods and meats may be preserved with sodium nitrite or nitrate. Healthy people rarely develop potassium deficiency. Almost all foods are rich in potassium. Whole grains, fruits, and vegetables are particularly good sources of potassium. Refined sugar, being acellular, contains no potassium. Costill (36), in studies on the effects of hypokalemia in humans, found significant difficulty in creating a low-potassium diet. The only way that he could create a potassium-deficient diet with enough calories for these runners was to feed them candy throughout the day. The kidneys and sweat glands were able to conserve potassium and the runners did not develop potassium deficiency.

By far, most potassium deficiency is induced by drugs such as diuretics or corticosteroids. Although rare, black licorice can cause sodium retention and significant potassium loss in the urine because of an aldosterone-like sodium-retaining agent. Prolonged diarrhea and vomiting can also cause the loss of large amounts of potassium. With diarrhea, potassium is lost in the stool, and with vomiting, hydrogen ion loss causes a metabolic alkalosis, which enhances potassium loss in the urine.

C. Salt

Most people do not need to consume extra salt when they exercise. The American diet contains so much extra salt that adding more is not necessary. Excess salt intake can be harmful. One out of every five people who ingests excess salt over a long period will develop high blood pressure. This is due in part to a genetic predisposition. Without exercise, salt needs are about 200 mg/day; with exercise, 3000 mg salt may be needed. Americans consume between 6000 and 18,000 mg salt/day; more than twice as much as they need even for hard exercise. Since salt enhances the taste of food, people add extra salt to their foods. In addition, manufacturers add salt to almost all prepared foods to help to keep them fresh. For example, canned peas contain 300 times as much salt as fresh peas. Even frozen vegetables may contain excess salt even though they are preserved by freezing, not by salting. Frozen peas contain 100 times as much salt as the fresh variety. In fact, one TV dinner contains all the salt you need for several days.

There is so much extra salt in prepared food that even if restricting salt by not salting food, not cooking with salt, and not eating anything that tastes salty, would still result in a total intake of 3000 mg salt/day. Some people can develop salt deficiency, which is related in general to a renal tubular defect in sodium reabsorption. They will develop tiredness and weakness and may develop painful muscle cramps. These individuals should have serum sodium and urine sodium levels assessed to determine if they are salt deficient.

D. Trace Minerals

There are 14 trace minerals that the body requires in small amounts. Diseases due to lack of trace minerals are virtually unheard of in this country. The only trace element deficiencies that are reported with any frequency throughout the world are those due to lack of iodine, selenium, cobalt, zinc, and fluorine. Protection from iodine deficiency is afforded by using iodized salt, and from fluorine deficiency by fluorinated drinking water. Plants absorb minerals and incorporate them into their cells. Eating plants or animals that have eaten the plants provides the necessary mineral intake. With the exception of the above five minerals, plants require the same minerals to grow as humans. Thus, by eating vegetable foods all of the required minerals should be obtained with the possible exception of these five trace elements.

The 25 Minerals Essential for Life

Carbon	Trace minerals
Hydrogen	Fluorine
Oxygen	Silicon
Nitrogen	Vanadium
Major minerals	Chromium
Calcium	Manganese
Phosphorus	Iron
Chlorine	Cobalt
Potassium	Nickel
Sulfur	Copper
Sodium	Zinc
Magnesium	Selenium
	Molybdenum
	Tin
	Iodine

However, ingestion of plants grown on soil that does not contain the above-mentioned five minerals may result in a deficiency in one or more of them. This situation is highly unlikely since the transportation and food delivery system is so efficient that foods come from a variety of locations and it is impossible for soil all over the world to be deficient in these minerals. For example, oranges may come from Florida, potatoes from Idaho, pecans from Texas, and apples from Washington.

VII. THE FOUR FOOD GROUPS

From the foregoing discussion, it should be clear that food supplements are not necessary. Rather, a well-balanced diet that supplies all essential nutrients should be established by varying foods as much as possible. The easiest system used to ensure adequate nutrition is the Four Food Plan developed by the Department of Agriculture in 1956.

Taking into account that almost all foods have a combination of nutrients, the plan, nevertheless, groups foods according to their predominate nutritional values. Each group supplies similar nutrients. Diet can be varied by substituting among foods within each group. All the necessary nutrients will be provided in this way.

The four food groups are (1) fruits and vegetables, (2) cereals and grains, (3) high protein foods, and (4) milk and milk products. At least four servings each of the first two groups and two servings each of the second two are needed each day. Although two foods seldom have the same nutritional values, foods within each group are related closely enough to provide good nutrition almost automatically. All that is necessary is a liberal use of the option to choose widely among the offerings in each group.

A. Fruits and Vegetables

All fruits and vegetables are excellent sources of carbohydrates, which are needed for muscle metabolism.

Dark green vegetables, deep yellow vegetables, and some fruits are good sources of vitamin A. Dark green vegetables are also an excellent source of vitamin B_2, folic acid, iron, and magnesium. Vitamins B_1, B_6, and C as well as iron, are abundant in citrus fruits and their juices, and in cantaloupes, strawberries, tomatoes, broccoli, and Brussels sprouts. Citrus fruits are also a good source of folic acid. Bananas are rich in potassium. Certain greens such as collards, kale, mustard greens, and turnip greens are good sources of calcium. Sixteen or more trace minerals are found in most vegetables and in many fruits. Leafy vegetables such as spinach, lettuce, cabbage, and celery are rich in fiber, a prevention against constipation. Nearly all vegetables and fruits are low in fat and none contains cholesterol.

Food and Nutrition Board, National Academy of Sciences–National Research Council Recommended Daily Dietary Allowances.[a] Revised 1980

Designed for the maintenance of good nutrition of practically all healthy people in the U.S.A.

Age (years)	Weight (kg)	Weight (lb)	Height (cm)	Height (in)	Protein (g)	Fat-soluble vitamins Vita-min A (µg RE)[b]	Vita-min D (µg)[c]	Vita-min E (mg α-TE)[d]	Water-soluble vitamins Vita-min C (mg)	Thia-min (mg)	Ribo-flavin (mg)	Niacin (mg NE)[e]	Vita-min B-6 (mg)	Fola-cin[f] (µg)	Vitamin B-12 (µg)	Minerals Cal-cium (mg)	Phos-phorus (mg)	Mag-nesium (mg)	Iron (mg)	Zinc (mg)	Iodine (µg)
Infants 0.0–0.5	6	13	60	24	kg × 2.2	420	10	3	35	0.3	0.4	6	0.3	30	0.5[a]	360	240	50	10	3	40
0.5–1.0	9	20	71	28	kg × 2.0	400	10	4	35	0.5	0.6	8	0.6	45	1.5	540	360	70	15	5	50
Children 1–3	13	29	90	35	23	400	10	5	45	0.7	0.8	9	0.9	100	2.0	800	800	150	15	10	70
4–6	20	44	112	44	30	500	10	6	45	0.9	1.0	11	1.3	200	2.5	800	800	200	10	10	90
7–10	28	62	132	52	34	700	10	7	45	1.2	1.4	16	1.6	300	3.0	800	800	250	10	10	120
Males 11–14	45	99	157	62	45	1000	10	8	50	1.4	1.6	18	1.8	400	3.0	1200	1200	350	18	15	150
15–18	66	145	176	69	56	1000	10	10	60	1.4	1.7	18	2.0	400	3.0	1200	1200	400	18	15	150
19–22	70	154	177	70	56	1000	7.5	10	60	1.5	1.7	19	2.2	400	3.0	800	800	350	10	15	150
23–50	70	154	178	70	56	1000	5	10	60	1.4	1.6	18	2.2	400	3.0	800	800	350	10	15	150
51+	70	154	178	70	56	1000	5	10	60	1.2	1.4	16	2.2	400	3.0	800	800	350	10	15	150
Females 11–14	46	101	157	62	46	800	10	8	50	1.1	1.3	15	1.8	400	3.0	1200	1200	300	18	15	150
15–18	55	120	163	64	46	800	10	8	60	1.1	1.3	14	2.0	400	3.0	1200	1200	300	18	15	150
19–22	55	120	163	64	44	800	7.5	8	60	1.1	1.3	14	2.0	400	3.0	800	800	300	18	15	150
23–50	55	120	163	64	44	800	5	8	60	1.0	1.2	13	2.0	400	3.0	800	800	300	18	15	150
51+	55	120	163	64	44	800	5	8	60	1.0	1.2	13	2.0	400	3.0	800	800	300	10	15	150
Pregnant					+30	+200	+5	+2	+20	+0.4	+0.3	+2	+0.6	+400	+1.0	+400	+400	+150	h	+5	+25
Lactating					+20	+400	+5	+3	+40	+0.5	+0.5	+5	+0.5	+100	+1.0	+400	+400	+150	h	+10	+50

[a] The allowances are intended to provide for individual variations among most normal persons as they live in the United States under usual environmental stresses. Diets should be based on a variety of common foods in order to provide other nutrients for which human requirements have been less well defined.

[b] Retinol equivalents. 1 retinol equivalent = 1 µg retinol or 6 µg β carotene. See text for calculation of vitamin A activity of diets as retinol equivalents.

[c] As cholecalciferol. 10 µg cholecalciferol = 400 IU of vitamin D.

[d] α-tocopherol equivalents. 1 mg d-α tocopherol = 1 α-TE. See text for variation in allowances and calculation of vitamin E activity of the diet as α-tocopherol equivalents.

[e] 1 NE (niacin equivalent) is equal to 1 mg of niacin or 60 mg of dietary tryptophan.

[f] The folacin allowances refer to dietary sources as determined by *Lactobacillus casei* assay after treatment with enzymes (conjugases) to make polyglutamyl forms of the vitamin available to the test organism.

[g] The recommended dietary allowance for vitamin B-12 in infants is based on average concentration of the vitamin in human milk. The allowances after weaning are based on energy intake (as recommended by the American Academy of Pediatrics) and consideration of other factors, such as intestinal absorption; see text.

[h] The increased requirement during pregnancy cannot be met by the iron content of habitual American diets nor by the existing iron stores of many women; therefore the use of 30–60 mg of supplemental iron is recommended. Iron needs during lactation are not substantially different from those of nonpregnant women, but continued supplementation of the mother for 2–3 months after parturition is advisable in order to replenish stores depleted by pregnancy.

B. Breads and Cereals

Like vegetables and fruits, grains and cereals are excellent sources of carbohydrates. They also supply almost all of the B vitamins, along with some iron and protein. Whole grain products contain a significant amount of fiber.

C. High Protein Foods

This groups includes meat, fish, poultry, and eggs along with dry beans, dry peas, seeds, and nuts. Meat, fish, poultry, and eggs supply all nine of the essential amino acids. In addition, all foods in the high protein group are rich sources of the B vitamins and of iron. Dry beans and peas, as well as soybeans and nuts, are also good sources of magnesium.

Menstruating female athletes should go out of their way to eat extra foods that contain iron. These include meats, whole grain and enriched breads and cereals, dry beans and dry peas, and various other vegetables. The iron in these foods is absorbed more completely if eaten at the same time that you take other foods that contain vitamin C, such as fruits.

D. Milk and Dairy Products

This group includes milk and milk derivatives. Milk, cheese, and yogurt are rich sources of protein, calcium, vitamin A, and vitamin B_2. In addition most milk is fortified with vitamin D.

REFERENCES

1. Saltin, B., Nazar, K., Costill, D. L., Stein, E., Jansson, E., Essén, B., and Gollnick, P. D. (1976). The nature of the training response. *Acta Physiol. Scand.* **96,** 289–305.
2. Hermansen, L., Hultman, E., and Saltin, B. (1967). Muscle glycogen during prolonged severe exercise. *Acta Physiol. Scand.* **71,** 129.
3. Christensen, E. H., and Hansen, O. (1939). Arbeitsfähigkeit und Ernähung. *Skand. Arch. Physiol.* **81,** 160–172.
4. Karlsson, J., and Saltin, B. (1971). Diet, muscle glycogen and endurance. *J. Appl. Physiol.* **31**(2), 203–206.
5. Åstrand, P. O. (1968). Something old and something new—very new. *Nutr. Today* **3**(2), 9–11.
6. Piehl, K. (1974). Time course for refilling of glycogen stores in human muscle fibers following exercise-induced glycogen depletion. *Acta Physiol. Scand.* **90,** 297–302.
7. Hultman, E., and Nilson, L. H. (1971). Liver glycogen on man: Effect of different diets and muscular exercise. *In* "Muscle Metabolism during Exercise" (B. Saltin and B. Pernow, eds.), pp. 143–152. Plneum, New York.
8. Foster, C., Costill, D. L., and Fink, W. F. (1979). Effects of preexercise feeding on endurance performance. *Med. Sci. Sports* **11**(1), 1–5.
9. Ahlborg, G., and Felig, P. (1977). Substrate utilization during prolonged exercise preceeded by the ingestion of glucose. *Am. J. Physiol.* **223,** 188.

10. Hunt, J. H., and Pathak, J. O. (1960). The osmotic effects of some simple molecules and ions on gastric emptying. *J. Physiol. (London)* **154,** 254.
11. Costill, D. L., and Saltin, B. (1974). Factors limiting gastric emptying during rest and exercise. *J. Appl. Physiol.* **37,** 679–683.
12. Fordtran, J. S., and Saltin, B. (1967). Gastric emptying and intestinal absorption during prolonged severe exercise. *J. Appl. Physiol.* **23,** 331.
13. Costill, D. L., Kammer, W. F., and Fisher, A. (1970). Fluid ingestion during distance running. *Arch. Environ. Health* **21,** 520–525.
14. Consolazio, C. F., Johnson, H. L., Nelson, R. Q., Dramise, J. G., and Skala, J. H. (1975). Protein metabolism of intensive physical training in the young adult. *Am. J. Clin. Nutr.* **28,** 29–35.
15. Wilson, H. E. C. (1932). The influence of muscular work on protein metabolism. *J. Physiol. (London)* **75,** 67–80.
16. FAO/WHO (1973). "Energy and Protein Requirements," Report of a joint ad hoc Expert Committee, Serial No. 522, pp. 5–118. FAO/WHO. Rome.
17. Goldberg, A. L., Etlinger, J. D., Goldspink, P. F., and Jablecki, C. (1975). Mechanism of work-induced hypertrophy of skeletal muscle. *Med. Sci. Sports* **7**(3), 185–198.
18. Serfass, R. C. (1977). Nutrition for athlete. *Contemp. Nutr.* **12.**
19. Anonymous (1975). Nutrition and Athletic performance. *Dairy Counc. Dig.* **46.**
20. National Research Council (1980). "Recommended Dietary Allowances." Nat. Acad. Sci., Washington, D.C.
21. Shils, M. E. (1973). Food and nutrition relating to work and environmental stress. *In* "Modern Nutrition in Health and Disease" (R. S. Goodhart and M. E. Shils, eds.), 5th ed., pp. 711–729. Lea, & Febiger, Philadelphia, Pennsylvania.
22. Herbert, V. (1980). "Nutrition Cultism," p. 77. Stickley Co., Philadelphia, Pennsylvania.
23. Berry, W. T. C., and Dark S. J. (1968). Vitamins in health and disease. *Practitioner* **201,** 305.
24. Dykes M. H. M., and Meier, P. (1975). Ascorbic acid and the common cold evaluation for its efficacy and toxicity. *JAMA, J. Am. Med. Assoc.* **231,** 1073–1079.
25. Karlowski, T. R., Chalmers, Frenkel, L. D., *et al.* Ascorbic acid for the common cold: A prophylactic trial. *JAMA, J. Am. Med. Assoc.* **231,** 1038–1042. 1975
26. Chalmers, T. C. (1975). Effect of ascorbic acid in the common cold—an evaluation of the evidence. *Am. J. Med.* **58,** 532.
27. Baird, I. McL., Hughes, R. E., Wilson, H. R. *et al.* (1979). The effect of ascorbic acid and flavinoids on the occurrence of symptoms normally associated with the common cold. *Am. J. Clin. Nutr.* **32,** 1686–1690.
28. Coulehan, J. L. (1979). Ascorbic acid and the common cold. *Postgrad. Med.* **66,** 153–160.
29. Pitt, H. A., and Costrini, A. M. (1979). Vitamin C prophylaxis in marine recruits. *JAMA, J. Am. Med. Assoc.* **241,** 908–911.
29a. Anderson, T. W., Beaton, G. H., Corey, P. M., and Spero. (1975). Winter illness and Vitamin C. The effects of relatively low doses. *Can. Med., Assoc. J.* **112,** 823; Anderson, T. W., Reid, D. B. W., and Beaton, G. H. (1972). Vitamin C and the common cold: A double blind trial. *ibid.* **107,** 503; Anderson, T. W., Suranyi, G. and Beaton, G. H. (1974). Effect on winter illness of large doses of Vitamin C. *ibid.* **111,** 31.
30. Girandola, R. N., Wiswell, R. A., and Bulbulian, R. (1980). A controlled trial of pangamic acid. *Med. Sci. Sports Exercise* **12**(2), 98.
31. Check, W. A. (1980). Vitamin B_{15}—whatever it is, it won't help. *JAMA, J. Am. Med. Assoc.* **243** (24), 2473–2480.
32. Nilson, K., Schoene, R. B., Robertson, H. T., Escourron, P., and Smith, N. J. (1981). The effects of iron repletion on exercise-induced lactate production in minimally iron-deficient subjects. *Med. Sci. Sports Exercise* **13**(2), 92.

33. Hubbard, R. W., Maser, M., Bowers, W. D., Lear, I., Angoff, G., Matthews, T., and Sils, I. V. (1981). Effects of a low-potassium diet on rats. Hyperthermia and heatstroke mortality. *J. Appl. Physiol.* **51**(1), 8–13.

34. Hazeyama, Y., and Sparks, H. (1979). Exercise hyperemia in potassium depleted dogs. *Am. J. Physiol.* **5**(3), H480–H486.

35. Knochel, J. P., and Schlein, E. M. (1972). On the mechanism of rhabdomyolosis in potassium depletion. *J. Clin. Invest.* **51**, 1750–1758.

36. Costill, D. (1978). Muscle water and electrolytes during acute and repeated bouts of dehydration. *In* "Nutrition, Physical Fitness, and Health" (J. Parizkova and V. A. Rogozkin, eds.), pp. 106–115. Univ. Park Press, Baltimore, Maryland.

II

Women, Youth, and the Elderly

CHAPTER 6

Physiological Aspects of Women and Exercise

RITA A. CAREY

Smith Kline and French
Laboratories
Philadelphia
Pennsylvania

I. INTRODUCTION

Currently medical science recognizes that physical exercise and conditioning are important for the physical and mental health of both women and men. Furthermore, the social climate of the United States today encourages both women and men to engage in sport for recreation and to improve health.

113

Exercise Medicine: Physiological Principles
and Clinical Applications

Prior to the 1960s the prevailing philosophy was that women's participation in sports and athletics was unusual and only marginally acceptable. The vast majority of women became totally sedentary at puberty when socially imposed sex roles forbid vigorous sports activity. Title IX of the Educational Act and the formation of the Association of Intercollegiate Athletics for Women contributed to establishing women's right to participation in sports and provided the organization for women's athletic competition. More important than legislation and structured competition, a marked attitudinal change occurred as the feminist movement of the 1960s influenced the American woman's view of sports activity. The modern woman feels free to participate in sports and athletics uninhibited by social taboos. She does not fear loosing her femininity, newly defined though femininity may be, by participation in physical conditioning and sports.

For women athletes the era of dramatically accelerated participation in sports and improvements in athletic performance has arrived. Previously established records in virtually all sports engaged in by women have been shattered. More significantly great numbers of women of all ages and with widely diverse backgrounds in physical conditioning are taking part in the quest for the enjoyment of athletic performance and for improved health and fitness through sport. Questions arise concerning the capacity of women to become conditioned for vigorous exercise and comparisons are inevitably made between the trainability and athletic achievements of female performers versus their male counterparts. Preventing and treating of athletic injury among sports women receives much attention.

One may question whether or not these comparisons between women and men are worthwhile since women's participation in sport should be evaluated on its own merit independent of how their achievements compare with men's. Nevertheless, our knowledge of training and conditioning in males provides a starting point for learning how women adapt to and benefit from exercise. What we have learned about safely enhancing physical fitness and improving athletic performance of men as well as our scientific understanding of exercise physiology and exercise biochemistry in males provides the basis for training and studying the female athlete. As more and more women participate in sports it is the responsibility of medical personnel to become informed about the female athlete, to disseminate accurate information about physical fitness and athletic training in women, and to treat the athletic female patient in a scientifically sound manner.

This chapter compares women and men with regard to their response to strength and endurance training, sports related injuries, performance in hot and cold environments, and the effects of exercise on the bone mineral metabolism, blood chemistry, and reproductive physiology. Only research studies in which human beings are subjects for investigation are cited with all experimental animal data omitted. It may be noted, however, that much of the basic exercise physiology and biochemistry research has been done on female experimental animals or in animal studies including both sexes. Much of what we know about exercise physiology has been derived from research in which the sex of the experimental animal was ignored.

Generally, many of the differences between women and men relative to their capacity to participate in sports and athletics have recently been found to be less than previously thought. The discrepancies between early studies and more recent research can be partially explained by noting the almost universal problem with early investigations in which the female subjects did not train or condition in the same manner as males to whom they were compared. Thus, the comparisons were biased in favor of males. With social influences allowing women to train more vigorously, recent scientific evidence about the capacity of women in sport contradicts earlier studies. Nevertheless physiological differences between women and men relative to conditioning and sports performance need to be clearly understood so that training programs are safe and to optimize the potential of the female participant for excellent athletic achievement.

II. RESPONSE TO STRENGTH AND ENDURANCE TRAINING: COMPARISON OF FEMALES AND MALES

How do the anatomical and physiological differences between women and men influence the way they adapt to strength training and to endurance training? Are there qualitative and/or quantitative differences in the way skeletal muscles of women respond to exercise stress compared to muscle tissue in males? What implications do sex differences in strength and endurance have for clinical medicine and athletic competition?

A. Strength

Skeletal muscle strength is defined and measured as the capacity of a muscle group to move a weight or to exert force against a stationary object. "Strength exercises" are those that are performed for a short time and that require nearly maximum effort over that relatively brief period. For example, wrestling, lifting the maximum weight possible, and sprinting are strength exercises. Success in these events depends primarily on skeletal muscle strength.

One can measure strength in the clinic or laboratory simply as the maximum pounds or kilograms moved. Alternatively, strength can be expressed as the force exerted per gram of lean body mass. In the latter instance the percentage of body weight which is fat is subtracted from total body weight and the force exerted divided by the remaining active tissue mass.

Although there have been few studies that compare the strength of adult men and women, it is generally agreed that when strength is measured in absolute terms, not per unit of lean body mass or cross sectional area of muscle, untrained women are about two-thirds as strong as untrained men. Hettinger (1), evaluating an average population in the early 1960s, compared the muscular strength of women and men and expressed his results as ratio of strength in women/men. The forearm flexor strength ratio for women/men was 0.55; finger flexor, 0.60; and for hip flexors combined with extensor, 0.80. Similarly a review by Laubach (2) in which he compiled data comparing the absolute strength of women and men determined that the upper extremity strength of females was 56% that of men. Lower extremity strength of females was 72% and trunk strength 64% that of males. Both hormonal differences between men and women and social influences discouraging women from strength-demanding activities account for these observations. The greater androgen level in the male accounts for his greater assimilation of protein into skeletal muscles compared to females. This hormonal difference and the resulting reduced capacity of the female to proliferate skeletal muscle limits the potential for strength development in women. Nevertheless, recent studies show that the differences in skeletal muscle strength in females and males is not as great when both sexes experience the same training program. Recently the U.S. Army began giving women and men the same basic training

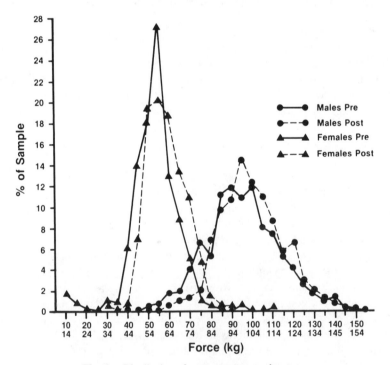

Fig. 1. Distribution of upper torso strength scores.

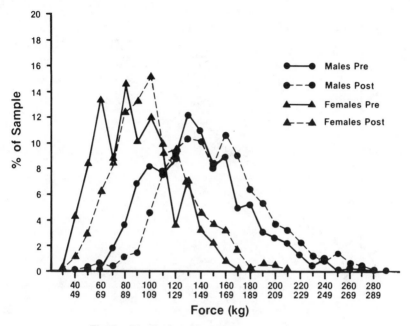

Fig. 2. Distribution of leg extensor strength scores.

including the same physical conditioning program. Knapik and co-workers (3) report the effects of army basic training on the muscular strength of men and women; 948 males and 496 females participated in the study. They were studied pre- and posttraining for percentage body fat and lean body mass, and maximum isometric strength of the upper torso, leg extensors, and trunk extensors. As shown in Figs. 1–3 there is considerable overlap in the strength values for women and men. Both males and females experienced increased strength after training. Females improved significantly ($p < 0.05$) more than males in upper torso strength (female = 9.3% and males = 4.2%) and trunk extensors strength development (female = 15.9% and male = 8.1%). Both improved about the same in leg extensors strength (female = 12.4%, males = 9.7%). Since the women started at lower strength values, the intensity of the work load stress stimulating training would be greater for the females and would account for their greater improvement compared to males.

Similar results were observed by Wilmore (4) in a study of university students participating in a 10-week strength training program. The females in this study improved more than males in their capacity to perform a bench press (female = 28.6%, male = 16.5%) and in grip strength (female = 12.8%, male = 5.0%) tests. Women and men increased leg strength by about the same amount (female = 29.5%, male = 28.6%) and men increased their forearm flexor strength,

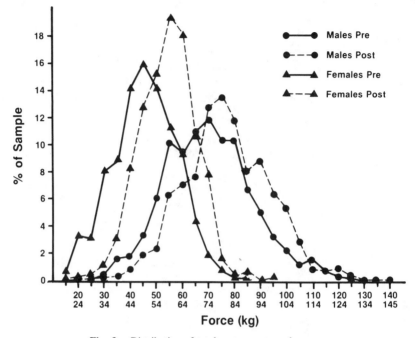

Fig. 3. Distribution of trunk extensor strength scores.

tested as an arm curl, more than women (female = 10.6%, male = 18.9%). The greater improvement of women, especially in upper body strength, was again related to their lower initial values.

There have been reports (5) of selected groups of female athletes (track and field throwing events) who are stronger than untrained males. Male athletes participating in the same or similar athletic events are, however, stronger than their female peers. Although absolute strength is of major interest in physically demanding labor and in some athletic events, it is of clinical and scientific interest that strength differences between women and men are considerably reduced and in some instances disappear when strength is expressed relative to body weight. In the study sited above (3) of women and men participating in U.S. Army Basic training, strength pre- and posttraining was also expressed relative to body weight and lean body mass (Table I). Differences between males and females are reduced when strength is normalized for body weight and the differences are less when strength is expressed per unit lean body mass. Following army basic training, the strength differences between women and men are less than before training.

The differences in the ratios of female/male strength relative to body weight compared to the female/male ratios relative to lean body mass are due to the greater percentage of body weight which is fat in the women than in men. Others (1,4,6) have reported similar decrease in the differences between strength of women and men when strength is expressed relative to lean body mass. In some instances (4) leg strength per unit lean body mass was greater in trained females than in trained males.

It is well recognized that hormonal differences between men and women account for an increased quantity of skeletal muscle mass in men compared to women. Researchers have studied muscle fiber composition and metabolism in an effort to determine if skeletal muscle in women and men are qualitatively different. Further, there is interest in determining if adaptive changes which occur as a result of training are different in women and men? If skeletal muscle in untrained women and men is qualitatively different and/or if females and males adapt to conditioning programs differently, then these factors together with differences in muscle mass would be important for designing training programs for women and men and could account for sex differences in athletic achievement.

In both women and men skeletal muscle can be simply classified as slow-twitch or fast-twitch (7), the classification refering not only to the time required for a single muscle contraction but also indicating different metabolic characteristics. Fast-twitch muscle fibers have higher glycogen content and higher activity of glycolytic enzymes compared to slow-twitch muscle. This fiber type is well suited for anaerobic function and is present in high concentration in athletes who perform at maximum effort for short periods of time such as sprinters and weight lifters. A major component of metabolism required for these athletic endeavors is anaerobic. Slow-twitch muscle fibers have greater density of mitochondria, higher content of myoglobin, and greater capacity to metabo-

TABLE I

Force/Weight (F/WT) and Force/Lean Body Mass (F/LBM) Ratios for Males and Females[a]

| | Site[b] | F/WT (kg/kg) | | | F/LBM (kg/kg) | | |
		Males	Females	Ratio F/M	Males	Females	Ratio F/M
Pretest	UT	1.39 ± 0.23	0.94 ± 0.21	0.68	1.66 ± 0.25	1.31 ± 0.27	0.79
	LE	2.04 ± 0.53	1.59 ± 0.50	0.78	2.43 ± 0.61	2.20 ± 0.68	0.91
	TE	1.04 ± 0.26	0.81 ± 0.22	0.79	1.24 ± 0.30	1.13 ± 0.29	0.91
Posttest	UT	1.43 ± 0.18	1.00 ± 0.16	0.70	1.67 ± 0.20	1.36 ± 0.20	0.82
	LE	2.22 ± 0.54	1.75 ± 0.50	0.79	2.59 ± 0.62	2.38 ± 0.68	0.92
	TE	1.11 ± 0.22	0.93 ± 0.18	0.84	1.29 ± 0.26	1.27 ± 0.24	0.98

[a] Values represent means ± SD.
[b] UT, upper torso; LE, leg extensors; TE, trunk extensors.

lize lipid as substrate for exercise than fast-twitch fibers. Slow-twitch fibers are adapted for aerobic metabolism and are predominate in athletes who perform at submaximal effort for long periods of time such as a long-distance runners, bicyclers, and distance swimmers. Metabolic processes are primarily aerobic in these events. An individual is likely to be genetically endowed with a greater proportion of one fiber type than the other. There is some controversy about whether athletic training can specifically develop either the fast-twitch or slow-twitch muscle fiber type required for a selected athletic event or if training simply increases the oxidative capacity of all fiber types.

In a study comparing muscle composition in women and men Costill *et al.* (8) found that in untrained female subjects the ratio of slow-twitch/fast-twitch fibers ranged from 0.60 to 1.82 and averaged 0.98; in untrained males the same ratio ranged from 0.88 to 1.27 and averaged 1.15. No statistically significant difference was observed. Edström and Nyström (7) observed the same phenomenon. Thus, the evidence to date is that sedentary individuals of either sex have the same skeletal muscle fiber composition.

Costill and co-workers (8) also studied the muscle fiber composition, fiber size and oxidative and glycolytic enzymes activities of 17 female and 23 males international-caliber track athletes. Six track and field events were studied including those that demand primarily anaerobic metabolism and others that require aerobic performance. Overall fiber composition for both female and male athletes was the same (50% slow-twitch). Closer examination of fiber type distribution of both women and men within the various athletic events show the expected preponderance of slow-twitch fibers in athletes who perform aerobically (62.3% in distance runners) and a relatively fewer of these fibers in those who perform anaerobically (38.3% in shot put and discus throwers). The female and male track athletes for each type of track and field event had similar muscle fiber composition. Differences in proportions of fiber types was related to the athletic event in which they participate and totally unrelated to sex. Further, insofar as training alters fiber-type composition, women and men appear to adapt to conditioning for any given track or field event in the same manner.

In another study (9) comparing lipid metabolism in female and male long-distance runners who trained the same amount (80–115 Km/week) and who had the same aerobic capacities ($\dot{V}o_2 = 60 \pm 6.2$ ml/kg/minute), it was found that both men and women had the same muscle fiber composition and derived similar fractions of their energy from lipids during a treadmill test that required 70% of maximal effort. *In vitro* studies of gastrocnemius muscle biopsies taken from these subjects suggest, however, that mitochondrial enzyme activities associated with lipid oxidation are lower in females than males. There is a discrepancy between the *in vitro* mitochondrial enzyme activity measurements of the capacity for lipid metabolism and the total body treadmill test measurement of lipid oxidation. It is evident that the phenomenon that limits the use of lipid during exercise includes factors in addition to mitochondrial enzyme activities. This study demonstrates that the major substrate utilized for exercise and the portion of energy derived from it are the same in females and males.

Other studies (10,11) of female athletes and sedentary females show that fiber-type distribution, fiber cross-sectional area, and enzymatic profiles change as a consequence of training in women in the same manner as in men.

Thus, it is evident that although men have more muscle mass, skeletal muscle is qualitatively the same in women and men. Women do benefit from strength training. They experience the same conditioning response as men. It is reasonable to expect that the positive effects of strength training on health and toward increased athletic prowess are the same in both sexes.

B. Endurance

Physical endurance refers to the capacity to perform submaximal physical work for a long period of time. "Endurance exercises" are those activities that one performs for an extended period of time and that require less than maximum effort. Running, bicycle riding, and swimming for long distances are examples of endurance exercises. These are in contrast to "strength exercises," the short bursts of maximum effort required for running a quarter mile, shot put, or lifting the maximum amount of weight possible.

In the clinic or laboratory the best measure an individual's endurance is their oxygen uptake. This is the amount of oxygen taken into the body, delivered to active tissue, and actually used in metabolic processes. Maximum oxygen uptake is determined during a standardized work load test. If a treadmill is used, for example, then the individual begins running slowly at zero grade and as the test continues the speed and elevation of the treadmill increase in small increments. The individual performs as long as possible with oxygen consumption measured during his maximum effort. Oxygen uptake is expressed as milliliters oxygen consumed per kilogram body weight per minute. The greater the person's maximal oxygen uptake, the more endurance capacity that person has, and as endurance conditioning occurs, maximal oxygen uptake values increase. It is recognized that there is a large cardiovascular component to endurance-type exercises serving to deliver oxygen to the working muscles. In addition there is a skeletal muscle component to endurance exercise in that the muscle cell must be capable of utilizing the oxygen available to synthesize the high energy phosphates necessary to perform work. The subcellular uptake of oxygen is thought to be the limiting factor in the capacity to perform endurance exercise. As a result of endurance training, changes occurs within the cell increasing the capacity of the cell for oxidative metabolism. Adaptations also occur in the cardiovascular system, including increased capillarization in skeletal muscle and perhaps some improvement of myocardial pump function.

In comparing the endurance capacity of adult women and men we compare their maximum oxygen uptake values. It is of interest to compare the absolute values and also to compare the responses of females and males to conditioning programs. Do women benefit from endurance training as much as men? Will women achieve the same maximal oxygen consumption values as men? Will they improve by the same percentage during a given training program?

Most of the studies comparing maximum oxygen consumption in women and men are survey studies of world-class athletes. The few studies of sedentary populations can be critized because at the time of these surveys sedentary females were far more inactive than their sedentary male peers. Nevertheless, these studies suggest that the maximum oxygen consumption of sedentary women is 70–75% of that observed in untrained men (12).

Comparisons of sedentary and athletic women with sedentary and athletic men show that the best male athletes have greater maximal oxygen uptake values than the best female athletes. There is, however, a great deal of overlap between the values in women and men. Hermansen and Andersen (13) reported in the mid-1960s that female and male athletes had maximum oxygen uptake values of 55 and 71 ml/kg/minute, respectively (Fig. 4). It can be seen that many of the values for females overlap with those observed in males. In a study of world-class competitors the maximal oxygen consumption among female and male members of the Swedish National Team revealed that for the same sport male athletes had greater maximal oxygen consumption values than their female peers (14) (Fig. 5). Untrained men and women are also included in this study. Somewhat in contrast to these studies, the highest reported value of oxygen uptake in a female is 74 ml/kg/minute for a cross-country runner (15).

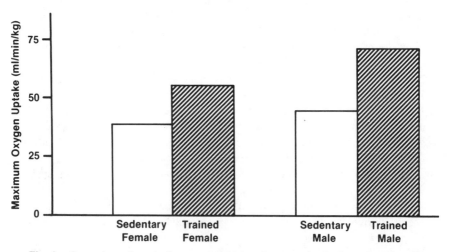

Fig. 4.   Comparison of maximal oxygen uptake in sedentary and trained women and men.

A.

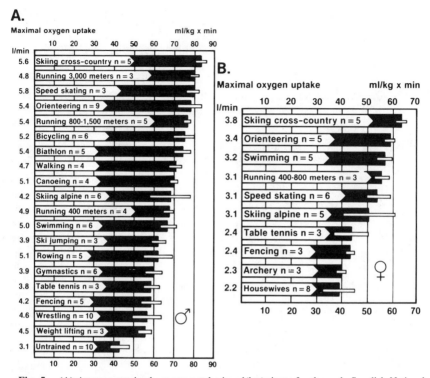

Fig. 5. (A) Average maximal oxygen uptake in ml/kg/minute for the male Swedish National Team in different sport events. The horizontal thin white bar in the middle of each blank bar denotes the range. To the left the average maximal oxygen uptake in liters/minute is given. (B) Average maximal oxygen uptake in ml/kg/minute for the female Swedish National Team in different sports. Symbols are the same as in (A).

As with strength measurement, oxygen uptake data can be experessed per unit lean body mass. The interest in doing so is to determine if the metabolically active tissue is equally efficient in women and men. It has been reported (16) that sex differences in maximum oxygen consumption disappear when data are expressed relative to lean body weight. At the cellular level the muscles of women and men have the same endurance capacity.

Studies comparing the training capacity of men and women show that women adapt to endurance training programs in a manner similar to males (17–21). In a recent study (18) of the effects of basic U.S. Army Basic training on maximal oxygen consumption in women and men, the conditioning response in women was the same as in men. The most poorly fit men and women increased their maximal oxygen consumption 13.6 and 10.5%, respectively. Men and women with higher initial values improved only 2.0 and 3.3%, respctively. Both sexes improved by about the same amounts and as expected those starting at the lowest levels of fitness showed the greatest improvement.

What implications do sex differences in strength and endurance have for health and for athletic performance? Insofar as skeletal muscle tone and strength, cardiovascular, and muscular endurance conditioning has positive effects on the health of men, conditioning programs of the same type are equally beneficial to the health of women. Coaches and women athletes are recognizing that appropriate training programs, similar to those employed by men, will markedly enhance athletic performance of women. Utilization of this increased factual knowledge, plus social changes, have resulted in dramatically improved sports performance by women. Recently, greater improvements have been made by women than by men. Between 1970 and 1980 the women's world track record for the 1500-meter run decreased by 25.8 seconds while the men's record for the same decade declined by only 1 second. Similar dramatic improvement by women occurred in other sports events. Over the short term these dramatic improvements will continue especially in long-distance running, swimming, and similar endurance events where the training process for women is just now becoming comparable to men's. Inevitably, it is asked if women's world record performances will ever surpass men's and should men and women compete against each other. It appears that the strength differences between men and women have a physiological basis that will prevent even world-class female athletes from out performing world-class males in those events that demand a great deal of strength for success. However, given a wide range of sports events from those that rely almost entirely on brute force to those in which success depends more and more on motor skill and endurance, there is every reason to expect the best women to compete equally with the best men. It has been argued that in the sport of running women are most likely to hold records surpassing men at the ultramarathon (greater than 26 miles) distances. The justification for this view is that at these distances endurance rather than strength is of prime importance and that given equal training women and men will perform this event equally well. In sports such as badminton and archery there is every reason to expect equal performance from both women and men. In these types of events there is no logical reason for women and men not to compete and there is every reason to expect either women or men to become champions.

Of far greater importance is the obvious fact that there are very few world-class athletes and that among the vast majority of females and males there is a wide overlap of physical capacity, again more in motor skill and endurance than in strength. This means that in the average community there will be female athletes who can out perform their male peers. Some high school girls will be good enough to qualify for the track, swimming, and other sports teams traditionally limited to boys. The girls may not be (but may be) the national champions. They will be valuable assets to their team and out perform the less than champion male who 20 years ago would have enjoyed the benefits of sports to the total exclusion of more talented women.

III. SPORTS RELATED INJURIES: COMPARISON OF FEMALES AND MALES

Are the anatomical and physiological differences between women and men such that the female athlete is more susceptible to injury than her male counterpart performing the same sport event? Are there athletic injuries unique to women that should preclude them from participation in any given sport?

With the implementation of Title IX more female high school and college students are participating in a greater variety of sports. Inevitably the absolute number of athletic injuries among these young women will increase. It is of interest to determine if a disproportionate number of injuries occur in young women compared with young men. Thus, survey research has been conducted to document the incidence of athletic injuries among high school and college female and male athletics.

Few studies have been conducted on the sports injuries of adult women. A recent investigation of girl's and boy's high school and college sports shows that the pattern of injury within a given sport is the same for girls and boys. Major differences in the frequency of injury between boys and girls are associated with different sports events. Garrick and Requa (22) studied four high school athletic programs for 2 years and examined 3049 participants in 19 sports. They found that overall injuries, considering all 19 sports, occurred in girls' sports at a rate of 22 per 100 participants whereas the boys' rate of injury was 39 per 100 athletes (Fig. 6). Upon closer examination it can be seen that boys contact sports have markedly higher rates of injury than any other athletic events. Boys football resulted in 81 injuries per 100 participants, and boys wrestling, 75 injuries per 100 performers. In contrast the highest rate of injury among girls was in softball where 43 per 100 athletes were injured. In other sports in which both girls and boys participated the injury rates for boys and girls were approximately the same.

Clarke and Buckley (23) reported on women's injuries in collegiate sports with data from more than 100 institutions gathered during 1975–1978. Only injuries that caused the athlete to miss 1 week or more of participation were reported. In their study they observed that the type of injuries which occur in women's and men's sports were essentially the same (Table II). The majority of injuries for both women and men were sprains and strains. For example 65% of the baseball injuries in men's collegiate baseball were sprains and strains compared with 52% of injuries of the same type of women's softball. In basketball 60% of men's and 62% of women's injuries were sprains and strains. Comparison of college men's soccer and women's field hockey showed that 61% of the men's and 58% of the

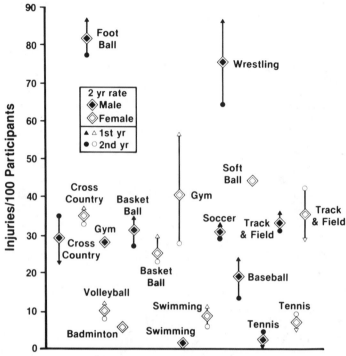

Fig. 6. Injury rate for two years of high school sports; injury rate was 10% lower during the second year of study.

women's injuries were sprains and strains. One dissimilarity occurred in comparison of men and women's gymnastics where women had a higher injury rate and conversely in track and field where men experienced more injuries. The difference between women's and men's injuries in gymnastics and track and field may occur because women and men do not participate in exactly the same events in these two sports.

In the same study it was shown that the occurrence of a major injury, defined as one that caused a disability of greater than 3 weeks duration, was nearly the same in men and women participants in basketball, gymnastics, and track and field. Women's softball participants, however, had more major injuries than men's baseball players. Also men's soccer players were more often seriously injured than women's field hockey participants. Again the differences between the sports events being compared may explain the discrepancy between men's and women's rate of major injury.

Also important is the relative inexperience of either men or women in their chosen sport. It has has been found (22) that more injuries occur during the first year of participation than in subsequent years. Thus, more injuries are likely in

TABLE II

Average Annual Rate (per 100 Cases) and Proportion of Significant Injuries in Selected Collegiate Sports by Types of Injury, 1975–1978

	Baseball	Softball	Basketball		Gymnastics		Soccer	Field hockey	Track and field	
	Men	Women	Men	Women	Men	Women	Men	Women	Men	Women
Neurotrauma	0.1	0.3	0.1	0.4	0.3	0.0	0.2	0.2	0.1	0.0
%	1	4	1	2	2	0	1	4	1	0
Sprains	3.4	3.5	11.1	11.8	6.8	18.8	6.5	2.0	1.8	2.0
%	37	40	54	58	41	66	49	37	18	16
Sprains	2.6	1.0	1.3	0.8	4.2	4.8	1.6	1.2	4.8	3.1
%	28	12	6	4	26	17	12	21	48	26
Fractures	0.6	2.2	2.9	3.0	2.8	3.7	1.2	0.4	0.5	2.2
%	7	25	14	15	17	13	9	7	5	19
Dental fractures	0.2	0.2	1.7	1.2	0.0	0.0	0.3	0.4	0.1	0.1
%	3	2	8	6	0	0	3	7	1	1
Chronic orthopaedic	0.5	0.3	1.3	1.1	0.6	0.9	0.3	0.5	0.8	0.7
%	5	4	6	6	3	3	3	9	8	6
Other	1.8	1.2	1.8	1.9	2.3	2.3	1.9	0.9	1.8	3.9
%	19	13	9	10	14	8	22	16	18	33

those sports in which women or men are novices rather than in those sports in which people are experienced.

These investigators and others (22,24,25) observed that for men and women more injuries occurred during competition than during practice. In some sports a greater percentage of injuries occurred while competing at other colleges rather than on the home field. It is important to note that there is no evidence of an excessively high incidence of athletic injuries or a disproportionate number of severe major sports related injuries in young women compared to men participants in the same sports. Some (26) have speculated that women's pelvic width and joint laxity would lead to higher incidence of chondromalacia and more joint sprains in women than in men. To date, the data do not support this position.

It has been demonstrated (27) in young adult men that the incidence of injury increases in parallel with increasing intensity of training. The duration of each training session and frequency of exercise periods are also important factors correlating positively with the rate of injury. It is reasonable that this general principle is also true for the female athlete. When designing a training program, it must be remembered that "intensity" is relative to each person's initial performance level. Thus, the relatively highly conditioned person training at 70% of his or her maximum capacity will perform more work than a poorly conditioned individual performing at 70% of his or her maximal capacity. Recent entrance of college age women into the United States Military Academy and their participation in vigorous physical training illustrate the need to consider the individuals initial fitness level before beginning a training program. It has been found (28,29) that initially women experience significantly more stress-related orthopedic injuries than men, participating in nearly identical physical training and sports. As women progressed into the second, third, and fourth years at the military academy the incidence of stress-related injury decreased to the same level as that of the male students. These data suggest that because their initial level of fitness was lower than their male peers, a more gradual training regimen is indicated for women upon entrance into the military academy. It also suggests that women, once achieving as high as a fitness level as men, are no more prone to injury than their male counterparts.

In addition to the high school and college women who are taking advantage of new opportunities to participate in organized sports, there is an increasingly large group of older women participation in a wide variety of athletic activity. These women are particularly noteworthy because of the nearly total lack of experience in exercise training or sports competition. Although it is nearly impossible to find a 30-year-old man who as had no experience in either varsity of intramural athletics during his school years, it is equally difficult to find a woman over 30 year of age who has had such experience. One might speculate that the older woman would be more susceptable to sports related injuries than her male peers. Her lack of experience may make her prone to overtrain and consequently develop some of the injuries characteristic of overuse. Also many middle-age women have been sedentary for a number of years and are now progressing toward improved health from a very low level of fitness. Her initial poor level of conditioning combined with inexperience in the training process increase her chances of overtraining even more. An example of this phenomenon is a report (29) of stress fractures in adult female and male athletes. This study found that the incidence of this injury is associated with a substantial increase in athletic activity and it was suggested that more women may suffer from stress fractures than men due to their very low initial level of activity. Almost any training represents a substantial increase in intensity of sports training for previously sedentary middle-aged women. Therefore, the previously sedentary individual should begin training at modest levels of strenuousness.

The possibility of injury to the breast and reproductive system has been emphasized and this argument has been used to discourage women from sports participation. There are no data to suggest that such injuries are common or of such severity that women should be excluded from athletics. The old wives' tale that breast injuries increase the risk of breast cancer is totally unfounded. Furthermore, if metal or heavy plastic supporters are satisfactory for preventing gonadal injuries in men engaged in contact sports, then protective gear made of similar material could be made available for women.

It is reasonable to conclude that women are not more susceptible to injury than men. Although relatively less fit men and women may be more likely to be injured than better fit individuals there are no anatomical or physiological reasons for excluding women from any sports endeavor, providing she is sufficiently conditioned to participate. If the sports event warrants protective gear for men or women it is obvious that it should be worn.

More studies, particularly involving older female and male athletes, will provide insight into the pattern of athletic injuries experienced by women. This additional knowledge will be useful in preventing future sports related injuries.

IV. PERFORMANCE IN HOT AND COLD ENVIRONMENTS: COMPARISON OF FEMALES AND MALES

Can women adapt to extremes of temperature as well as men? Are there anatomical or physiological differences between women and men which prevent women from adapting to heat as well as men, thus making athletic endeavors in a hot environment more hazardous for women than for men? Is heat more limiting to the athletic achievement of women than men? Is performance in the cold more dangerous or more limiting to women than men?

Effective thermoregulation in a hot environment keeps the body core temperature low during strenuous exercise. Further, perfect thermoregulation would allow an athlete to perform as well in a hot environment as in moderate temperature and humidity. The capacity for efficient thermoregulation in a hot environment is closely linked to other factors in which sex differences are often, although not always, observed. Researchers have not always separated the physiology of thermoregulation from other conditioning effects. The most important of these is cardiovascular fitness. Early investigators (30–32) of heat tolerance in women compared to men were not cognizant of the importance of cardiorespiratory fitness in determining the capacity to perform in the heat. In these studies no attempt was made to select female and male subjects of equal cardiovascular capacity or to factor out the effects of varying fitness levels. Since the females in these studies were relatively sedentary and poorly conditioned, the women appeared to be less tolerant of heat stress than men. More recent investigations (33,34) compared heat tolerance of women and men, taking into consideration fitness level and employing equal relative work loads for both sexes. These studies show that women's adaptation to heat is not inferior to men, and it has been suggested that women have some advantages over men for working in a hot environment.

Intricately associated with the capacity for effective thermoregulation is body surface area relative to exercising tissue mass, body weight, and body fat. The surface area to lean body mass ratio is generally greater in women than men (34). The exercising male, with relatively greater working muscle mass, produces more heat than a woman performing at the same relative workload but the male has proportionally less body surface area over which heat loss can occur. Thus, the female has the advantage of somewhat less heat production and relatively greater surface area over which heat can be dissipated. Greater vasodilitation has been observed in women than in men exposed to a hot environment (31,35). Delivering a greater volume of blood to the body surface would be expected to facilitate cooling.

Early investigations (36–38) demonstrated that women have markedly lower sweat rates than men. Initially this observation was interpreted to mean that women were less able to tolerate heat exposure than men. However, it is now recognized that the reduced sweating rate has the advantage of conserving body fluids while working in the heat. The loss of body fluids during exercise in the heat leads to reduced plasma volume resulting in a decrease in venous return to the heart and a fall in stroke volume. Heart rate will reflexly increase. The elevated heart rate is often used to indicate physiological stress and lack of tolerance to heat exposure. Following prolonged work in the heat Senay and Kok (39) found that men who are acclimatized have a significantly higher sweat rate than women who are acclimatized. After prolonged heat exposure the mens' heart rates were significantly greater than that observed in the female subjects. The elevated heart rate was associated with the loss of fluid volume. The women were able to dissipate metabolic heat at the same rate as men but with less sweat produced. Women have therefore been referred to as more efficient regulators of body temperature than men (38–40).

Further evidence of the detrimental effects of a high sweat rate is provided by Avellini *et al.* (34) in a study of heat tolerance in acclimatized women and men of comparable cardiovascular fitness. Women were studied pre- and postovulation since hormonal fluctuation may alter heat tolerance. Male subjects' sweat rate was 42–50% greater than the sweat rate of female subjects (Fig. 7). These investigators distinguished between evaporated sweat production, associated with cooling, from unevaporated sweating not related to cooling. Males were found to have significantly greater unevaporated sweat production than women. The unevaporated sweat increases fluid loss with no beneficial effect for cooling. The rectal temperature, skin temperature, and heart rate of men and women were identical for 90 minutes of walking on a treadmill in a hot environment. After 3 hours of exercise in the heat, however, the men had significantly higher core temperature and significantly greater heart rate than the women subjects. In this study the sweating response of the women was more purposeful than that of the male subjects and was associated with maintaining core temperature and heart rate at lower values.

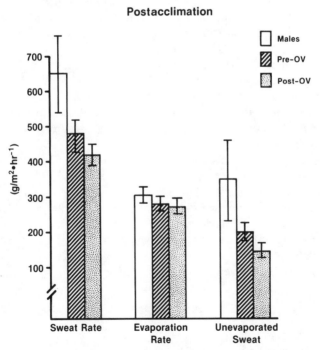

Fig. 7. Comparison of mean ± SE of sweat rate, evaporation rate, and rate of unevaporated sweat production for men and women after acclimation.

Others (41,42) have also observed that despite the lower sweat rates of women, women regulate their internal temperature during a combination of heat and exercise stress as well or better than men.

The perponderance of evidence indicates that, due to the reduced sweating rate and greater vasodilitation characteristic of the physically fit and acclimatized female compared to equally fit and acclimatized males, women tolerate working in the heat better than men. There is further evidence of an advantage to women over men in the capacity to work or perform athletic events in the heat as a result of conserving more body fluid and maintaining core temperature with lower heart rate. Paolone and co-workers (43) measured oxygen uptake of men and women exercising at 50% of their maximum capacity in neutral, warm, and hot environments. Oxygen uptake determined the metabolic cost of exercise, and it can be inferred that the lower the metabolic cost, the longer the exercise can be maintained. Consistent with other research cited previously, these investigators found sweat rates to be greater in male subjects than females performing the same relative work load. Measurements of body weight indicated that males lost slightly more body fluid per degree increase in rectal temperature than females. Heart rates were higher in male subjects during exercise than in females. In turn the increased metabolic cost of exercise in the heat compared to a neutral environment was 10% for women and 22% for men. It is reasonable to expect that the relative work or athletic achievement of men would be decreased more than that of women performing in the heat.

The physiological data indicate that performance in a hot environment is no more hazardous but instead probably less dangerous for women than for men. Measurements of metabolic cost of exercise in the heat suggest that a hot environment limits the athletic performance of women less than men. There is some evidence, therefore, to suggest that women have some advantage over men while performing in the heat.

Although the difference in sweat rate in men and women is well recognized, there are many more physiological adaptations to heat stress that are common to both sexes. Heat acclimatization in both women and men include more rapid onset of sweating upon exposure to heat, increased sweat rate with accompanying evaporation heat loss, and decreased loss of salts. Lower internal body temperature and heart rate are thus better maintained following heat acclimatization in women and men.

Further, it is well established that in both men and women tolerance to heat is closely correlated with cardiovascular fitness (40,43). Sedentary women and sedentary men with poor cardiovascular fitness are at great risk when working in the heat while individuals who are physically fit and acclimatized to the heat are in much less jeopardy.

Physiological adaptations to cold exposure do not occur in humans as in some other animal species. There is no evidence that athletic performance in a cold environment is hindered more in men or women or that cold exposure is more hazardous to either men or women. Some have argued, however, that the greater amount of subcutaneous fat in women (15% of body weight) compared to men (12% of body weight) is protective for women. This small difference, if important at all, is probably offset by the lower lean body mass of women which is in turn responsible for lower metabolic heat production in women compared to men. Future studies may define differences between the capacity for women and men to work in the cold.

V. DOES EXERCISE INFLUENCE OSTEOPOROSIS IN AGED WOMEN AND MEN?

Decreased mineral content of bone is known to occur in senescent women and men (44–48). Since the skeletal mass of females is generally less than that of males at any age, and since their rate of bone mineral loss with age is greater than that of males (49), postmenopausal osteoporosis is a more common problem in women than in men of the same age. Major orthopedic problems related to bone demineralization occur in 25–30% of postmenopausal women (50). Interest in maintaining the health of these individuals must include attention to prevention or attenuating the commonly observed decline in bone mineral mass.

Nutritional considerations are important in correcting the negative calcium balance characteristics of individuals in their fourth decade of life and older. Hormone therapy has been suggested as treatment for postmenopausal osteoporosis (51), but has not received universal approval.

There is evidence that exercise plays a role in increasing and/or maintaining mineral content of bone. Several years of participation in exercise has been associated with increased bone mineralization in athletes (52) and with reversal of mineral loss from bone in middle-aged (53) subjects placed on a training program.

Aloia and colleagues (54) conducted a study to determine if exercise could prevent bone loss in 18 postmenopausal women. Nine of the subjects exercised 1 hour 3 days a week for 1 year. The other nine women remained sedentary. Total body calcium increased in the exercise group and decreased in each subject in the sedentary group. The daily calcium balance was significantly ($p < 0.001$) different in the two groups. Although one can argue that it is impossible to account for all the variables that control bone mineralization, it appears that in this study exercise was influential in reversing the involutional bone loss.

In another study of 13 men ages 65.2 ± 5.4 years and 25 women ages 64.8 ± 4.3 years enrolled in a 4 hours per week endurance exercise program for 1 year, Sidney *et al.* (55) found reduced body fatness, increased lean body mass, and improved aerobic power in these exercising men and women. In these subjects mineral content of bone did not change over the time of the study. The normally observed age-related calcium loss was halted. Exercise was associated with avoiding the variations in bone pathology often encountered in inactive elderly people.

The perponderance of evidence suggests that exercise plays a role in attentuating or reversing, mineral loss from bone. A life-style that includes modestly strenuous physical exercise is likely to be important for prevention of the demineralization of bone in postmenopausal women. This benefit of exercise is likely to be more important for women than for men.

VI. ARE THE EFFECTS OF PHYSICAL ACTIVITY ON BLOOD LIPID CHEMISTRY DIFFERENT IN WOMEN THAN MEN?

Reports assessing the effects of physical conditioning on serum cholesterol and triglyceride content have reached conflicting conclusions with some (56,57) observing lowering of blood lipid following endurance training and others (58–60) seeing no change. The amount of obesity before training and weight loss during training, intensity of exercise bouts, type of exercises performed (dynamic versus static), diet, and smoking habits are among the factors responsible for the discrepancies in studies of blood chemistry. It appears that endurance exercise of sufficient intensity has a beneficial effect on lowering serum cholesterol in men, especially if there is a concomitant weight loss (59,61–63).

The same beneficial effects on serum lipid content may not occur in premenopausal women. It is important to note that young women normally have a lower serum cholesterol than men of the same age (64,65). Cholesterol is the substrate for the synthesis of estrogens. In the relatively few studies on the influence of exercise on blood chemistry in women, exercise alone has not been found to lower the concentrations of serum cholesterol or triglyceride (58,64,65). Exercise may not have the same beneficial effects of lowering serum cholesterol or triglycerides in women which are sometimes observed in men. This finding, however, must be interpreted with the knowledge that the blood chemistry of premenopausal women includes relatively lower serum lipid content.

Recent scientific evidence (66–71) supports the view that elevated concentrations of high-density lipoproteins (HDL) in plasma exert a protective effect against coronary artery disease. HDL is thought to transport cholesterol from the tissues including the arterial wall for catabolism in the liver (72) and HDL may inhibit cholesterol deposition (73). There have been numerous reports that males have elevated HDL following endurance exercise training (74,75). The data, however, are not unanimous (76). It has further been reported that the HDL levels of females do not change with training (77). To place this disparate response of men and women into the proper perspective, however, it is important to note that sedentary premenopausal women normally have a markedly higher HDL than their male peers. The HDL levels in male athletes do not differ significantly from levels in nonathletic females of the same age (75,78). Hormonal influences are responsible for the higher base line HDL values in women (79). Thus again, the difference in the effects of exercise on blood lipid chemistry in women and men is complicated by the different values in the nonexercising populations.

VII. ARE FEMALE ATHLETES MORE LIKELY TO HAVE GYNECOLOGICAL PROBLEMS THAN NONATHLETES? DOES ATHLETIC PERFORMANCE HAVE AN IMPACT ON FEMALE SEXUALITY?

This section presents an overview. Chapter 7 will address these questions in depth. In general, the age at menarche is delayed a few months in athletes compared to nonathletes. This has been shown for high school and college age (80) as well as Olympic (81) athletes. Further, a positive correlation exists between the level of athletic achievement and the length of time by which menarche is delayed. A survey of female participants in the 1976 Olympic games revealed the trend for delayed menarche in women from 27 countries and in all sports events except swimmers (82). A delay in the onset of menstruation was not found in female swimmers (81,82). In an effort to explain the later menarche, Maline (80) notes that the body build associated with later maturation is the same physique as that associated with athletic achievement. Girls who have matured later characteristically have a leaner physique, longer legs, narrower hips, and less weight for height with lower body fatness than those who matured earlier. These same physical characteristics are commonly found in athletes. Sports may select out those girls who would mature late regardless of their athletic endeavors. An additional consideration, perhaps more important 10–15 years ago than today, is that of the social pressure on girls whose maturation is early may be such that they may be directed away from sports during early adolescence.

Frisch (83) developed a method for predicting the age at menarche from height and weight and determined also that the ratio of lean body mass to fat can be used in determining sexual maturation. According to this study, 22% of body weight is fat at the age of menarche. Although this exact percentage of fatness has been disputed (84), nevertheless some claim that low body fatness induced by athletic training is responsible for delayed menarche. The importance of body fatness has been overemphasized. It is the hypothalamic secretion that leads to rising levels of estrogens that causes the onset of menstruation and that also is related to an increase in body fatness. Increased body fatness occurs concomitantly with onset of menarche but increased fatness is not to be emphasized as a determining factor in the age at menarche. Although it is possible that extremely low body fatness may be a factor in delayed menarche, the exact role if any of lowered body fatness secondary to sports training in delaying sexual maturity is yet to be defined. It is important to note that there is no evidence that the few months delay in menarche common in female athletes has any detrimental short- or long-term medical consequence. Delayed maturity does not imply that sports participation should cease.

Menstrual dysfunction in adult female athletes is a controversial topic. There is a great deal of evidence that menstrual problems diminish in physically active women (85–89). The strenuousness of exercise reported in these studies would be considered moderate by today's standards. With the increasing participation of women in long-distance running, as well as other intense training programs, the incidence of amonorrhea has grown. It has been estimated that 15–20% of those who train strenuously experience short-term amenorrhea. Recognizing that excessive weight loss in pathological states such as anorexia nervosa will cause amenorrhea, it has been suggested that low body fat in athletes is responsible for cessation of menstruation (90). Other data, however, do not support this hypothesis. Feicht and colleagues (91) surveying 400 women on 15 collegiate track and field and cross country teams found that amenorrheoic and menstrually regular women were of equal weight and height. The relationship between body fatness and normal menstrual cycles is not clear. Fatness per se is probably not the key determining factor.

A second theory put forth to explain amenorrhea in female athletes is that stress, both physical and psychological, of intense training and competition leads to depressed hypothalamic function and menstrual irregularities. Some (91) have claimed that running 60 or more miles per week is a critical stress level above which menstrual problems develop. Further, it is known that stress from other causes unrelated to sports such as entering college, death of family members, divorce, and career crises result in depressed hypothalamic function leading to amenorrhea. There is, however, probably no single amount of stress, i.e., number of miles run per week, hours of training, or psychological desire to win or fear of failure, that will induce amenorrhea in female athletes. Each individual probably has a threshold of stress for cessation of menstruation which is determined by numerous physical and psychological factors. Reduced intensity of training (92) or adaptation to the strenuousness of the exercise (87) is accompanied by return of normal menstrual cycles. Perhaps the only medical risk of brief periods of amenorrhea is that a serious health problem could be ignored in the belief that cessation of menstruation was secondary only to sports training. Additional research will resolve some of the controversies about gynecological problems in athletes. Individual differences in length of "normal" cycle and the large numbers of sedentary young women who have irregular menstrual cycles makes it nearly impossible to separate the effects of exercise stress from other causes of menstrual irregularities. Minor menstrual irregularities do not warrant dropping out of sports.

A question often asked by athletic coaches and athletes is whether or not the phase of the menstrual cycle experienced by the athlete effects athletic performance? Again conflicting information abounds. Some believe that peak performances are reached during preovulation or immediately after menses. It has been reported that tolerance to heat is altered during different phases of the menstrual cycle (34); others refute this finding (89,93). One study (94) reports decreased efficiency during the few days before menstruation. The misinformation concerning advantages of athletic performance at various phases of the menstrual cycle have led to questionable coaching procedures and extreme measures by athletes. Women have taken oral contraceptives, altering their normal menstrual cycle, so they could perform in Olympic competition immediately after menses. They believed their performance would be best at this time. Others believe that delaying menses for prolonged time periods with oral contraceptives, taken out of the proper sequence, may increase hematocrit, inducing a form of "blood doping" which will improve athletic performance (95). The advantages, if any, of these practices has not been documented.

In addition to the potential medical hazards of using or misusing oral contraceptives, these practices are unsound because they may not effect athletic performance. Females have performed at their own personal best at all phases of their cycle (92). Nevertheless, the advantages or lack of advantages of sports performance at any given phase of the menstrual cycle are yet to be fully documented.

VIII. DOES PHYSICAL TRAINING HAVE ANY EFFECT ON FERTILITY OR PREGNANCY IN WOMEN?

Insofar as fertility is influenced by body fatness and predictable menstrual cycles, sports training may have an adverse effect on fertility. All evidence to date (92) shows that the amenorrhea secondary to strenuous sports training as well as weight loss is reversible when exercise is moderated. Long-term ill effects of amenorrhea on fertility has not been found in female athletes.

Investigations (96–99) of the effects of athletic activity on pregnancy indicate that there are no undesirable consequences of continued exercise. Numerous anecdotes of women who exercise throughout their pregnancy reveal that the health benefits of exercise continue throughout their pregnancy. The normal pregnancy is not a disease requiring rest therapy.

Menopause in women is characterized by physiological changes, which may be accompanied by psychological upset. General anxiety is often experienced by perimenopausal women. Since it has been demonstrated in Olympic caliber (100) and novice (101,102) female athletics, that exercise performed regularly has a positive effect on mental health, perimenopausal women would be likely to benefit from athletic endeavor. Advising women to stop exercising because of menopause is not indicated, conversely, initiating a condition program at this time may have positive psychological as well as physical effects.

IX. IS MALE SEXUALITY AFFECTED BY ATHLETIC PERFORMANCE?

Sports related changes in the female menstrural cycle are obvious, whereas males may have hormonal changes and be unaware they exist. Bloom (103) discussed a study of hormonal changes in male marathon runners and Morville *et al.* (104) studied 19 men running 100 km races. Statistically significant reductions in plasma testosterone levels were found following participation in their respective running events. Recovery to normal androgen concentrations occurred in the days following the long runs. Further, it has also been proposed (103) that low body fatness in men resulting from athletic training leads to fertility problems. It is reasonable to postulate that reproductive hormone levels in males, especially at the age of puberty, can be altered in much the same manner as in females. The physical stress of exercise or emotional stress of training and competition and/or low body fatness may alter reproductive endocrinology in both sexes. Additional studies of the effects, or lack of effects, of exercise on female and male reproduction are warranted.

REFERENCES

1. Hettinger, T. (1961). "Physiology of Strength." Thomas, Springfield, Illinois.
2. Laubach, L. L. (1976). Comparative muscular strength of men and women: A review of the literature. *Aviat., Space Environ. Med.* **47,** 534–542.
3. Knapik, J. J., Wright, J. E., Kowal, D. M., and Vogel, J. A. (1980). The influence of U.S. Army basic initial entry training on the muscular strength of men and women. *Aviat., Space Environ. Med.* **51,** 1086–1090.
4. Wilmore, J. (1974). Alterations in strength, body composition and anthropometric measurements consequent to a 10-week weight training program. *Med. Sci. Sports* **6,** 133–136.
5. Wilmore, J. (1974). Alterations in strength, body composition and anthropometric measurements consequent to a 10-week weight training program. *Med. Sci. Sport* **6,** 136–138.
6. Rodahl, L., and Horvatz, S. M., eds. (1962). "Muscle as a Tissue." McGraw-Hill, New York.
7. Edström, L., and Nyström, B. (1969). Histochemical types and sizes of fibres in normal human muscles. *Acta Neurol. Scand.* **45,** 257–269.
8. Costill, D. L., Daniels, J., Evans, W., Fink, W., Krahenguhl, G., and Saltin, B. (1976). Skeletal muscle enzymes and fiber composition in male and female track athletes. *J. Appl. Physiol.* **40,** 149–154.

9. Costill, D. L., Fink, W. J., Getchell, L. H., Ivy, J. L., and Witzmann, F. A. (1979). Lipid metabolism in skeletal muscle of endurance-trained males and females. *J. Appl. Physiol.* **47**, 787–791.
10. Prince, F. P., Hikida, R. S., and Hagerman, F. C. (1977). Muscle fiber types in women athletes and non-athletes. *Pflüegers Arch.* **371**, 161–165.
11. Gregor, R. J., Edgerton, V. R., Perrine, J. J., Campion, D. S., and Debus, C. (1979). Torque-velocity relationships and muscle fiber composition in elite female athletes. *J. Appl. Physiol.* **47**, 388–392.
12. Astrand, P. O., and Cristensen, E. H. (1964). Aerobic work capacity. *In* "Oxygen in the Animal Organism" (F. Dickens, E. Neil, and W. R. Widdas, eds.), p. 295. Pergamon, Oxford.
13. Hermansen, L., and Andersen, K. L. (1965). Aerobic work capacity in young Norweigan men and women. *J. Appl. Physiol.* **20**, 425–431.
14. Saltin, B., and Åstrand, P.-O. (1967). Maximal oxygen uptake in athletes. *J. Appl. Physiol.* **23**, 353–358.
15. Drinkwater, B. L. (1975). Aerobic power in females. *J. Phys. Educ. Rec.* **46**, 36–38.
16. Daries, C. T. M. (1971). Body composition in children: A reference standard for maximum aerobic power output on a stationary bicycle ergometer. *Acta Paediatr. Scand., Suppl.* **217.**
17. Pollack, M. L. (1973). The quantification of endurance training programs. *Exercise Sport Science Review* (J. Wilmore, ed.). Academic Press, New York.
18. Patton, J. F., Daniels, W. L., and Vogel, J. A. (1980). Aerobic power and body fat of men and women during army basic training. *Aviat., Space Environ. Med.* **51**, 492–496.
19. Feldin, S. M., Morganroth, J., and Rubler, S. (1978). Cardiac hypertrophy in response to dynamic conditioning in female athletes. *J. Appl. Physiol.* **44**, 849–852.
20. Kollias, J., Barlettt, H. L., Mendez, J., and Franklin, B. (1978). Hemodynamic responses of well-trained women athletes to graded treadmill exercise. *J. Sports Med. Phys. Fitness* **18**, 365–372.
21. Davies, C. T. M., and Thompson, M. W. (1979). Aerobic performance of female marathon and male ultramarathon athletes. *Eur. J. Appl. Physiol.* **41**, 233–245.
22. Garrick, J. G., and Requa, R. K. (1978). Injuries in high school sports. *Pediatrics* **61**(3), 465–469.
23. Clarke, K. S., and Buckley, W. E. (1980). Women's injuries in collegiate sports. *Am. Sports Med.* **8**(3), 187–191.
24. Garrick, J. G., and Requa, R. K. (1978). Girl's sports injuries in high school athletics. *JAMA, J. Am. Med. Assoc.* **239** (21), 2245–2248.
25. Calvert, R. (1979). "Athletic Injuries and Deaths in Secondary Schools and Colleges, 1975–76." National Center for Education Statistics, Department of Health, Education, and Welfare, U.S. Govt. Printing Office, Washington, D.C.
26. Drinkwater, B. L., Horvath, S. M., and Wells, C. L. (1975). Aerobic power of females, ages 10 to 68. *J. Gerontol.* **30**, 385–394.
27. Pollock, M. L., Gittman, L. R., Milesis, C. A., Bah, M. D., Durstine, L., and Johnson, R. B. (1977). Effects of frequency and duration of training on attrition and incidence of injury. *Med. Sci. Sports* **9**(1), 31–36.
28. Belkin, S. C. (1980). Stress fractures in athletes. *Orthop. Clin. North Am.* **11**(4), 735–741.
29. Haycock, C. E., and Gillette, J. V. (1976). Susceptibility of women athletes to injury. *JAMA, J. Am. Med. Assoc.* **236**(2), 163–165.
30. Drinkwater, B. L., Kupprat, I. C., Denton, J. E., and Horvath, S. M. (1978). Heat tolerance of female distance runners. *Ann. N.Y. Acad. Sci.* **301**, 777–792.
31. Nadel, E. R., Roberts, M. R., and Wenger, C. B. (1978). Thermoregulatory adaptation to heat and exercise: Comparative responses of men and women. *In* "Environmental Stress: Individual

Human Adaptations'' (L. J. Folinsbee, J. A. Wagner, J. F. Borgia, B. L. Drinkwater, J. A. Gliner, and J. F. Bedi, eds.), pp. 29–38. Academic Press, New York.

32. Wells, C. L., and Paolone, A. M. (1977). Metabolic responses to exercise in three thermal environments. *Aviat., Space Environ. Med.* **48,** 989–993.

33. Wells, C. L. (1980). Responses of physically active and acclimatized men and women to exercise in a desert environment. *Med. Sci. Sports Exercise* **12,** 9–13.

34. Avellini, B. A., Kamon, E., and Krajewski, J. T. (1980). Physiological responses of physically fit men and women to acclimation to humid heat. *J. Appl. Physiol.* **49,** 254–261.

35. Brouh, L., Smith, P. E., DeLanae, R., and Maxfield, M. E. (1961). Physiological reactions of men and women during mascular activity and recovery in various environments. *J. Appl. Physiol.* **16,** 133–140.

36. Fox, R. H., Lofstedt, B. E., Woodward, P. M., Erikkson, E., and Werkström, B. (1969). Comparison of thermoregulatory function in man and women. *J. Appl. Physiol.* **26,** 444–453.

37. Hertig, B. A., and Sargent, F., III (1963). Acclimatization of women during work in hot environment. *Fed. Proc., Fed. Am. Soc. Exp. Biol.* **22,** 810–813.

38. Wyndham, C. H., Morrison, J. F., and Williams, C. G. (1965). Heat reaction of male and female caucasians. *J. Appl. Physiol.* **20,** 357–364.

39. Senay, L. C., and Kok, R. (1977). Effect of training and heat acclimatization on blood plasma contents of exercising men. *J. Appl. Physiol.* **43,** 591–599.

40. Dill, D. B., Soholt, L. F., McLean, D. C., Drost, D. F., Jr., and Loushran, M. T. (1977). Capacity of young males and females for running in desert heat. *Med. Sci. Sports* **9,** 137–142.

41. Weinman, K. P., Slabochova, Z., Bermauer, E. M., Morimoto, T., and Sargent, F., II (1967). Reactions of men and women to repeated exposure to humid heat. *J. Appl. Physiol.* **22,** 533–538.

42. Morimoto, T., Salbochova, Z., Naman, R. K., and Sargent, F., II (1967). Sex differences in physiological reaction to thermal stress. *J. Appl. Physiol.* **22,** 526–532.

43. Paolone, A. M., Wells, C. L., and Kelly, G. T. (1978). Sexual variation in thermoregulation during heat stress. *Aviat. Space Environ. Med.* **49,** 715–719.

44. Norris, A. H., Lundy, T., and Shock, N. W. (1963). Trend in selected indices of body composition in man between the age of 30 and 80 years. *Ann. N.Y. Acad. Sci.* **110,** 623.

45. Steinbach, H. A. L. (1965). Symposium on problems in geriatric radiology. Roentgenology of the skeleton of the aged. *Radiol. Clin. North Am.* **3,** 277.

46. Newton-John, H. F., and Morgan, D. B. (1968). Osteoporosis: Disease senescence? *Lancet* **1,** 232.

47. Exton-Smith, A. N., Millard, P. H., Payne, P. H., and Wheeler, E. F., Pattern of development and loss of bone with age. *Lancet* **2,** 1154.

48. Nordin, B. E. C. (1971). Clinical significance and pathogenesis of osteoporosis. *Br. Med. J.* **1,** 571.

49. Avioli, L. V. (1977). Osteoporosis: Pathogenesis and therapy. *In* ''Metabolic Bone Disease'' (L. V. Avioli and S. M. Krane, eds.), Vol. I, pp. 307–370. Academic Press, New York.

50. Avioli, L. V. (1981). Postmenopausal osteoporosis: Prevention versus cure. *Fed. Proc., Fed. Am. Soc. Exp. Biol.* **40,** 2418–2422.

51. Laroche, C., Detilleux, M., and Sereni, D. (1979). Current research in therapy of postmenopausal osteoporosis. *Sem. Hop.* **55,** 325–329.

52. Rockwell, D., Kulund, D. N., and Harrison, R. B. (1980). Bone mass in lifetime tennis players. *JAMA, J. Am. Med. Assoc.* **244,** 1107–1109.

53. Smith, E. L., and Babcock, S. W. (1973). Effects of physical activity on bone loss in the aged. *Med. Sci. Sports* **5,** 68.

54. Aloia, J. F., Cohn, S. H., Ostuni, J. A., Cane, R., and Ellis, K. (1978). Prevention of involutional bone loss by exercise. *Ann. Intern. Med.* **89,** 356–358.

55. Sidney, K. H., Shephard, R. J., and Harrison, J. E. (1977). Endurance training and body composition of the elderly. *Am. J. Clin. Nutr.* **30**, 326–333.
56. Naughton, J., and Balke, B. (1964). Physical working capacity in medical personnel and the response of serum cholesterol to acute exercise and to training. *Am. J. Med. Sci.* **247**, 286.
57. Holloszy, J. O., Skinner, J. S., Toro, G., and Cureton, T. K. (1964). Effects of a six month program of endurance exercise on the serum lipids of middle-aged men. *Am. J. Cardiol.* **14**, 753.
58. Lewis, W. L., Haskell, D., Wood, P. D., Manoogian, N., Baildy, J. E., and Pereira, M. (1976). Effects of physical activity on weight reduction in obese middle-aged women. *Am. J. Clin. Nutr.* **29**, 151–156.
59. Goode, R. C., Firstbrook, J. B., and Shephard, R. J. (1966). Effects of exercise and a cholesterol free diet on human serum lipids. *Can. J. Physiol. Pharmacol.* **44**, 575.
60. Lehtonen, A., and Viidari, J. (1978). Serum triglycerides and cholesterol and serum high-density lipoprotein cholesterol in highly physically active men. *Acta Med. Scand.* **204**, 111–114.
61. Weltman, A., Matter, S., and Stamford, B. A. (1980). Caloric restriction and/or mild exercise: Effects on serum lipids and body composition. *Am. J. Clin. Nutr.* **33**, 1002–1009.
62. Olefsky, J., Reaven, G. M., and Farquhar, J. W. (1974). Effects of weight reduction on obesity. Studies of lipid and carbohydrate metabolism in normal and hyperlipoproteinemic subject. *J. Clin. Invest.* **53**, 64.
63. Oscai, L. B., Patterson, J. A., Bogard, D. L., Beck, R., and Rothermel, B. L. (1972). Normalization of serum triglycerides and lipoprotein electrophoretic patterns by exercise. *Am. J. Cardiol.* **30**, 775.
64. Getchell, L. H., and Moore, J. C. (1974). Physiological responses of middle-aged women to physical training. *Med. Sci. Sports* **5**, 75.
65. Kilbom, A. (1971). Physical training in women. *Scand. J. Clin. Lab. Invest.* **28**, Suppl. 119, 1.
66. Miller, G. J., and Miller, N. E. (1975). Plasma-high-density-lipoprotein concentration and development of ischaemic heart disease. *Lancet* **1**, 16.
67. Carlson, L. A., and Ericsson, M. (1975). Quantitative and qualitative serum lipoprotein analysis. *Atherosclerosis* **21**, 435.
68. Nikkila, E. A. (1976). Serum high-density-lipoprotein and coronary heart disease. *Lancet* **2**, 320.
69. Rhoads, G. G., Gulbrandsen, C. L., and Kanganl, A. (1976). Serum lipoproteins and coronary heart disease in a population study of Hawaii Japanese men. *N. Engl. J. Med.* **294**, 293.
70. Roseman, R. H., Jenkins, R. J., Jenkins, D. C., Friedman, M., Straus, R., and Wurm, M. (1975). Coronary heart disease in the western collaborative group study. *JAMA, J. Am. Med. Assoc.* **233**, 872.
71. Gordon, T., Castelli, M. C., and Hjortland, M. C. (1977). High density lipoprotein as protective factor against coronary heart disease. *Am. J. Med.* **62**, 707–714.
72. Glomset, J. A. (1968). The plasma lecitin: Cholesterol acyl-transferase reaction. *J. Lipid Res.* **9**, 155.
73. Carem, T. E., Koschinsky, T., Hayes, S. B., and Steinberg, D. A. (1976). A mechanism by which high-density lipoproteins may slow the atherogenic process. *Lancet* **1**, 1315.
74. Wood, P. D., Klein, H., Lewis, S., and Haskell, W. L. (1974). Plasma lipoprotein concentrations in middle-aged runners. *Circulation* **50**, 115.
75. Wood, P. D., Haskell, W., Klein, H., Lewis, S., Stern, M. P., and Farquhar, J. W. (1976). The distribution of plasma lipoproteins in middle-aged male runners. *Metab., Clin. Exp.* **25**, 1249–1257.

76. Vodak, P. A., Wood, P. D., Haskell, W. L., and Williams, P. T. (1980). HDL-Cholesterol and other plasma lipid and lipoprotein concentrations in middle-aged male and female tennis players. *Metab., Clin. Exp.* **29,** 745–752.

77. Moll, M. E., Williams, R. S., Lester, R. M., Quarfordt, S. M., and Wallace, A. G. (1979). Cholesterol metabolism in non-obese women. *Atherosclerosis* **34,** 159–166.

78. Enger, S. C., Herbjornse, K., Erikssen, J., and Fretland, A. (1977). High density lipoproteins (HDL) and physical activity—The influence of physical exercise, age and smoking on HDL-cholesterol and the HDL-total cholesterol ratio. *Scand. J. Clin. Lab. Invest.* **27,** 251.

79. Bradley, D. D., Wingard, J., Petitti, D. B., Krauss, R. M., and Ramcharan S. (1978). Serum high-density lipoprotein cholesterol in women using oral contraceptives, estrogens, and progestins. *N. Engl. J. Med.* **299,** 17.

80. Malina, R. M., Spirduso, W. W., Tate, A., and Baylor, A. M. (1978). Age at menarche and selected menstrual characteristics in athletes at different competitive levels and in different sports. *Med. Sci. Sports* **10,** 218–222.

81. Malina, R. M., Bouchard, C., Shoup, R. F., Demirjian, A., and Larivere, G. (1979). Age at menarche, family size, and birth order in athletics at the Montreal Olympic Games, 1976. *Med. Sci. Sports* **11,** 354–358.

82. Astrand, P. O., Erikkson, B. O., Nylander, I., Engström, L., Karlberg, P., Saltin, B., and Thoren, C. (1963). Girl swimmers, with special reference to respiratory and circulating adaptation and aynaecological and psychiatric aspects. *Acta Paediatr. Scand., Suppl.* **147.**

83. Frisch, R. E. (1974). A method of prediction of age of menarche from height and weight at ages 9 through 11 years. *Pediatrics* **53,** 384–390.

84. Hayock, C. E. The female athlete and sports medicine in the 1970's. (1980). *J. Fla. Med. Assn.,* 411–414.

85. Wearing, M. P., Yuhosz, M. D., Campbess, R., and Love, E. T. (1972). The effect of the menstrual cycle on tests of physical fitness, England. *J. Sports Med. Phys. Fitness* **12,** 38–41.

86. Doolittle, J. L., and Engebretsen, J. (1972). Performance variations during the menstrual cycle, England. *J. Sports Med. Phys. Fitness* **12,** 54–58.

87. Women at the Military Academies (1979). *Symp., Physician Sportsmed.* **7,** 41–80.

88. Erdelyi, G. J. (1976). Gynecological survey of female athletes. *Physician Sportsmed.* **4,** 79–80.

89. Wells, C. L., and Horvath, S. M. (1974). Responses to exercise in a hot environment as related to the menstrual cycle. *J. Appl. Physiol.* **36,** 299–302.

90. Dale, E., Gerlach, D. H., and Wilhite, A. L. (1979). Menstrual dysfunction in distance runners. *Obstet. Gynecol. (N.Y.)* **54,** 47–53.

91. Feicht, C. G., Johnson, T. S., Martin, B. J., Sparkes, K. E., and Wagner, W. W. (1978). Secondary amenorrhoea in athletes. *Lancet,* 1145–1146.

92. Haycock, C. E. (1980). The female athletic and sportsmedicine in the 70's. *J. Fla. Med. Assoc.* **67,** 411–414.

93. Wells, C. L., and Horvath, S. M. (1973). Heat stress responses related to the menstrual cycle. *J. Appl. Physiol.* **35,** 1–5.

94. Fraccaroli, G. (1980). Li rendimento sportivo della donna durante il ciclo menstruale. *Minerva Med.* **71,** 3557–3566.

95. Ekblom, B., Goldbarg, A. N., Gullbring, B. (1972). *J. Appl. Physiol.* **33,** 175–179.

96. Hale, R. W. (1979). Women and sports: Keeping up with female athlete's needs, cont. *Obstet. Gynecol.* **13,** 84–95.

97. Fressendorfer, R. N. (1978). Physical training during pregnancy and lactation. *Physician Sportsmed.* **6,** 74–80.

98. Shangold, M. (1980). "Pregnancy and the Athlete: Sportsmedicine for the Athletic Female," Chapter 25. Medical Economics, Oradell, New Jersey.

99. Ferrarese, C., and Fraccaroli, G. (1980). Attivita sportive e maternita. *Minerva Med.* **71,** 1321–1328.
100. Jones, R. D., and Weinhouse, S. (1979). Running as self therapy. *J. Sports Med.* **19,** 397–404.
101. Bortz, W. M., Angwin, P., Medford, I. N., Boarder, M. R., Noyce, N., and Barchas, J. B. (1981). Catecholamines, dopamine, and endorphin levels during extreme exercise. *N. Engl. J. Med.* **305,** 466–467.
102. Balaza, E., and Nickerson, E. (1976). A personality needs profile of some outstanding female athletes. *J. Clin. Psychol.* **32,** 45–49.
103. Bloom, M. (1978). Running as birth control? *Runner* **1,** 21.
104. Morville, R., Pesquies, P. L., Guezennec, C. Y., Serrurier, B. D., and Guignard, M. (1979). Plasma variations in testicular and agrenal androgens during prolonged physical exercise in man. *Ann. Endocrinol.* **40,** 501–510.

CHAPTER 7

Gynecological and Obstetrical Aspects of Exercise

MONA M. SHANGOLD

Department of Obstetrics and
Gynecology
Cornell University Medical
College
New York, New York

I. INTRODUCTION

Increasing interest in female reproductive physiology has arisen among sports medicine specialists as a result of the growth in women's athletic participation.

145

Exercise Medicine: Physiological Principles
and Clinical Applications

The main issues that have received much publicity are menstrual irregularity and amenorrhea, puberty, pregnancy, menopause, menstrual cramps, heavy bleeding, premenstrual syndrome, contraception, infertility, urinary incontinence, pelvic and vaginal infections, sanitary protection, breast concerns, and postoperative training. All these topics are addressed in this chapter. Attention will be directed toward identification and explanation of each issue, as well as recommendations for the management of athletes with these problems.

In caring for women athletes, it is essential to remember the importance of exercise in the life-style of each athlete. Women who are advised to cease exercising in order to correct their problems will either seek another physician or avoid medical care altogether. Both competitive and casual athletes are susceptible to a number of gynecological problems. In many cases, exercise may be related to the condition, but often the exercise may be totally unrelated. It is dangerous to assume that exercise is causative; a thorough evaluation is always warranted. Even when serious pathology has been ruled out, many athletes require treatment. Therapy always should be individualized and goal oriented and sometimes should be modified because of the athlete's training needs.

It has been claimed casually and incorrectly by some that women athletes should disregard gynecological problems and continue exercising. It is appropriate for women to keep exercising, but it is inappropriate and dangerous to disregard these problems. Despite these glib claims to the contrary, most women athletes are genuinely concerned about these issues and want answers to their questions. They have concerns about their own health and future fertility. Since women athletes are particularly in tune with their bodies, any dysfunction is distressing. Those that pertain to the sensitive areas of sexuality and reproduction can be even more worrisome.

Women athletes at all degrees of participation need the understanding of informed and concerned physicians and coaches. This chapter is intended to provide the background needed for the provision of optimal care.

II. BASIC REVIEW OF MENSTRUAL PHYSIOLOGY

The reproductive system of a woman depends on a delicate balance of carefully timed events, involving integration between the hypothalamus, pituitary gland, and ovaries. The external environment plays a role because the brain produces hormones in response to the signals it perceives from the outside world, and these hormones, in turn, affect the hypothalamus, pituitary, and ovaries. Hence, stress and anxiety may modify the hormone production of all these glands. The intricacies of hormonal timing and availability that are necessary for normal menstrual function make it much more surprising that women ever ovulate and menstruate so regularly.

The events taking place in the ovary are divided into two phases. The *follicular phase* is dominated by the follicle (the egg-containing structure) and lasts from the first day of menstruation until ovulation. The *luteal phase* is dominated by the corpus luteum (that which remains of the follicle after the egg has been expelled during ovulation) and lasts from ovulation until the first day of the next menstrual period.

The hypothalamus produces and secretes several releasing factors and inhibiting factors that stimulate or suppress pituitary hormone production and secretion. Among these, the factor of greatest importance in menstrual physiology is a decapeptide called by the following names: gonadotropin-releasing hormone (GnRH), luteinizing hormone-releasing hormone (LH-RH), and luteinizing hormone-releasing factor (LRF). Generally, GnRH stimulates the production and secretion of the pituitary glycoproteins, follicle-stimulating hormone (FSH) and luteinizing hormone (LH). FSH promotes growth of the follicle and production of estrogen from androgen precursors. LH promotes production of androgens by all parts of the ovary and production of progesterone by the corpus luteum. GnRH can also affect ovarian steroid production directly, in addition to indirectly via the pituitary gonadotropins.

Estrogen is produced by the ovaries throughout the menstrual cycle. The blood concentration of estrogen is low in the early follicular phase of the menstrual cycle and high in the late follicular phase. The high estrogen level in the late follicular phase triggers a surge of LH, which causes ovulation. The estrogen produced by the ovarian follicle leads to the ovarian production of a small amount of progesterone, which causes an important FSH surge at midcycle and which enhances the important LH surge at the same time. After ovulation, the corpus luteum produces large amounts of both estrogen and progesterone.

Estrogen stimulates the endometrium (the inner lining of the uterus) to grow. Progesterone acts on an endometrium that has already been stimulated by estrogen and converts such an endometrium into a stable, mature structure. In the absence of pregnancy, a normal corpus luteum lives about 14 days. As it approaches the end of its lifetime, a corpus luteum stops producing estrogen and progesterone. The decline in the concentrations of these two hormones, near the end of the menstrual cycle, leads to shedding of the endometrium in the process of menstruation.

III. MENSTRUAL IRREGULARITY AND AMENORRHEA: CAUSES, EVALUATION, AND TREATMENT

Some women produce very little estrogen and do not achieve a blood concentration of estrogen high enough to trigger an LH surge. The endometrium of such a woman would get very little stimulation, and she would bleed rarely, if at all. The other parts of her body also would lack estrogen stimulation, much of which is beneficial. Thus, her bones may be more susceptible to osteoporosis than are the bones of a regularly menstruating athlete. Her vagina similarly is more susceptible to atrophic vaginitis than is the vagina of a regularly menstruating woman. Although exercise tends to enhance bone density, it has not yet been shown to be beneficial enough to compensate for an estrogen deficiency.

The cause of inadequate estrogen production in these women appears complex and variable. In some cases it may be related to weight loss, low weight, loss of body fat, or low body fat. Acute and chronic hormone alterations may also play a role and may result from the exercise itself, from the stress and anxiety of training or competition, or from both. Because hypoestrogenic amenorrhea is so common among athletes, it may be tempting to assume the problem is related to the exercise. Such an assumption is dangerous and can lead to a failure to recognize other, serious problems. Athletes are not immune to the development of pituitary, adrenal, or ovarian tumors, which can also lead to amenorrhea. Premature menopause may also present with this same picture. Hence, all athletes with irregular periods or amenorrhea require thorough evaluation, in order to detect serious pathology. The hazards of an estrogen deficiency make replacement therapy indicated for women with low estrogen levels.

Another common cause of oligomenorrhea (infrequent periods) and amenorrhea among athletes is a deficiency of progesterone. This results whenever estrogen is produced without ovulation taking place. Before this condition (anovulation) develops, many women first develop a shortened luteal phase, due to diminished progesterone production. Although the cause of this problem is not serious, the result can be. A progesterone deficiency can lead to endometrial cancer because progesterone normally protects the endometrium from overstimulation by estrogen. Infertility can also result from a progesterone deficiency. The risk of endometrial cancer makes progesterone therapy indicated for women with endogenous or exogenous estrogen stimulation without progesterone protection.

The most common cause of amenorrhea among women of reproductive age is pregnancy. Athletes are not immune to this condition either, even if they have been amenorrheic for some time. Pregnancy usually can be detected by a pelvic examination. Several blood and urine tests are available for the diagnosis of very early pregnancy. Athletes who do not want immediate fertility should be advised to use appropriate contraception, even for those who are temporarily amenorrheic.

Evaluation of the oligomenorrheic or amenorrheic athlete should begin with a thorough history and physical examination. Pelvic examination usually reveals pregnancy and indicates a woman's estrogen level. Women with low estrogen levels have very scanty cervical mucus, whereas women with adequate estrogen levels have moderate or profuse cervical mucus that is clear, colorless, watery, and stretchable. Women who have adequate levels of both estrogen and progesterone have white, opaque, sticky cervical mucus, and they will bleed within 2 weeks unless they are pregnant or lack an endometrium. Absence of a functioning endometrium should be suspected from a history of prior endometrial curettage, instrumentation, or infection. Such women are incapable of responding to endogenous or exogenous hormone stimulation.

Unless pregnancy is suspected, all oligomenorrheic or amenorrheic athletes should undergo the following serum tests: prolactin concentration, thyroid-stimulating hormone (TSH) concentration, and thyroid function tests (thyroxine concentration and T_3 resin uptake); a progesterone challenge test should also be done. Hyperprolactinemia is a cause of both hypoestrogenic and euestrogenic oligomenorrhea and amenorrhea. An elevated TSH indicates primary hypothyroidism (due to thyroid insufficiency), even before thyroxine levels fall. A low thyroxine concentration in the face of a low or normal TSH concentration indicates secondary or tertiary hypothyroidism (due to pituitary or hypothalamic insufficiency, respectively). The T_3 resin uptake reflects the amount of binding and permits interpretation of the thyroxine value, since nearly all thyroxine circulates in the bound form. Hypothyroidism of any etiology can lead to oligomenorrhea or amenorrhea, with or without hyperprolactinemia.

Administration of progesterone to a woman with an estrogen-stimulated endometrium will lead to bleeding when the progesterone is withdrawn (usually within 2–5 days of the last dose of medroxyprogesterone acetate). If withdrawal bleeding does not follow progesterone ingestion, a low estrogen level is diagnosed in any woman with a functioning endometrium. If her prolactin and TSH concentrations and her thyroid function tests are normal, lack of progesterone-induced withdrawal bleeding should be followed by measurement of her serum FSH concentration. An elevated FSH level indicates ovarian failure (menopause); a low or normal value suggests hypothalamic or pituitary dysfunction. Menopause before the age of 30 should be evaluated with a blood karyotype to rule out a chromosomal etiology. The presence of a Y chromosome in a cell line warrants gonadectomy because of the risk of gonadal malignancy in intra-abdominal gonads bearing a Y chromosome.

Further evaluation of hypoestrogenic athletes with low or normal FSH levels, normal prolactin and TSH levels, and normal thyroid function tests should include a coned-down roentgenogram of the sella turcica, to seek a sizable non-prolactin-producing pituitary tumor. No further diagnostic evaluation is necessary if this roentgenogram is normal, If the prolactin concentration is elevated and/or if the coned-down skull film is abnormal, high-resolution computed axial tomography of the brain is warranted to identify and localize pituitary tumors.

Athletes with clinical signs of androgen excess (i.e., acne, hirsutism) need evaluation of androgen levels. Mild androgen excess can lead to oligomenorrhea or amenorrhea without acne or hirsutism, but much less commonly. Identification of this condition generally is of interest and of importance only for counseling purposes; it rarely affects patient management. Hence, it is worthwhile to assess androgen status only if acne or hirsutism is noted. Hyperandrogenism can be detected most conveniently by measurement of blood concentrations of dehydroepiandrosterone sulfate (DHEAS) and testosterone. Collection of 24-hour urine for measurement of 17-ketosteroid (17KS) excretion is more cumbersome but reflects the blood DHEAS level reasonably well. If blood DHEAS concentration is not available to the clinician, the urinary 17KS may be substituted.

Any athlete who has been unable to achieve a pregnancy within 1 year of unprotected intercourse at least two to three times per week should undergo a thorough infertility evaluation with her partner. This type of evaluation, and those for most other specific problems described here, should be carried out by specialists who are familiar and comfortable with these conditions.

Therapy for any oligomenorrheic or amenorrheic athlete must be individualized and should respect the importance of exercise in the life-style of the athlete. Hypoestrogenic athletes with normal examinations, normal concentrations of prolactin and TSH, and normal thyroid function tests should be treated with estrogen and progesterone replacement for protection against osteoporosis and atrophic vaginitis. This may be administered most conveniently as follows: conjugated estrogens (0.625 mg daily on days 1–25 of every calendar month) and medroxyprogesterone acetate (2.5–10 mg daily on days 16–25 of this estrogen therapy). Until recently, it was thought that 10 mg medroxyprogesterone acetate was needed daily for adequate endometrial protection, but recent evidence suggests that as little as 2.5 mg daily is sufficient (1).

Euestrogenic athletes with normal examinations, normal concentrations of prolactin and TSH, and normal thyroid function tests should be treated with progesterone for endometrial protection. A 10-day regimen of medroxyprogesterone acetate should be employed every month or two for those women who have developed this condition recently. For those women who have had this condition for one year or longer, this 10-day regimen should be administered every month.

Management of hyperprolactinemic women with or without radiographic evidence of pituitary tumors has changed greatly during the past few years. Surgery and radiation therapy are indicated much less commonly for the removal of pituitary tumors than was formerly true. Expectant management for mild hyperprolactinemia and/or small tumors is considered acceptable, and medical management with bromocryptine currently is advisable for all women with hyperprolactinemia, with or without radiographic evidence of tumors.

Hypothyroid athletes should be treated with thyroid hormone replacement therapy. Management of hyperandrogenic athletes should be individualized and varies with the underlying cause. Therapeutic options for women without androgen-producing tumors (which are a very rare cause) include oral contraceptives, glucocorticoids, cimetidine, and spironolactone. Treatment of the infertile couple depends on the cause or causes of the problem. Most infertile amenorrheic women will require ovulation induction, and many of their male partners may require therapy as well.

For those women who developed oligomenorrhea or amenorrhea when they began exercising, the option of reducing activity may be suggested as a means of correcting the problem. However, most athletes appreciate the benefits of exercise and are unwilling to select this therapeutic modality. The choice remains with the patient herself. Encouragement of less exercise by some physicians has led to patient distrust and alienation, which obviously are undesirable.

IV. HORMONE CHANGES RELATED TO EXERCISE

The preceding discussion of the evaluation and management of athletes with oligomenorrhea or amenorrhea also applies to nonathletes. Although the same conditions occur in athletes and nonathletes, and although similar, individualized management is appropriate, specific hormone alterations do occur with acute and chronic exercise. It is worth mentioning some of these for academic interest, even though clinical management remains the same.

Acute increases in plasma prolactin (2,3), estrogen (4,5), progesterone (4,5), testosterone (3), prostaglandins (6), β-endorphin (7), and melatonin (8) have been observed following exercise. The mechanisms for these alterations may include increased production, decreased clearance, decreased metabolism, or a combination of these. Chronic alterations include reduced luteal progesterone levels and shortening of the luteal phase (9,10). Current investigators have identified altered responsivity of the pituitary gland to hypothalamic stimulation in association with training. The mechanisms for these changes and the effects of repetitive acute increases remain to be elucidated.

V. OTHER MENSTRUAL PROBLEMS

Although oligomenorrhea and amenorrhea in athletes have received greatest publicity and attention, other menstrual problems occur in athletes too. Heavy bleeding, menstrual cramps, and premenstrual syndrome warrant special mention because these are both so common and so disabling.

A. Heavy Bleeding

Heavy bleeding at the expected time (menorrhagia) or at an unexpected time (metrorrhagia) may represent significant causative pathology and may lead to both anemia and inconvenience. Heavy bleeding includes an increased rate of menstrual blood flow and/or a prolonged duration of flow. Many women who bleed heavily are anovulatory and bleed from endometria stimulated by only estrogen. Such bleeding may occur more often or more seldom than the generally accepted normal interval: 25–32 days (counting from the first day of one menstrual period to the first day of the next menstrual period). Anovulatory bleeding also may occur at normal intervals.

Anovulatory women less than 25 years of age can be treated with monthly progesterone. If bleeding occurs only after withdrawal of the progesterone and to a lesser (and normal) extent, no further evaluation is necessary. Monthly progesterone for 10 days is appropriate treatment for such young women.

Heavy and/or irregular bleeders over age 25 require endometrial sampling prior to institution of progestational therapy, in order to rule out endometrial carcinoma. Curettage may be curative if endometrial polyps are the cause of the abnormal bleeding. If progesterone does not correct the problem in a woman under age 25, curettage is indicated, for detection of polyps or other pathology.

Heavy bleeding can lead to iron deficiency, which can impair performance. Thus, hematological assessment of heavily menstruating athletes is always incidated. The inconvenience of heavy menstruation can be alleviated by the use of higher absorbency tampons and/or sanitary napkins (see Section VI,C).

B. Dysmenorrhea

Dysmenorrhea (menstrual cramps) is caused by prostaglandins, which are produced by the endometrium and which cause the myometrium (uterine muscle) to contract. When a myometrial contraction exceeds a certain threshold, it is painful.

Many athletes report less pain acutely during exercise and/or chronically since exercising regularly. However, others note no change or worsening. Several potent prostaglandin inhibitors are available and may be prescribed with impunity. These include naproxen (250 mg every 12 hours), ibuprofen (400 mg every 6 hours), mefenamic acid (250 mg every 8 hours), and naproxen sodium (275 mg every 8 hours). Aspirin (2 tablets every 4 hours), although much less potent, is sufficiently effective for many women. Medication for true, physiological dysmenorrhea should be required for only the first 24–36 hours of the menstrual period. It is advisable to take any of these on a full stomach, to decrease their potential for gastrointestinal discomfort or ulcers. If one of these does not provide adequate relief or promotes undesirable side effects (usually gastrointestinal), another one should be tried. If all fail to provide relief, pelvic pathology (e.g., endometriosis or infection) should be sought. Prostaglandin inhibitors are contraindicated in individuals with known sensitivity to aspirin and aspirinlike compounds.

C. Premenstrual Syndrome

This complex entity remains poorly understood, although it has become better defined recently. Premenstrual syndrome includes several symptoms that occur during the few days immediately preceding the beginning of each menstrual period. These symptoms fall into four main categories: anxiety, depression, edema, and increased appetite. Although these symptoms are prevalent among both athletic and nonathletic women, many report fewer or milder symptoms since they have been exercising regularly. Despite the vague definition of this entity, symptoms are real and are undoubtedly due to hormonal alterations.

Vitamin B$_6$ (pyridoxine) may be helpful for some who have this condition, beginning with 50 mg/day throughout the cycle and increasing to 200 mg/day if symptoms persist. If this regimen fails, spironolactone should be tried, beginning with 25 mg/day throughout the cycle and increasing to 50 mg/day if symptoms persist.

VI. OTHER GYNECOLOGICAL PROBLEMS

A. Stress Urinary Incontinence

The term "stress urinary incontinence" refers to the symptom of involuntary urine loss when intra-abdominal pressure is increased. This commonly affects athletes, who often strain during exertion, but exercise does not promote this underlying anatomic defect. True stress incontinence results from loss of the posterior vesicourethral angle, often due to obstetrical trauma.

Women who leak urine involuntarily require urological evaluation to rule out neurological or infectious etiologies. Although some may benefit from Kegel exercises, which strengthen the muscles of the pelvic floor, others require a surgical procedure (e.g., anterior vaginal colporrhaphy, Marshall–Marchetti–Krantz procedure, fascia lata sling procedure) to restore urinary continence.

Athletes should be reassured that although exercise may exacerbate symptoms, it does not cause or worsen the problem. Similarly, exercise does not promote uterine prolapse either.

B. Pelvic and Vaginal Infections

Pelvic infections commonly cause pelvic pain and tenderness, fever, and leukocytosis. These infections are more prevalent among women who are sexually active, those with multiple partners, and those with intrauterine devices. Although athletes are no more susceptible than the general population, these disorders can impair the performance and training of any athlete very significantly. Prompt diagnosis by cervical and intraperitoneal (via culdocentesis) Gram's stain and culture is needed, and this should be followed by appropriate antibiotic therapy. Urgency and/or inadequate diagnostic facilities often require that empirical therapy be initiated before a definitive diagnosis can be made.

Vaginal infections commonly produce pruritus and/or discharge. Although these infections are no more prevalent among athletes than among the general population, and although athletic underwear and perspiration do not promote these disorders, the discomfort from these problems may impede athletic training and competition. The most common vaginal pathogens are *Candida vaginalis, Trichomonas vaginalis,* and *Gardnerella vaginalis,* all of which may be quickly and accurately diagnosed by wet prep examinations of the vaginal discharge in saline and KOH. Cultures are equally accurate but require more time for diagnosis and are inappropriate for symptomatic women in need of immediate relief. *Candida vaginitis* is treated optimally with topical nystatin or one of its more potent derivatives. *Trichomonas* vaginitis requires oral treatment of the patient and her partner(s) with metronidazole. *Gardnerella* vaginitis may be treated with metronidazole or, less reliably, with ampicillin or tetracycline.

C. Sanitary Protection

Recent publicity about toxic shock syndrome (TSS) alarmed many women and discouraged many from using tampons. Athletic and other active women are particularly dependent on internal sanitary protection for comfort, convenience, and mobility. The facts should be considered in perspective.

TSS is a very rare disease and is caused by a bacterial toxin, produced by *Staphylococcus aureus*. Even among regularly menstruating women, the risk of developing TSS is less than the risk of being hit by a car while a pedestrian. The disease also occurs in non-tampon users, nonmenstruating women, and men.

Women athletes remain aware of the convenience of tampons and should not be discouraged from using them. They should be advised to follow the instructions of the manufacturer, which are enclosed with every package, and they should be informed of the symptoms of TSS: fever, headache, nausea, vomiting, diarrhea, rash, sore throat, and myalgias. Any woman who develops these symptoms should call her doctor immediately and, if wearing a tampon, should remove the tampon also. If a woman wants to reduce an already small risk even further, she may consider alternating tampon use with sanitary napkin use.

D. Contraception

Choice of an optimal contraceptive should include consideration of a woman's medical history, physical examination, coital frequency, fertility plans, motivation, and personal preference. Rarely is the selection affected by the fact that she is an athlete. Oral contraceptives are now available in lower doses. In contrast to previously popular higher doses, these offer fewer risks and side effects, and they provide excellent protection and convenience. Absolute contraindications to oral contraceptives include liver disease, breast cancer, history of thromboembolic disease, and undiagnosed abnormal uterine bleeding. Relative contraindications include age over 35, cigarette smoking, diabetes mellitus, migraine headaches, hypertension, sickle cell disease, familial hyperlipidemia, strong family history of coronary heart disease, and xanthomatosis. Regular exercise may decrease some of the cardiovascular and thromboembolic risk factors associated with oral contraceptive use (e.g., improved HDL/LDL cholesterol ratio, enhanced fibrinolytic activity). Coital frequency of weekly or less often does not justify the small risks and minor side effects of daily hormone ingestion for most women.

Intrauterine devices (IUDs) carry a small risk of pelvic infection that may lead to infertility. Although they afford excellent convenience and protection, they are not recommended for women who plan to have children in the future. The pain and increased bleeding that occasionally are associated with their use may impair athletic performance in some women, particularly if anemia results. Those athletes who have completed child bearing, who have coitus at least once or twice each week, and who experience neither pain nor excessive bleeding in association with IUD use may select this form of contraception as a reasonable option.

Many athletes prefer mechanical contraception (foam, condoms, diaphragm), which impose fewer side effects and risks, offer adequate protection, and require motivation and discipline for successful use. Some women report pelvic or vaginal discomfort when they exercise while wearing a diaphragm. No medical hazards have been found in connection with this problem, which usually is mild and easily tolerated. Mechanical contraception is recommended for those who practice coitus less often than weekly, who have contraindications to hormonal contraception, and who have not completed child bearing.

Athletes who have completed child bearing and who require contraception should consider tubal sterilization. Male partner sterilization may be preferred by some couples.

E. Infertility

Infertile couples should consult a specialist for evaluation of both partners and their interaction and for appropriate therapy. As mentioned previously, most oligomenorrheic or amenorrheic infertile athletes will require ovulation induction.

F. Postoperative and Postpartum Training

Athletes who have undergone major surgery or vaginal delivery usually can resume training when no pain results. Pain generally indicates incomplete healing. Thus, lack of pain during exercise generally reflects that sufficient healing has occurred. For some women, this may require only a few days, particularly following a vaginal delivery without an episiotomy. For others, this may require as long as 6–8 weeks. Fatigue and some loss of training should be anticipated, and exercise should be modified accordingly.

G. Breast Concerns

Since the breast is composed mostly of fat tissue and contains no muscles, no exercises can augment breast size. However, increased pectoral musculature may give the illusion of a fuller chest. A reduction in body fat often leads to a diminution in breast size. Exercise does not reduce breast tone, which probably occurs with increasing age. However, gravity appears to promote stretching of the skin overlying the breast in all women with weighty breasts. Observations of different populations reveal such stretching and loss of desirable breast contour in women who do not wear breast support (11). Most women with large breasts find exercise more comfortable when wearing a bra that provides good support, whereas many small-breasted women find exercise more comfortable when braless. There are no medical contraindications to the latter (11), and each athlete should be guided by her own comfort in choosing any bra or none.

VII. PUBERTY

Athletic girls have been noted to experience menarche at a later age than nonathletic controls (12,13). In many cases this may be related to decreased weight and/or body fat in athletes. In other cases it may be related to stress and/or exertion alone. It remains unclear whether exercise actually delays puberty or a delay in puberty promotes increased athletic success and perseverance. Increased estrogen production at the time of puberty promotes epiphyseal closure and fat deposition. Short stature and fatness generally have a detrimental effect on athletic skills. Thus, women who experience puberty at an earlier age may become discouraged in athletic endeavors and encouraged in sociosexual interests. This issue remains complex and unresolved.

Any 16-year-old who has not begun to menstruate should be examined by a gynecologist. If examination reveals axillary and pubic hair, some breast development, a uterus, and estrogenic cervical mucus, the girl should be reassured that menarche probably will occur within 6 months and that no further evaluation is necessary unless it does not. Evaluation at that time should follow the protocol in the section on oligo-/ amenorrhea. If examination reveals axillary and pubic hair, a uterus, and no cervical mucus, evaluation should follow the protocol in Section III. Those patients in whom no uterus can be palpated or visualized require pelvic sonography, blood testosterone concentration, and blood karyotype. Results of these tests will determine further management. There are no harmful effects from a constitutional delay in puberty, except for possible psychological problems.

VIII. MENOPAUSE

Menopause is the cessation of menstruation that occurs when the ovaries are depleted of functioning follicles. When this condition (ovarian failure) takes place prior to the earliest age generally accepted as normal (forty), it is considered premature. The most reliable way to diagnose the menopause is a measurement of the plasma FSH concentration, but it is rarely necessary to do this in women of menopausal age.

The main problems associated with menopause are related to the aging process and estrogen deficiency. These include vasomotor symptoms (hot flushes), osteoporosis, cardiovascular disease, atrophic vaginitis, and depression. Abnormal uterine bleeding occasionally occurs as the menopause is being approached and always should be evaluated by adequate endometrial sampling. Postmenopausal bleeding always requires adequate endometrial sampling (i.e., by curettage) for evaluation.

Vasomotor symptoms can be very incapacitating, particularly if associated with chronic sleep deprivation, which can promote several psychiatric and behavioral disorders. The cause of vasomotor symptoms remains to be determined. However, these can be relieved with estrogen therapy or, less reliably, with progestin therapy. Exercise has not been shown to be helpful (14).

Osteoporosis is the most serious problem of the menopause because 25% of all Caucasian women over the age of 60 experience osteoporotic bone fractures, and 17% of all elderly patients die within 3 months of a hip fracture. Bone density is lost with aging in both sexes, although at a younger age and to a greater extent in women. Estrogen administration improves bone density by inhibiting bone resorption, increasing renal tubular reabsorption of calcium, and enhancing intestinal absorption of calcium. Exercise increases bone density when dietary calcium is adequate (15). For most adults, this requires 800–1000 mg daily. Postmenopausal women require 1.5 gm of calcium daily, in order to maintain optimal bone density (16). The beneficial effects of exercise on bone density suggest that all postmenopausal women should be so encouraged. Women who are thin, Caucasian, smokers, alcoholics, or expected to be long-lived or who have a family history of osteoporosis are at higher risk of developing osteoporosis. Such women will benefit from estrogen (and progestin) therapy also, unless contraindicated (17).

The increased risk of cardiovascular disease in older women probably is associated with increasing age and detrimental life-style, rather than estrogen deficiency. The beneficial effects of exercise on reduction of these risks are well known. HDL cholesterol levels have been shown to increase with physical activity (18), and high levels of HDL cholesterol are associated with a protective effect against ischemic heart disease (19). Physical conditioning also can enhance the augmentation of fibrinolytic activity that occurs in response to venous occlusion (20). Thus, the risks of cardiovascular and ischemic heart disease are decreased by exercise in several ways.

Postmenopausal estrogen deficiency is the cause of atrophic vaginitis and urethritis, which should be treated by estrogen replacement therapy.

Depression is a significant problem in older women and is associated with decreased brain concentrations of norepinephrine (21). With increasing age, there are decreases in the catecholamine synthesizing enzymes, tyrosine hydroxylase, and dopa decarboxylase, and an increase in the catecholamine catabolizing enzyme, monoamine oxidase. Also, aging is associated with reduced synthesis and enhanced catabolism of serotonin (22), a mood-elevating chemical. Rats that have been exercised have higher brain concentrations of both norepinephrine and serotonin (23) than do sedentary rats. The augmenting effect of exercise on these two hormones may explain the successful treatment and prevention of depression by exercise. This represents another beneficial effect of exercise for older women.

Obesity is associated with several diseases and risk factors, and older women often tend to acquire this problem. Because exercise promotes a loss of weight and body fat and suppression of appetite, it helps to prevent cardiovascular disease, diabetes mellitus, gallbladder disease, and several forms of cancer.

Most older women were not encouraged to exercise when they were young and need guidelines to do so. Most were taught that a sedentary life-style was desirable. Thus, reeducation of these women is necessary.

Previously sedentary older women should be encouraged toward brisk walking, stationary bicycling, and swimming, which offer endurance activity with little risk of injury. To achieve cardiovascular fitness, they should exercise three to five times per week, at a heart rate of at least 110–120 beats per minute, and sustained for 15–60 continuous minutes (24). Appropriate warming up, cooling down, and nutrition should be taught also, probably in group sessions that offer camaraderie and emotional support as well.

IX. PREGNANCY

The issue of training during pregnancy has become controversial because maternal benefits of exercise are known but are offset by potential fetal risks.

Women who are physically fit and their fetuses tolerate the work load of labor and delivery better than women who are not (and their fetuses), with less lactic acidosis in the former (25). During exercise, hepatic (26) and renal (27) blood flow decrease, although to a lesser extent in trained individuals. It is not known how much exercise can be performed without decreasing uterine blood flow, which supplies the fetus. Strenuous, prolonged, and repetitive exercise in some animal species is associated with an increased incidence of intrauterine growth retardation, prematurity, and perinatal morbidity and mortality (28–31). There are differences between animal species, and it is not known whether extrapolation to humans is applicable.

Women should be encouraged to acquire fitness before becoming pregnant and to maintain fitness during pregnancy. Because pregnancy involves work even at rest, and because exercise with the added weight of pregnancy involves even more work, pregnant athletes should exercise more slowly. They should avoid fatigue and hyperthermia, the latter of which is associated with an increased risk of teratogenicity (32,33) in the first trimester and with an increased risk of premature labor subsequently. Sports should be avoided if they involve trauma to the abdomen, reduced oxygen availability, or excessive heat accumulation. Nutritional requirements for the pregnant athlete are not greater than for her sedentary counterpart, except for greater caloric needs.

An obstetrician should be consulted before any athlete undertakes exercise during pregnancy, in order to ensure that the pregnancy appears normal and uncomplicated. If pain, bleeding, rupture of membranes, or absence of fetal movement develops, exercise should cease immediately and an obstetrician should be consulted. In the absence of complications, pregnant athletes can expect to continue participation throughout pregnancy.

X. CONCLUSION

Women of all ages should be encouraged to exercise. Among the benefits they should anticipate from such exercise are cardiovascular, skeletal, psychological, and body composition and resultant reduction in disease risk. If any gynecological problems arise, they should be dealt with on an individual basis, respecting the importance of exercise in the athlete's life-style.

REFERENCES

1. Gibbons W. (1982). Personal communication.
2. Brisson, G., Volle, M., De Carufel, D., Desharnais, M., and Tanaka, M. (1980). Exercise-induced dissociation of the blood prolactin response in young women according to their sports habits. *Horm. Metab. Res.* **12**, 201.

3. Shangold, M., Gatz, M., and Thysen, B. (1981). Acute effects of exercise on plasma concentrations of prolactin and testosterone in recreational women runners. *Fertil. Steril.* **35,** 699.
4. Jurkowski, J., Jones, N., Walker, W., Younglai, E., and Sutton, J. (1978). Ovarian hormonal responses to exercise. *J. Appl. Physiol.* **44,** 109.
5. Bonen, A., Ling, W., MacIntyre, K., Neil, R., McGrail, J., and Belcastro, A. (1979). Effects of exercise on the serum concentrations of FSH, LH, progesterone and estradiol. *Eur. J. Appl. Physiol. Occup. Physiol.* **42,** 15.
6. Demers, L., Harrison, T., Halbert, D., and Santen, R. (1981). Effect of prolonged exercise on plasma prostaglandin levels. *Prostaglandins Med.* **6,** 413.
7. Carr, D., Bullen, B., Skrinar, G., Arnold, M., Rosenblatt, M., Beitins, I., Martin, J., and McArthur, J. (1981). Physical conditioning facilitates the exercise-induced secretion of beta-endorphin and beta-lipotropin in women. *N. Engl. J. Med.* **305,** 560.
8. Carr, D., Reppert, S., Bullen, B., Skrinar, G., Beitins, I., Arnold, M., Rosenblatt, M., Martin, J., and McArthur, J. (1981). Plasma melatonin increases during exercise in women. *J. Clin. Endocrinol. Metab.* **53,** 224.
9. Shangold, M., Freeman, R., Thysen, B., and Gatz, M. (1979). The relationship between long-distance running, plasma progesterone, and luteal phase length. *Fertil. Steril.* **31,** 130.
10. Bonen, A., Belcastro, A., Ling, W., and Simpson, A. (1981). Profiles of selected hormones during the menstrual cycles of teenage athletes. *J. Appl. Physiol.* **50,** 545.
11. Haycock C. (1982). Personal communication.
12. Malina, R., Harper, A., Avent, H., and Campbell, D. (1973). Age at menarche in athletes and non-athletes. *Med. Sci. Sports* **5,** 11.
13. Warren, (1980). The effects of exercise on pubertal progression and reproductive function in girls. *J. Clin. Endocrinol. Metab.* **51,** 1150.
14. Wallace, J. (1981). Serum concentrations of sex hormones during exercise in pre-, peri-, and post-menopausal women. Doctoral Thesis, Pennsylvania State University.
15. Albanese, A. (1981). Personal communication.
16. Albanese, A., Lorenze, E., Edelson, A., Wein, E., and Carroll, L. (1981). Effects of calcium supplements and estrogen replacement therapy on bone loss of postmenopausal women. *Nutr. Rep. Int.* **24**(2), 403.
17. Henneman, P., and Wallach, S. (1957). A review of the prolonged use of estrogens and androgens in postmenopausal and senile osteoporosis. *Arch. Intern. Med.* **100,** 715.
18. Lopez, S., Vial, R., Balart, L., and Arroyave, G. (1974). Effect of exercise and physical fitness on serum lipid and lipoproteins. *Atherosclerosis* **20,** 1.
19. Gordon, T., Castelli, W., Hjortland, M., Kannel, W., and Dawber, T. (1977). High density lipoprotein as a protective factor against coronary heart disease: The Framingham study. *Am. J. Med.* **62,** 707.
20. Williams, R., Logue, E., Lewis, J., Barton, T., Stead, N., Wallace, A., and Pizzo, S. (1980). Physical conditioning augments the fibrinolytic response to venous occlusion in healthy adults. *N. Engl. J. Med.* **302,** 987.
21. Robinson, D. (1975). Changes in monoamine oxidase and monoamines with human development and aging. *Fed. Proc., Fed. Am. Soc. Exp. Biol.* **34,** 103.
22. Robinson, D., Nies, A., and Davis, J. (1972). Aging, monoamines and monoamine oxidase levels. *Lancet* **1,** 290.
23. Brown, B., Payne, T., Kim, C., Moore, G., Krebs, P., and Martin, W. (1979). Chronic response of rat brain norepinephrine and serotonin levels to endurance training. *J. Appl. Physiol.: Respir., Environ. Exercise Physiol.* **46,** 19.
24. American College of Sports Medicine (1978). Position statement on the recommended quantity and quality of exercise for developing and maintaining fitness in health adults. *Med. Sci. Sports* **10**(3), vii.

25. Erkkola, R., and Rauramo, L. (1976). Correlation of maternal physical fitness during pregnancy with maternal and fetal pH and lactic acid at delivery. *Acta Obstet. Gynecol. Scand.* **55,** 441.

26. Rowell, L., Blackmon, J., and Bruce, R. (1964). Indocyanine green clearance and estimated hepatic blood flow during mild to maximal exercise in upright man. *J. Clin. Invest.* **43,** 1677.

27. Radigan, L., and Robinson, S. (1949). Effects of environmental heat stress and exercise on renal blood flow and filtration rate. *J. Appl. Physiol.* **2,** 185.

28. Emmanouilides, G., Hobel, C., Yashiro, K., and Klyman, G. (1972). Fetal responses to maternal exercise in the sheep. *Am. J. Obstet. Gynecol.* **112,** 130.

29. Longo, L., Hewitt, C., Lorijn, R., and Gilbert, R. (1978). To what extent does maternal exercise affect fetal oxygenation and uterine blood flow? *Fed. Proc., Fed. Am. Soc. Exp. Biol.* **37,** 905.

30. Gilbert, R., Cummings, L., Juchau, M., and Longo, L. (1979). Placental diffusing capacity and fetal development in exercising or hypoxic guinea pigs. *J. Appl. Physiol.* **46,** 828.

31. Wilson, N., and Gisolfi, C. (1980). Effects of exercising rats during pregnancy. *J. Appl. Physiol.* **48,** 34.

32. Smith, D., Clarren, S., and Harvey, M. (1978). Hyperthermia as a possible teratogenic agent. *J. Pediatr.* **92,** 878.

33. Harvey, M., McRorie, M., and Smith, D. (1981). Suggested limits to the use of the hot tub and sauna by pregnant women. *Canadian Med. Assoc. J.* **125,** 50.

CHAPTER 8

Exercise in the Young

BONITA FALKNER
Department of Pediatrics
Hahnemann University
School of Medicine
Philadelphia, Pennsylvania

I. INTRODUCTION

Exercise may be considered beneficial and therapeutic for children when the exercise activity results in an improved level of cardiovascular and neuromuscular fitness. Development of a greater body fitness and body skills generally achieve another goal for the child, that of an improved self-image. These are compelling reasons to encourage exercise programs for the child whether healthy or a patient. Optimally, exercise activities should augment the normal childhood phases of growth and development and avoid undue physical injuries as a result of misguided direction or poor supervision.

Injury prevention is generally relegated to the area of supervised sports programs in schools and communities. The physician, however, may contribute significantly to improved general fitness levels of both normal children and many children with medical limitations.

Studies have been performed in children to determine the cardiovascular response to exercise (1,10). From these studies normal values are available for maximal endurance time and maximal work load for children according to age

163

Exercise Medicine: Physiological Principles
and Clinical Applications

and sex. Standards in children for exercise response to the Bruce protocol have been developed by Cummings *et al.,* (1978). According to their data the maximal heart rate for both boys and girls 4–18 years is 190–200 beats/minute. However, differences do exist in endurance time. By treadmill testing mean values for endurance time are slightly lower in girls than boys with a progressive increase in endurance time for both sexes until age 11–12 years. Following 12 years boys have a progressive increase in endurance time until late adolescence. However, girls demonstrate a progressive decline in mean endurance time following age 12 and this decline then persists into adulthood. Thus, it would seem that girls peak in their fitness level at age 12 years and decline thereafter. Whether the decline in female endurance performance at the onset of adolescence is determined by endocrine physiology or reflects socially directed behavior patterns remains to be documented. However, the observations of much greater endurance performance levels in girls engaged in competitive activities such as track, gymnastics, swimming, skating, and other sports indicate that the endurance time potential for females is greater than that demonstrated on average groups of female adolescents. Therefore, as a group adolescent females should be encouraged to develop a life-style involving regular exercise simply to maintain the cardiovascular fitness that they have achieved at the onset of puberty.

Medical disorders in pediatrics which may involve exercise as a component of therapy include pulmonary disorders, cardiovascular disorders, and obesity. Orthopedic and neuromuscular disorders have traditionally used exercise to improve strength and flexibility and will not be discussed in this chapter. The rationale for involving exercise prescriptions is to restore or increase cardiovascular reserves and also counteract further degeneration.

II. ASTHMA

Children who experience respiratory distress related to exercise tend to withdraw from exercise activities. This reduction in physical activity then results in a lower level of cardiovascular fitness. Many asthmatic children experience acute and sometimes severe airway obstruction during or after strenuous physical exertion.

In susceptible children exercise induced asthma occurs following several minutes of strenuous exercise and then continues or worsens several (5–10) minutes after completion of strenuous exercise. In some patients the postexertion bronchospasm may become progressively worse for 30–60 minutes before it spontaneously improves (7).

The incidence of exercise-induced asthma appears to be greater in children than adults. Patients with exercise-induced asthma do not develop postexertional bronchospasm after every strenuous physical activity. Therefore, standardized laboratory testing is necessary to clarify the relationship of physical activity as an inductor in the acute bronchospasm. Some investigators have demonstrated that exercise-related bronchospasm can be demonstrated in the majority of asthmatic children. Cropp has observed that 25–30% of children with chronic asthma develop mild, often subclinical, exercise-induced asthma; 25–30% develop moderate attacks; and 15–25% will develop severe attacks (6–8). A further observation is that occurrence of the severe postexertion bronchospasm is greater in boys than girls.

Previous studies have described the alterations in pulmonary function during exercise-induced asthma. The evidence indicates that the exercise-provoked airway obstruction in asthmatics is associated with bronchospasm of large and small airways. This results in increases in airway resistance and reduction in specific airway conductance and forced expiratory flow rates. Also present is hyperinflation, maldistribution of inspired air, and slowed volume emptying (2,3,24,28).

In affected children some types of exercise are more asthmagenic whereas others are better tolerated. Intermittent activities are better tolerated than prolonged endurance activities. Therefore, football, tennis, or weight lifting may be better tolerated than running, soccer, or basketball. Of all activities swimming is particularly well tolerated (19).

It is appropriate to prevent the occurrence of exercise-induced bronchospasm so that asthmatics can participate in activities enabling them to achieve optimal physical fitness. Standardized exercise stress testing is indicated to determine the degree of functional impairment and the response to medication (12,19). Preexercise prophylactic medication with selective β-sympathomimetic agents or cromolyn sodium before beginning intense exercise will reduce or abate exercise-induced asthma in the majority of asthmatics (18).

Asthmatic children should not be restricted from exercise simply because the exercise provokes attacks. Rather the child should be evaluated and placed on an appropriate treatment regimen along with guidance in types of activities in which to participate.

Physical conditioning programs for asthmatic children will improve their exercise tolerance as it does in nonasthmatics (19). Training programs will not prevent the occurrence or the severity of bronchospasm after intense exercise. However, conditioning programs will raise the exertion threshold for bronchospasm (20).

III. CYSTIC FIBROSIS

Children with chronic and progressive pulmonary disease will have significant impairment in their physical endurance capacity. There is no evidence that long-term exercise therapy will improve pulmonary function in these patients. A few studies have been performed in which children with cystic fibrosis participated in general endurance activities over a period of a few months. In some the endurance training resulted in an increase in work capacity with proportionate increase in peak ventilatory capacity (22,23). It is suggested that because acute exercise increases sputum expectoration in many patients, repeated daily exercise training may complement postural drainage in their treatment. Although the long-term effects of endurance training on the prognosis in children is unknown, two areas warrant further exploration. There is considerable variation in severity of the pulmonary pathology in the early phases of the disease. Exercise programs directed toward achieving and maintaining cardiovascular fitness should be developed at early and milder stages. Good nutrition and muscle mass concur with more favorable courses in cystic fibrosis. Therefore, another area to be explored is the possible advantages of isometrics or weight training programs directed toward improving strength of upper body muscles and, in particular, accessory muscles of respiration. Intense exercise programs must be used with extreme caution in patients with cystic fibrosis. However, regular moderate exercise should be encouraged for its potential to slow the progression of degenerative processes.

IV. CARDIAC DISEASE

Children with structural cardiac lesions must be evaluated on an individual basis to determine those who should be encouraged to exercise and those who should be restricted from exercise.

In general, a large portion of children with congenital heart defects are able to participate in exercise activity; however, a majority will not be able to achieve levels of cardiovascular endurance of normal children. Cummings (9) has studied exercise endurance by treadmill testing in children with cardiac lesions. A striking observation of this study was the variability of exercise endurance in children with significant shunts. Children with ventricular septal defects, atrial septal defects, and patient ductus arteriosus generally had better exercise capacity. Children with tetralogy of Fallot, severe valvular disease, and cyanotic heart disease were most impaired in their exercise capacity. Cummings has postulated that the healthy myocardium of the young child with a structural cardiac lesion has some capacity to compensate for the extra cardiac work load required during exercise. In some cases, the burden of the mechanical defect may lessen with exercise. In case of aortic regurgitation the reguritant fraction lessens with an increased heart rate occurring with exercise (26). Some patients with atrial septal defect have a reduction in the left to right shunt during exercise (11).

Other studies have demonstrated that patients who have had surgical correction of their cardiac defects and have achieved normal resting hemodynamics may continue to have impaired exercise capacity (16). These studies have been performed in older individuals and it is not clear whether the exercise impairment is related to intrinsic cardiac impairment or whether it is due to lack of cardiovascular conditioning.

With some cardiac lesions strenuous exercise may be dangerous and should be restricted. This group of lesions consist of those with a high risk for lethal arrhythmias. Children with idiopathic hypertrophic subaortic stenosis have a high risk for sudden death (29). Also, children with severe aortic stenosis and high gradient are at risk for severe arrhythmias (32) as are children with tetralogy of Fallot and right bundle branch block (30). Another group of concern is patients who develop syncope with exercise. Such individuals may develop dangerous tachycardias and should receive careful cardiac evaluation before they are allowed to engage in strenuous exercise (4).

The role of the physician in the area of cardiac lesions of childhood is twofold: (1) to develop appropriate exercise programs for children with identified lesions, and (2) to identify those children engaging in sports programs who have as yet undetected lesions.

Relative levels of physical activity and noncompetitive exercise may be encouraged in most children unless symptomatic or cyanotic. Conditions in which strenuous exercise should be restricted are severe valvular lesions including mitral stenosis, aortic stenosis, and idiopathic hypertrophic subaortic stenosis. Other cardiac lesions in which exercise must be limited are active myocarditis, pulmonary hypertension, and conditions with significant arrhythmias (32).

Guidelines for cardiac screening of children participating in school sports programs have been published by Schell (31). These guidelines provide screening measures to identify children who warrant a cardiac evaluation prior to participation in strenuous sports. In addition to resting tachycardia, significant cardiac murmurs, or elevated blood pressure, any child with symptoms of syncope, chest pain, or palpation with physical exertion should be evaluated before encouraging vigorous exercise.

Children with identified cardiac lesions may be limited in their capacity to engage in strenuous or competitive sports. However, in many cases exercise programs may be developed which will enable them to improve their fittness level and, more importantly, enjoy the physical activity.

V. HYPERTENSION

Hypertension is a recognizable entity in childhood as well as adulthood. Standards are now available for normal and abnormal blood pressure of children and adolescents (33). Young children with significant blood pressure elevation generally will have some underlying cause of their hypertension. These children warrant careful clinical evaluations to identify the cause of the hypertension which will then direct treatment of the cause and control of the blood pressure. In adolescents essential hypertension may be diagnosed with greater frequency (25).

The hemodynamic response to exercise in hypertensive juveniles is similar to that of adult hypertensives. With progressive exercise systolic blood pressure and heart rate rise until peak exercise effort is achieved in both normotensive and hypertensive. However, hypertensive juveniles will have higher systolic blood pressure and heart rate at each exercise level. During aerobic exercise diastolic pressure remains stable or decreases in both normotensive and hypertensive adolescents (17). During isometric exercise, the diastolic pressure increases (21). However, whether this response to isometric exercise is detrimental in young hypertensives is as yet undetermined.

When identified, hypertension in juveniles should be monitored for consistency. If the blood pressure elevation is persistent, the youngster should be evaluated for secondary causes and also for evidence of target organ injury of the hypertension itself. In cases of essential hypertension, endurance types of exercise should be encour aged. The reasons for such recommendations are the secondary benefits of aerobic endurance types of exercise such as decrease in resting heart rate, improved cardiovascular fittness, and weight control. Those hypertensive adolescents who wish to engage in strenuous weight training programs should be monitored closely to determine if the intense isometric exercises have an adverse effect on the diastolic blood pressure.

VI. OBESITY

A very common childhood disorder in which exercise may be directly therapeutic is obesity. Obesity is due to an imbalance between caloric intake and energy expenditure. In childhood the balance of energy intake and expenditure must also adapt to normal growth and developmental processes. Energy expenditure includes the basal metabolic and physiological processes and voluntary work. Exercise then is a major voluntary form of energy expenditure. The issue of aerobic exercise and body weight has been extensively reviewed by Epstein and Wing (15). These authors demonstrate that exercise has a positive benefit or weight reduction and weight control although the weight loss from exercise alone may be small.

The overall problem in childhood obesity is that of instituting permanent behavior or life-style changes. In addition to inappropriate caloric intake obese children are more sedentary. Activity levels of thin and obese girls were compared during camp activities such as volley ball, tennis, or swimming by Bullen et al. (5). Their results reliably showed that obese girls were less active during the same activities compared to thin girls.

Inducing variations in activity level are thought by some to have an effect beyond increasing caloric expenditure. Mayer *et al.* (27) have hypothesized a relationship among activity, caloric intake, and weight which suggests that increases in caloric expenditure in sedentary obese persons may also result in decreases of food intake. This hypothesis has been supported by Epstein *et al.* (13,14) in their work in obese children. Obese children decreased their caloric intake as much following prelunch exercise as during diet (14). They also demonstrated that the amount of exercise change was inversely related to the decrease in caloric intake. Obese children with the greatest increase in expenditure showed the greatest decrease in intake (13). Therefore, there is evidence that exercise in obese children not only increases energy expenditure but may also contribute to the achievement of decreases in caloric intake.

In addition to dietary counseling, an exercise program for obese children should be designed. Appropriate dietary patterns should be developed and reinforced. Exercise should be begun at a modest level which will not result in discouragement or injury. Aerobic exercises such as walking, biking, or swimming are recommended. As some weight reduction is achieved and improvement in the child's self-image develops the child should spontaneously move toward exercises involving more social interaction such as team or competitive sports. The necessary component in achieving weight reduction in children is motivation. Essential to maintaining any weight reduction is achieving permanent changes in behavior patterns including activity levels.

VII. SUMMARY

Normal children, especially girls, should be encouraged to participate in exercise or athletic programs. Most children with cardiovascular or respiratory disorders can also enjoy involvement in athletic activities to some degree. Any child considered for restriction from exercise activity should receive a medical evaluation to determine if exercise does incur a risk. The benefit of medical management and optimal development of physical capacity will then be achieved. The common problem of childhood obesity is an area in which exercise programs should be strongly encouraged.

REFERENCES

1. Alpert, B. S., Dover, E. V., Booker, D. L., Martin, A. M., and Strong, W. B. (1981). Blood pressure response to dynamic exercise in healthy children. Black vs white. *J. Pediatr.* **99,** 556–560.
2. Anderson, S. D., McEvoy, J. D. S., and Bianco, S. (1972). Changes in lung volumes and airway resistance after exercise in asthmatic subjects. *Am. Rev. Respir. Dis.* **106,** 30–37.

3. Benatar, S. R., and König, P. (1974). Maximal expiratory flow and lung volume changes associated with exercise induced asthma in children and the effect of breathing a low density gas mixture. *Clin. Sci. Mol. Med.* **46,** 317–329.
4. Bernuth, G., Long, D., and Hofstetter, R. (1977). Exercise induced tachyarrhythmic syncope with sinus brachycardia and normal QT interval at rest. *Z. Kardiol.* **66,** 55–60.
5. Bullen, B. A., Reed, R. B., and Mayer, J. (1964). Physical activity of obese and non-obese adolescent girls appraised by motion picture sampling. *Am. J. Clin. Nutr.* **14,** 211–223.
6. Cropp, G. J. A. (1975). Relative sensitivity of different pulmonary function tests in the evaluation of exercise induced asthma. *Pediatrics* **56,** 860–867.
7. Cropp, G. J. A. (1975). Grading time course, and incidence of exercise induced airway obstruction and hyperinflation in asthmatic children. *Pediatrics* **56,** 868–879.
8. Cropp, G. J. A. (1975). Exercise induced asthma. *Pediatr. Clin. North Am.* **22,** 63–76.
9. Cummings, G. R. (1978). Maximal exercise capacity of children with heart defects. *Am. J. Cardiol.* **42,** 613–619.
10. Cummings, G. R., Everatt, D., and Hastman, L. (1978). Bruce treadmill test in children: Normal values in a clinic population. *Am. J. Cardiol.* **41,** 69–75.
11. Davies, H., and Gazetopoulos, N. (1966). Hemodynamic changes on exercise in patients with left to right shunts. *Br. Heart J.* **28,** 579–589.
12. Eggleston, P. A. (1975). The cycloergometer as a system for studying exercise induced asthma. *Pediatrics* **56,** 899–903.
13. Epstein, L. H., Masek, B. J., and Marshall, W. R. (1978). The effects of pre-lunch exercise on lunch time caloric intake. *Behav. Ther.* **1,** 3–15.
14. Epstein, L. H., Masek, B. J., and Marshall, W. R. (1978). A nutritionally based school program for control of eating in obese children. *Behav. Ther.* **9,** 766–778.
15. Epstein, L. H., and Wing, R. R. (1980). Ahrobic exercise and weight. *Addict. Behav.* **5,** 371–388.
16. Epstein, S. E., Beiser, G. D., Goldstein, R. E., Rosing, D. R., Redwood, D. R., and Morrow, A. G. (1973). Hemodynamic abnormalities in response to mild and intense upright exercise following correction of ventricular septal defect in tetrology of Fallot. *Circulation* **47,** 1065–1075.
17. Falkner, B., and Lowenthal, D. T. (1980). Dynamic exercise response in hypertensive adolescents. *Int. J. Pediatr. Nephrol.* **1,** 161–165.
18. Fitch, D. D., and Godfrey, S. (1976). Asthma and athletic performance. *JAMA, J. Am. Med. Assoc.* **236,** 152–157.
19. Fitch, K. D. (1975) Comparative aspects of available exercise systems. *Pediatrics* **56,** 904–907.
20. Fitch, K. D. (1975). Exercised induced asthma and competitive athletics. *Pediatrics* **56,** 942–943.
21. Fixler, D. E., Laird, W. P., Browne, R., Fitzgerald, V., Wilson, S., and Vance, R. (1979). Response of hypertensive adolescents to dynamic and isometric exercise stress. *Pediatrics* **64,** 579–583.
22. German, K., Orenstein, D., and Horowitz, J. (1980). Changes in oxygenization during exercise in cystic fibrosis. *Med. Sci. Sports Exercise* **12,** 105 (abstr.).
23. Godfrey, S., and Mearns, M. (1971). Pulmonary function and response to exercise in cystic fibrosis. *Arch. Dis. Child.* **46,** 144–151.
24. Jones, R. S. (1966). Assessment of respiratory function in the asthmatic child. *Br. Med. J.* **2,** 972–975.
25. Kilcoyne, M. M., Richter, R. W., and Alsup, P. A. (1974). Adolescent hypertension and prevalence. *Circulation* **50,** 758–764.
26. Marshall, R. J., and Shepherd, J. T. (1968). "Cardiac Function in Health and Disease," Lippincott, Philadelphia, p. 286.

27. Mayer, S., Roy, P., and Mitra K. P. (1956). Relation between caloric intake, body weight, and physical work: Studies in an industrial male population in West Bengal. *Am. J. Clin. Nutri.* **4,** 169–175.
28. McNeil, R. S., Nairn, J. R., Miller, J. S., and Ingram, C. G. (1966). Exercise induced asthma. *Q. J. Med.* **35,** 55–67.
29. Orinius E. (1979). Prognosis in hypertrophic obstructive cardiomyopathy. *Acta. Med. Scand.* **206,** 289–292.
30. Quattlebaum, T. G., Varghese, J., and Neill, C. A. (1979). Sudden death among postoperative patients with tetrology of Fallot: A follow-up study of 243 patients for an average of twelve years. *Circulation* **54,** 289–293.
31. Schell, N. B. (1978). Cardiac evaluation of school sports participants. *N.Y. State J. Med.* **78,** 942–943.
32. Starek, P. J. K. (1982). Athletic performance in children with cardiovascular problems. *Physician Sportsmed.* **10,** 78–89.
33. Task Force on Blood Pressure Control in Children (1977). Report of the Task Force. *Pediatrics* **59,** Suppl., 797–820.

CHAPTER 9

Exercise in the Elderly

ALFRED A. BOVE

Cardiovascular Division,
and Department of
Physiology
Mayo Foundation
Rochester, Minnesota

Although there has been a trend toward increased physical activity in older individuals, the majority of elderly people do not exercise and indeed are often discouraged from participating in regular exercise. Although physical capacity is known to decline with age (1–3), it is unclear whether the loss of physical capacity is related to age or to the reduction in physical activity common in older individuals and to some extent caused by social factors that relegate physical activity and exercise to the younger population. Because of this continuing reduction in the amount of physical activity experienced by older individuals, there tends to be a deconditioning effect associated with age, not because of age itself, but because of the decline in physical activity as age progresses. These observations lead to the question whether the reduced state of physical conditioning associated with the elderly is a result of age, a result of deconditioning, or a combination of the two. Several studies have examined older athletes and found marked physiological differences in these individuals when they are compared to age-matched, nontrained persons (4–6). These findings again suggest that the decline in physical capacity with age can be minimized by continued physical training. Indeed some of the alterations in body structure and physiological responses considered to occur because of age appear to be altered or reduced in older individuals who remain in good physical condition. From these observations one would postulate that physical activity may be important for the elderly

173

Exercise Medicine: Physiological Principles
and Clinical Applications

to provide improved physical capacity, and improved function of tissue and organ systems. Thus, recommendations for exercise in the elderly should be provided when chronic or acute illness does not preclude such physical activity. This chapter reviews some of the changes in physiological responses known to occur with aging, and based on these concepts, provides some recommendations for exercise in the elderly.

I. CARDIOVASCULAR RESPONSES WITH AGING

It is generally accepted that systolic and diastolic blood pressure rise with age (2). Thus, the standard accepted range of normal blood pressures is known to increase slowly with age so that at age 70, for example, and acceptable high limit for normal systolic blood pressure would be higher than the acceptable high level of normal in a 20- to 30-year-old individual. Although diastolic pressure often rises with age, the alteration in diastolic pressure is not marked in normal individuals, and the finding of elevated diastolic pressure in elderly individuals should be considered evidence for hypertension. Blood pressure elevation in the elderly is due in part to alterations in the compliance or stiffness of the aorta. As the collagen and elastic tissues of arteries stiffen with age (7), aortic compliance falls and larger peaks in systolic pressure are transmitted through the aorta as the ventricle empties in systole. The effects of exercise on aortic compliance are not well documented. Clinical observations (8) and experimental studies (9) with exercise suggest that reduced aortic smooth muscle tone would occur following prolonged exercise training. The finding of reduced aortic strip tension following exercise found in experimental studies (9) also suggests that a continuous exercise program might reduce peripheral vascular resistance and increase aortic compliance, thus lowering blood pressure even in elderly subjects.

Peripheral vascular resistance is also known to increase with age. This increase may be caused by a reduction in skeletal muscle mass (10,11); however, this change is probably caused by multiple factors and is not necessarily related to long-standing hypertension. Since most of the systemic vascular resistance is produced by the vasculature of skeletal muscle, it is possible that the increase in peripheral vascular resistance found in elderly individuals is a result of combined increased hormonal sensitivity (12) and reduced muscle mass with partial loss of microvascular channels in the peripheral vascular bed. Studies in hypertensive populations suggest that peripheral vascular resistance is lowered with chronic endurance exercise (13,14). A program of endurance exercise training in elderly hypertensives reduces blood pressure because of changes in peripheral vascular resistance, and possibly changes in the vascular tone of the large distributing arteries. Blood pressure response to ácute exercise in older individuals is known to be altered by chronic endurance training (2,4,15); however, elderly individuals with apparently mild hypertension may develop marked elevation of blood pressure during acute exercise. If exercise produces a significant elevation of blood pressure (diastolic > 110; systolic > 210 mm Hg), it may be necessary to provide antihypertensive treatment prior to instituting an exercise program.

Cardiac performance in the elderly is also a topic of interest. Studies in experimental animals and in patients (16–19) indicate that a reduction in contractile performance of the myocardium occurs with age. This reduction is small and generally of minimal consequence; however, it can be detected in studies designed specifically to examine the contractile characteristics of the myocardium (20). Catecholamine responses in the elderly are enhanced (12,21); however, it is unclear whether catecholamine receptors in the elderly have the same sensitivity as receptors in younger age population (22). Some studies (12) have demonstrated increased blood catecholamine levels in response to exercise in the elderly, suggesting that the control system that stimulates the heart during exercise requires release of greater amounts of catecholamines to obtain a cardiac response appropriate for the exercise level. The myocardium in the elderly is also known to have increased stiffness (23,24). Thus, diastolic ventricular relaxation in the elderly is impaired, and high heart rates are presumably less well tolerated in the older age groups than in younger individuals. A well-known alteration in cardiac performance associated with age is the decline of maximum heart rate with age (3,25). A variety of graphical relationships and formulas (for example, maximum heart rate = 220 − age) have been provided for estimating the maximal heart rate response to standard diagnostic exercise stress tests and for development of exercise programs in the elderly. The cause for this alteration in heart rate response in the elderly is not clear; however, changes in autonomic tone or in the state of innervation of the heart through the autonomic system are possible reasons for this altered heart rate response (22). In addition to reduced maximal heart rate with aging, maximum oxygen uptake also declines with age beyond the late twenties (1,17,26). Reduction in maximum oxygen uptake with age may occur rapidly or slowly depending on the state of physical condition and the continuity of endurance training over many years. Thus, the decline of maximal oxygen uptake with age described from early studies was found to be associated with a state of poor physical conditioning, and a program of physical activity continuing over several decades has been found to reduce the decline of oxygen uptake originally thought to be age related (27,28). This information again provides evidence that alterations in physical work capacity, oxygen uptake, and other indices of physical capacity are not only age related, but are also due to inactivity or detraining. Loss of physical strength with age may also result from detraining (29). Because of the decline in maximal oxygen uptake with age, maximal work capacity is reduced in older individuals when compared to individuals in the third and fourth decades; similar changes occur in both male and female populations (30). The superimposition of chronic illness adds further to the decline of work performance in the elderly. Thus, in prescribing activities for the elderly which require physical exertion, one should consider this diminution in physical performance, since the elderly individual will experience a greater amount of physical stress when exercising at a given level in comparison to a younger individual, even when the state of physical training is approximately equivalent in the two individuals.

Other contributing factors for consideration of exercise in the elderly include age related alterations in the metabolic state (31). Older individuals may have more glucose intolerance that younger individuals (32), and appropriate nutrition in the older individual should be considered to avoid large swings in blood sugar associated either with meals or prolonged exercise. Other endocrine systems may be changed with age. The activity of the thyroid gland may be diminished and the elderly individual, therefore, will be less tolerant to alterations in temperature. Elderly persons are noted to have reduced basal metabolic rates when compared to younger individuals (11), and these differences in metabolism also should be considered when prescribing exercise programs for older individuals. This population may also have a reduced corticosteroid response to stress. In general elderly persons will not be able to withstand the prolonged exertion required in some team sports and long-distance events.

In addition to known cardiovascular, endocrine, metabolic, respiratory, and nervous system changes with age, connective tissue structure also changes. As age progresses, collagen polymerizes from a relatively soluble form to a relatively insoluble form which is stiffer than the younger nonpolymerized collagen (33). The changes in collagen structure results in increased stiffness of tendons, ligaments, and joints. Because of the increased stiffness, the elderly individual is more prone to injuries associated with excess stress on ligaments and tendons. Current data suggest that alterations in collagen structure cannot be avoided in the elderly. Thus, the known increase in stiffness of joints and tendons in the elderly must be taken into account when prescribing exercise programs. Careful attention to preexercise stretching activities should be emphasized in the elderly so that some compensation can be made for the elasticity changes and to avoid ligament or tendon injury. It is not clear at the present time whether the alterations in collagen stiffness that are usually associated with age can be slowed or reversed by long-term endurance exercise. Endurance exercise strengthens ligaments and tendons by stimulating growth of collagen, resulting in a greater mass of tissue in the ligament or tendon.

Another important consideration in dealing with the elderly for exercise is alterations in neurological function (21). Normally with age a slowing of certain central nervous system functions can be noted. There is a lengthening of reflex time, and somewhat less precise motor control when compared to younger individuals. Because of these changes, it is important to provide exercises that can be performed appropriately in the elderly and that do not generate excess frustration because of the inability to perform an exercise due to lack of specific motor skills or speed.

II. SPECIAL CONSIDERATIONS IN PRESCRIBING EXERCISE IN THE ELDERLY

When dealing with elderly normals or elderly patients who wish to exercise, physical capacity must be determined. Often, this evaluation will reveal that physical capacity is significantly reduced compared with individuals of younger age, although elderly individuals who have continuously exercised may have surprisingly good physical capacity. One should also consider the increased incidence of chronic disease. The elderly individual is more likely to have coronary disease, which may be undiagnosed. Pulmonary function may be reduced, there may be endocrine metabolic disorders either manifest or undiagnosed, renal function may be impaired, and blood flow to the central nervous system may be impaired because of arterial stenosis. Peripheral vascular disease also may be present in the elderly and should be searched for prior to providing exercise prescriptions. All of the alterations that occur in the elderly as part of the aging process, part of detraining, or as a result of chronic illness must be considered in prescribing exercise programs for the aged.

The reduced work capacity of older individuals requires lower level exercise programs for these persons. The general principle mentioned in previous chapters of testing the patient for exercise capacity using a standard exercise test, then designing an exercise prescription based on that test, is still valid. In exercise testing, elderly individuals in general do not achieve the same levels of exercise capacity found in younger individuals, and when chronic illnesses are present, exercise tolerance may be severely limited in comparison to younger individuals. However, it is unreasonable to reject out of hand a request by an elderly individual for advice concerning exercise. The elderly individual may tire more quickly from physical exertion, and exercise programs should provide for appropriate rest periods and not demand prolonged continuous exercise, which will lead to severe exaustion.

The known reduction in thermal tolerance (both hot and cold) also must be considered when designing exercise programs for the elderly. Exercise in extreme heat or cold is normally difficult for any individual, and in the elderly person who wishes to participate in an exercise program, exposure to extremes of temperature during exercise may result in severe hyper- or hypothermia following exercise. Prolonged outdoor exercise exposure such as long-distance running in cool temperatures is known to produce hypothermia in some individuals, and this response will be more evident in older individuals who exercise in the cold (see Chapter 10). Careful instructions concerning reduced work capacity and altered cardiovascular responses in extremes of temperature should be provided to the individual prior to the institution of exercise activities. By considering these factors, exercise prescriptions can be provided for the elderly in many climates, provided appropriate instructions are given for handling thermal alterations and for maintaining a work capacity that is within tolerable limits.

Chronic diseases known to be of higher incidence in the elderly present special problems when developing exercise programs. A significant and important problem in the elderly is the high incidence of cardiovascular disease. Alterations in the vascular system can affect flow to the brain, heart, kidneys, or skeletal muscle such as the legs. Many times these arterial obstructions are undetected and the high flow demands induced by exercise may result in inadequate oxygen supply and abnormal function of a tissue or organ. Because these disorders are higher in frequency in the elderly it is important to search carefully by physical examination, history, and appropriate laboratory studies to rule out the possibility of significant atherosclerosis. Of most importance is the presence of coronary atherosclerosis with proximal coronary artery obstruction which limits flow to the myocardium. Flow demands in the myocardium increase substantially with exercise, and in the presence of severe atherosclerosis with impaired blood flow, myocardial infarction, serious arrhythmias, or sudden death may follow. Avoidance of serious cardiac problems with exercise in the elderly can be achieved through appropriate screening evaluation (34), and an exercise stress test with electrocardiographic and blood pressure monitoring which identifies the capacity of the patient as well as the possibility of underlying coronary artery disease. The value of an exercise stress test in this population cannot be emphasized too greatly, and since this test provides both diagnostic screening for coronary disease, and the information needed to prescribe an exercise program, a study of this type is essential in elderly individuals prior to instituting exercise activity.

In most cases, well-controlled metabolic diseases will not seriously impair the exercise capacity at any age. Patients with insulin-dependent diabetes mellitus can exercise appropriately. In these patients, however, one should recall that exercise reduces insulin requirements. This change in response is also present in the elderly (see Chapter 15). Thus when prescribing exercise programs for elderly patients who are diabetic, the dependence on insulin and more rapid utilization of glucose should be taken into account.

Considerations of exercise training in the elderly must also take into account the alterations in bone and joint structure and strength to avoid musculoskeletal injury during exercise. The osteoporosis of the elderly can be a significant problem if a subject in an exercise program is injured and reduced bone strength leads to a fracture. As in all exercise prescriptions, poorly trained individuals beginning a program of endurance exercise should be instructed in the initial phase of exercise to avoid extremes, which are likely to result in injury to bones, joints, or tendons while these structures are relatively weak. As training procedes and ligaments and tendons strengthen, subjects can increase their physical activity to match the capacity of their cardiovascular systems. For individuals poorly conditioned and who have not exercised for long periods of time, the initial exercise can result in a significant musculoskeletal injury, which precludes further exercise for several months. In this case many individuals become discouraged and do not return to exercise activities because of fear of further injury. The occurrence of injuries can be reduced by careful evaluation of bones and joints for detection of previous abnormalities, and then careful monitoring of individual activities to prevent excess that would injure bones and joints not strengthened by continuous exercise.

In conclusion, it is not only reasonable but desirable for physicians dealing with the elderly to provide advice and encouragement for exercise programs in this population. Programs for the elderly require special considerations because of the reduced physical capacity and alterations in the neurological, cardiovascular, pulmonary, and endocrine systems which, in general, alter the type and intensity of exercise that the elderly person can withstand. The basic principle of exercise testing in a controlled environment with electrocardiographic and blood pressure monitoring is still valid, and guidelines for maximal heart rate response in the elderly are available for proper exercise testing (see Chapter 19). With a careful evaluation, an elderly individual can be given an appropriate exercise prescription and obtain significant benefit from a continuous program of exercise. In the initial period of this exercise program, however, the physician must be aware of the potential for injury to bones, joints, and muscles due to the sudden increase in physical activity and relative weakness of these structures which requires several weeks to months to strengthen in response to continuous exercise. Taking into account all of these variables, it is possible and desirable to provide exercise prescriptions to elderly individuals.

REFERENCES

1. Dehn, M. M., and Bruce, R. A. (1972). Longitudinal variations in maximal oxygen intake with age and activity. *J. Appl. Physiol.* **33,** 805–807.
2. Raven, P. B., and Mitchell, J. (1980). The effect of aging on the cardiovascular response to dynamic and static exercise. *In* "The Aging Heart" (M. L. Weisfeldt, ed.), pp. 269–296. Raven Press, New York.
3. Bruce, R. A., Fisher, L. D., Cooper, M. N., and Gey, G. O. (1974). Separation of effects of cardiovascular disease and age on ventricular function with maximal exercise. *Am. J. Cardiol.* **34,** 757–763.
4. Ordway, G. A., and Wekstein, D. R. (1979). The effect of age on selected cardiovascular responses to static (isometric) exercise. *Proc. Soc. Exp. Biol Med.* **161,** 189–192.
5. Currens, J. H., and White, P. D. (1961). Half a century of running: Clinical, physiological, and

autopsy findings in the case of Clarence De Mar ("Mr. Marathon"). *N. Engl. J. Med.* **265**, 988–993.

6. Cantwell, J. D., and Watt, E. W. (1974). Extreme cardiopulmonary fitness in old age. *Chest* **65**, 357–359.

7. Cox, R. H. (1977). Effects of age on the mechanical properties of rat carotid artery. *Am. J. Physiol.* **233**, H256–H263.

8. Pulik, G., and Frenkle, R. (1975). Sensitivity to catecholamines and histamine in the trained and untrained human organism. *Eur. J. Appl. Physiol.* **34**, 199–204.

9. Thorp, G. D. (1976). The effects of exercise training on blood pressure and aortic strip tension of normal and spontaneously hypertensive rats. *Fed. Proc., Fed. Am. Soc. Exp. Biol.* **35**, 796 (abstr.).

10. Sidney, K. H., Shephard, R. J., and Harrison, J. E. (1977). Endurance training and body composition in the elderly. *Am. J. Clin. Nutr.* **30**, 326–333.

11. Suominen, H., Heinkken, E., Liesen, H., Michel, D., and Hollmann, W. (1977). Effects of 8 weeks' endurance training on skeletal muscle metabolism in 56–70 year old sedentary men. *Eur. J. Appl. Physiol.* **37**, 173–180.

12. Palmer, G. J., Ziegler, M. G., and Lake, C. R. (1978). Response of norepinephrine and blood pressure to stress increases with age. *J. Gerontol.* **33**, 482–487.

13. Boyer, J. L., and Kasch, F. W. (1970). Exercise therapy in hypertensive men. *JAMA, J. Am. Med. Assoc.* **211**, 1668–1671.

14. Hansen, J. S., and Nedde, W. H. (1970). Preliminary observations on physical training for hypertensive males. *Circ. Res.* **26**, Suppl., 49–53.

15. Montgomery, D. L., and Ismail, A. H. (1977). The effect of a four-month physical fitness program on high- and low-fit groups matched for age. *J. Sports Med.* **17**, 327–333.

16. Gerstenblith, G., Lakatta, E. G., and Weisfeldt, M. L. (1976). Age changes in myocardial function and exercise response. *Prog. Cardiovasc. Dis.* **19**, 1–21.

17. Becklake, M. R., Frank, H., Dagenais, G. R. Ostiguy, G. L., and Guzman, C. A. (1965). Influence of age and sex on exercise cardiac output. *J. Appl. Physiol.* **20**, 938–947.

18. Yin, F. C. P., Spurgeon, H. A., Weisfeldt, M. L., and Lakatta, E. G. (1980). Mechanical properties of myocardium from hypertrophied rat hearts. *Circ. Res.* **46**, 292–300.

19. Dock, W. (1966). How some hearts age. *J. Am. Med. Assoc.* **195**, 148–150.

20. Mann, D. L., Mackler, P. T., and Bove, A. A. (1981). Reduced left ventricular contractile reserve in aged subjects. *Clin. Res.* **29**, 220A (abstr.).

21. Eisdorfer, C. (1980). Neurotransmitters and aging: Clinical correlates. *In* "Neural Regulatory Mechanisms During Aging" (R. C. Adelman *et al.*, eds.), pp. 53–69. Alan R. Liss, Inc., New York.

22. Lakatta, E. G. (1980). Age related alterations in the cardiovascular response to adrenergic mediated stress. *Fed. Proc., Fed. Am. Soc. Exp. Biol.* **39**, 3173–3177.

23. Weisfeldt, M. (1981). Left ventricular function. *In* "The Aging Heart" (M. L. Weisfeldt, ed.), pp. 297–316. Raven Press, New York.

24. Templeton, G. H. Platt, M. R. Willerson, J. T., and Weisfeldt, M. L. (1979). Influence of aging on left ventricular hemodynamics and stiffness in beagles. *Circ. Res.* **44**, 189–194.

25. Sidney, K. H., and Shephard, R. J. (1977). Maximal and submaximal exercise tests in men and women in the seventh, eighth, and ninth decades of life. *J. Appl. Physiol.* **43**, 280–287.

26. Saltin, B., and Grimby, G. (1968). Physiological analysis of middle-aged and old former athletes. *Circulation* **38**, 1104–1114.

27. Montoye, H. J., Block, W. D., and Gayle, R. (1978). Maximal oxygen uptake and blood lipids. *J. Chronic Dis.* **31**, 111–118.

28. DeVries, H. A. (1970). Physiologic effects of an exercise training regimen upon men aged 52 to 88. *J. Gerontol.* **25**, 325–336.

29. Petrofsky, J. S., and Lind, A. R. (1975). Aging, isometric strength and endurance, and cardiovascular responses to static effort. *J. Appl. Physiol.* **38,** 91–95.
30. Petrofsky, J. S., Burse, R. L., and Lind, A. R. (1975). Comparison of physiological responses of men and women to isometric exercise. *J. Appl. Physiol.* **38,** 863–868.
31. Sartin, J., Chaudituri, M., Obenrader, M., and Adelman, R. C. (1980). The role of hormones in changing adaptive mechanisms during aging. *Fed. Proc., Fed. Am. Soc. Exp. Biol.* **39,** 3163–3167.
32. Montoye, H. J. Block, W. D., Metzner, H., and Keller, J. B. (1977). Habitual physical activity and glucose tolerance. *Diabetes* **26,** 172–176.
33. Versar, F. (1964). Aging of the collagen fiber. *Int. Rev. Connect. Tissue. Res.* **2,** 243–300.
34. Camm, A. J. Evans, K. E., Ward, D. E., and Martin, A. (1980). The rhythm of the heart in active elderly subjects. *Am. Heart J.* **99,** 598–603.

III

Medical Aspects of Sports and Exercise

CHAPTER 10

Neurology of Sports and Exercise

OTTO APPENZELLER
*Departments of Neurology
and Medicine
University of New Mexico
School of Medicine
Albuquerque, New Mexico*

RUTH ATKINSON
*Departments of Neurology
and Pediatrics
University of New Mexico
School of Medicine
Albuquerque, New Mexico*

Exercise Medicine: Physiological Principles
and Clinical Applications

I. INTRODUCTION

Although the adaptation of the human body to endurance training and athletic activity is better understood from recent studies, there are still large gaps in our knowledge of the effect of physical activity on the normal and diseased nervous system. For example, the effect of vigorous exercise on cerebral oxygen consumption is controversial (11). One study suggests that this is increased; others found it unchanged. Brain glucose utilization also seems unaffected by exercise. Animal studies indicate that brain stem and hypothalamic monoamines decrease with acute exertion and serotonin increases in the same area. The net result of these changes is not known. Positron emission tomography (PET) of the human brain will undoubtedly provide useful insights into brain metabolism and neurotransmitter physiology and perhaps will elucidate focal alterations produced by exercise. Moreover, various manipulations of athletic performance may become correlated with changes in PET scans.

It is known that cerebral blood flow and metabolism may change focally in response to motor or sensory activation, but blood flow to the whole brain does not change with exercise. Thorough studies of cerebral blood flow in endurance-trained persons or the effect of exercise at altitude on cerebral blood flow have not been published.

Repetitive stimuli in the peripheral and, perhaps, central nervous system alter function of the nerves and brain. It is controversial whether the repetitive stimulation of prolonged exertion affects central or peripheral nervous system function. Moreover, the question of exertional fatigue in normal individuals remains unresolved. Although it is generally assumed that fatigue originates in muscles, it is clear that the central nervous system plays an important role in this area since incentive, stress, temperature, and other psychological factors affect fatigue. Perceived exertion correlates closely with heart rate and peripheral lactate accumulation. It is even more exciting that the only individuals who were unable to rate their degree of exertion appropriately were severely depressed or schizophrenic. Measurements of brain and peripheral nerve electrical activity suggest that function is unaffected by fatigue. Visual evoked responses, somatosensory evoked responses, brainstem auditory evoked responses, and peripheral nerve conduction velocities usually are unchanged after prolonged exertion. The autonomic nervous system is important in adaptation to exercise stress. Parasympathetic overactivity leads to the bradycardia of endurance-trained subjects, and blockade of the sympathetic nervous system causes impaired exertional performance. Moreover, mobilization of free fatty acids, glycogen utilization, and catecholamine secretion are important in the physiological adaptation to exertion.

Telemetric electroencephalographic recordings during exercise show an influence on α rhythm. The amount of α activity in the EEG is usually related to alertness, and α "reactivity" (blocking of α rhythms by attention, eye opening, and mental activity) is also influenced by exertion. In epileptics, the interictal epileptiform activity is markedly decreased with exercise and fatigue, and inactivity has the opposite effect. The influence of exercise on sleep stages is controversial primarily because of the diversity of the subjects studied. In endurance-trained individuals, deep sleep seems to be increased after a marathon. Altitude and exertion also influence sleep stages depending on the subject's level of training, the duration of altitude exposure, the degree of exertion, and sex. In general, endurance-trained individuals and altitude-acclimated persons have more deep sleep after exertion at altitude than those who are less adapted to these stresses.

Intellectual performance is decreased by fatigue, but endurance training in disturbed children improves behavior. Exercised subjects may perform better on specific cognitive tests. In these studies only relatively mild exercise was used. The effects of more strenuous endurance events on intellectual function have not been fully investigated. Academic achievement improves with sustained endurance training, but whether this results from the training itself or the personality traits that contribute to the initiation and maintenance of a conditioning program is not clear. Endurance-trained subjects are self-sufficient, intelligent, sober, shy, imaginative, and reserved. This might account for the suggestion that psychological aging is slowed by a higher level of physical training if it is maintained. The effect of other factors on intellectual function, such as dietary modification, frequently practiced by exercising individuals, has not been excluded.

Nothing is known of the nervous system's role in the acquisition of athletic skills and selection of athletic disciplines. Unquestionably, training influences establishment of appropriate motor and sensory circuits and causes adaptation of muscle fibers' contractile properties for specific events. Learning undoubtedly plays a major role in development of skills and proceeds through adaptation of proper circuitry in the central and peripheral nervous system. However, genetic factors are important in achieving excellence in certain sports because of the advantage offered by body size, limb length, and weight. Thus, certain racial groups are particularly suited to some sports whereas others excel in entirely different disciplines. Whether a less obvious genetically determined nervous system role exists that makes it advantageous for persons to pursue certain athletic disciplines is not known. Could specific synapses in one or other hemisphere make it easier for an individual to excel in track and field, swimming, tennis, or other sports, as it is easier for some individuals to acquire language skills?

II. PHYSICAL ACTIVITY AND NERVOUS SYSTEM AGING

Athletic participation by age groups has led to eager anticipation of entry in the next older bracket by weekend competitors in the hope that performance will not decline but will, even if static, be comparatively better than in the just departed 5-year segment. The anticipation of competing in an older age bracket and performing better in comparison with other members of the group seems to remove the sense of passing time and the sadness of old age. The common flattery addressed to elderly joggers (you look wonderful) motivates those who frequent our parks and promenades. It also encourages the old to exercise regularly.

All measurable functions of the nervous system deteriorate with age, e.g., visual evoked responses, brainstem auditory evoked responses, somatosensory evoked responses, and peripheral nerve conduction velocities. Investigations of endurance-trained elderly individuals showed shortened visual evoked response times and faster peripheral nerve conduction velocities, but these may have been related to the increased body temperatures of the subjects at the time of the tests. Many more studies are necessary to fully appreciate the effect of training on nervous system aging. For example, temperature regulation or the capacity to maintain constant body temperatures with cold exposure and with excessive heat loads deteriorates with advancing years. This has not been studied in age-matched, endurance-trained individuals. Similarly, baroreceptor function progressively fails in old age, but endurance exercise effects on this autonomic nervous system activity have not been studied. Coordination, which can now be measured with posturography, has also not been evaluated. It is, nevertheless, remarkable that when world marathon records are considered between the ages of 30 and 70, only 1% deterioration in performance occurs per decade. This, of course, refers to record times in various age groups, but must depend, among many other things, also on adaptation of the nervous system to stress and its relative preservation by endurance training.

III. TEMPERATURE REGULATION

The thermoregulatory system has appeared on the evolutionary scene relatively recently and has been investigated in detail. Since physical activity stresses thermoregulation, the effects of excessive heat loads, either environmental or from physical activity, have been studied. Since many sporting activities are performed in inclement weather, hypothermia has been investigated also.

Debate exists about how the thermoregulatory system works and on the nature of its regulation or set point on which temperature homeostasis is based. Evidence indicates that thermosensitive neurons in the anterior and preoptic hypothalamus respond to blood temperature changes. These same neurons are also activated by impulses from the periphery and cervical spinal cord. Several systems are involved in implementing appropriate heat loss or preservation. Behavioral changes are also important in thermoregulation and include use of climate adjusted apparel.

A. Exercise and Temperature Regulation

A number of organs share the demand for increased blood supply during physical activity. Importantly, the heart must supply adequate blood to its own contracting muscle, to the contracting skeletal muscles, and to the skin for transfer of excessive heat. In thermally neutral conditions, the oxygen uptake during exercise is directly proportional to cardiac output, which is then reflected in blood flow to muscles. Cutaneous blood flow, on the other hand, is largely determined by body temperature. Nevertheless, if cardiac output is insufficient to satisfy the demands of muscle and hypotension occurs, then skin vessels constrict reflexly. This may interfere with heat dissipation during prolonged exercise.

At the onset of exercise, metabolic heat increases at a rate directly proportional to the exercise intensity, and far in excess of the body's capacity to dissipate it. Because of this imbalance, body temperature rises until heat loss predominantly through the skin by increased blood flow and sweating equals the heat produced.

When a new balance is reached, a new set point at a higher internal body temperature occurs and is maintained until heat loads again change the set point upward or a decreased work load lowers body temperature. Skin temperature is closely related to environmental temperature and the circulatory demands of muscles and skin are determined not only by the body temperature, but also by the average skin temperature. Strenuous exercise in high ambient temperatures increases the circulatory demands considerably. In this circumstance, the heart must provide sufficient blood flow to muscles and skin or compromise delivery to one or the other. If exercise is so intense that the contracting muscles demand a disproportionately large part of the cardiac output, blood is shifted away from the skin. This limits heat dissipation from the body core to the skin and heat loss by convection and radiation. In turn, the rise in body temperature limits exercise capacity. If, on the other hand, an adequate skin blood flow is ensured at the expense of contracting muscles, the muscles must work under anaerobic conditions and synthesis of adenosine triphosphate (ATP) is decreased along with the ability for continued muscle activity. To allow proper distribution of the cardiac output to tissues crucial for successful physical activity in hot environments, the splanchnic blood flow is progressively reduced. In extremes of exercise and heat, the body is unable to maintain adequate circulation to both skin and muscle and hyperthermia with heatstroke may result (2).

Other complicating features of the circulation during exercise in the heat include increased venous volume in the skin. This, in part, results from vasodilatation of skin veins because of high compliance and reduced tone. It helps to transfer additional heat because of cutaneous decreased flow velocity and increased time for heat exchange. The increased peripheral blood volume, however, reduces central volume and compromises cardiac stroke volume. In order to maintain cardiac output under these circumstances, the heart rate must increase. Loss of plasma water to the extravascular compartment compromises central blood volume under these conditions. Significant fluid losses from the intravascular compartment occur even during short periods of exercise because of relative hyperosmolality of contracting muscle cells and transcapillary movement of fluid. Nevertheless, the absolute fluid loss from the intravascular compartment is more closely related to exercise intensity than to ambient temperature. Another factor depleting central blood volume and reducing cardiac output is body fluid loss through sweating directly related to ambient temperature and exercise intensity. Sweat rates may exceed 1–1½ liters/hour during exertion in a hot environment. Eventually, reduced central blood volume compromises cardiac filling and stroke volume, and tissue perfusion for a given level of exertion is inadequate. When systemic blood pressure falls, cardiac output becomes more dependent on heart rate, which is controlled by baroreceptor reflexes. At very high heart rates and shortened cardiac filling times, cardiac output cannot be maintained. Failure of brain perfusion then leads to syncope.

During exercise in the heat when near maximal heart rate for age occurs and cardiac output is falling due to reduced filling pressure, cutaneous vessels constrict in spite of the firmly established heat load mediated vasodilator drive. This compromises the already marginal heat transfer from the core to the surface resulting in further heat storage. It, nevertheless, helps maintain arterial blood pressure, cardiac filling, and thus, indirectly, the capacity of muscles to continue to contract. Vasoconstriction during decreasing systemic blood pressure is activated by baroreflexes, which override the thermoregulatory activity. Thus, if ambient temperatures and exercise are moderate, the cardiac output can be above that found with similar exercise under cool conditions. However, with heavy exercise in the heat, it is difficult to further increase cardiac output because heart rates are already near their maximum and stroke volume is therefore limited. Under such conditions, the cardiac output is maintained just as under cooler ambient temperatures, but this can only be achieved by relative cutaneous vasoconstriction, and this, in turn, leads to further heat storage.

B. Thermoregulation and Hydration

Dehydration affects body temperature both at rest and during exercise. Under experimental conditions, dehydrated subjects have a higher body temperature for a given intensity of work than the same subjects when properly hydrated. Sweating and forearm blood flow (muscle blood flow) are reduced in dehydrated subjects, changes that are attributed to a higher internal body temperature and impaired temperature regulation. The impaired cardiac output during exercise and dehydration depends, at least in part, on the initial blood volume. Exercise with a high initial blood volume lessens the exercise-induced fall in plasma volume and therefore decreases the circulatory strain. Circulatory adjustments are necessary if physical activity is to continue in hypovolemic (dehydrated) subjects. Studies on volunteers show that heat transfer through the cutaneous circulatory bed is as responsive per unit of central temperature change in hypovolemic as in normovolemic subjects. However, the vasoconstrictor influence superimposed on heat-induced cutaneous vasodilatation occurs at very much lower blood flows during dehydration. Consequences of dehydration are an increased central temperature threshold for vasodilation and a relative vasoconstriction at higher internal temperature in hypovolemic individuals. This, in turn, causes a much greater elevation in body temperature in such subjects than in those who exercise well hydrated even though the total heat production is the same (3).

During extremes of heat and dehydration, compromises in cutaneous circulation and thermoregulation occur. Increased body temperature due to the increased metabolism of exerising muscles is perceived in the central nervous system where a temperature threshold for cutaneous vasodilation exists, allowing for increased blood flow proportional to the increased temperature. When skin blood flow is high, venous return and cardiac filling are reduced. The fluid loss from the vasculature during exercise also decreases plasma volume and cardiac filling. At that point, cutaneous vasoconstriction redirects some of the blood back to the heart, and heat transfer from the core to the surface is reduced. If cardiac filling improves sufficiently, cutaneous vasoconstriction is immediately abolished and the core-to-skin transfer of heat again improves. However, if the decreased heat transfer during cutaneous vaso- constriction leads to a progressive increase in body temperature, heatstroke may occur.

C. Physical Fitness

Heat acclimatization improves performance in both fit and unfit subjects. Heart rates and rectal temperatures are lower in acclimatized than in nonacclimatized individuals for a given amount of work. Moreover, there is also better cardiovascular function in the heat in endurance-trained individuals than in those who are not endurance trained. In unacclimatized subjects, skin temperatures are very much higher than in acclimatized individuals although sweat evaporative rates do not differ in the two groups, implying that unacclimatized persons have greater cutaneous blood flows for a given heat and work load. This, of course, is a disadvantage since it causes an increase in heart rate, a lower stroke volume, and greater difficulties in maintaining cardiac output. Endurance training does not increase sweating, but endurance-trained individuals sweat at lower central temperatures and continuous aerobic activity enhances sweating sensitivity. Heat acclimatization of both fit and unfit subjects is associated with lower central temperatures for a given amount of work in hot ambient conditions. A smaller fraction of the cardiac output, therefore, need go to the skin to maintain normal central temperature. Heat acclimatization, therefore, decreases work strain in hot environments and endurance training offers an added advantage particularly when long-duration, high metabolic and external heat loads are present. Heat- and exercise-acclimatized individuals are capable of dissipating thermal loads more efficiently, decreasing peripheral circulatory demands and resulting in better cardiovascular and skeletal muscle performance.

D. Acclimatization

Heat acclimatization results in 10–25% expansion of plasma volume and isotonic expansion of the interstitial fluid. Close correlations exist between increased plasma volume and thermoregulatory and cardiovascular adaptation to heat and performance. Increased plasma volume enhances physical performance in hot conditions by decreasing core body temperature. Endurance training also increases blood volume mainly through its effect on plasma volume. Hypervolemia found in acclimatized and endurance-trained individuals is associated with decreased heart rate, increased stroke volume during both rest and exercise, and reduced hematocrit. All these are conducive to an increased maximum oxygen uptake and maximum cardiac output. Close similarities, therefore, exist between adaptive thermoregulatory responses to a hot environment and those that occur with exercise training. These are an increased sweat rate, decreased heat storage, and decreased core temperature for given work loads. Adaptive plasma volume expansion diminishes significantly within a week when heat or exercise stress no longer exists.

Heat acclimatization and endurance training are also associated with hyperproteinemia. The cause of this is not understood, and the relationship of the hyperproteinemia, the plasma electrolyte, osmotic, and endocrine responses to the hypervolemia associated with exercise alone or with heat exposure are very complex. The angiotensin and vasopressin increase during exercise is larger than during heat exposure alone. Hyperosmolality associated with prolonged exercise appears to be the main stimulus for angiotensin and vasopressin release and the hypervolemia is a secondary stimulus. During exercise, plasma renin also increases, but the vasopressin release during exertion does not stimulate a further increase in plasma renin implying that renin levels are already optimally high to produce maximum sodium retention and protect against stress-associated plasma volume losses. During heat acclimatization or endurance training, elevated plasma renin enhances sodium retention, which, in turn, increases plasma osmolality and vasopressin and thus promotes fluid retention. Whether sufficient stimuli are left after intermittent exposure to stress to account for the well-documented progressive chronic hypervolemia of endurance training, heat acclimatization, or both is not clear. It is, however, assumed that the depletion of intracellular fluid is the main stimulus for the chronic hypervolemia and not the depletion of extracellular fluid volume which occurs in either heat acclimatized or endurance-trained individuals.

It is important to advise those who embark on endurance training, heat acclimatization, or both not to rely on thirst alone as a stimulus to fluid intake. Thirst is an unreliable indicator of dehydration under conditions of stress. One complication of dehydration is urinary tract infection in the male runner who attempts to acclimatize to heat for competition in hot environments. Such an individual may never have had a urinary tract infection previously and does not require extensive studies to exclude mechanical obstruction or other abnormalities. He needs treatment for the acute infection and advice concerning fluid intake. A practical yardstick that can be given the patient is that his urine should always be almost the color of water (colorless). If that is the case, then hydration is adequate.

E. Temperature Regulation during Long-Distance Events

Thermoregulatory responses during events lasting more than 20 minutes have been studied and athletic performance depends, to a great extent, on the capacity to lose the excess metabolic heat produced during long exertion. In these circumstances, as in situations discussed previously, heat transfer from the body core to the surface and its dissipation through sweating, convection, and radiation are important. Anything that reduces cutaneous blood flow or decreases sweat evaporation lessens the efficiency of temperature regulation and increases the risk of overheating and cardiovascular collapse. Core temperatures in marathoners, for example, may reach 40°C or higher even in cool weather, but these are well tolerated in trained persons. During long distance events, the body temperature depends on the metabolic rate, which in turn, is affected by work load and body weight. Heavier athletes have higher rectal temperatures than lighter competitors even when performing at the same pace. In order to prevent excessive body temperatures, large sweat losses occur and athletes with inadequate hydration prior to competition have inordinate rises in body temperature, thus limiting performance and increasing the risk of heat illness. In animals during high speed running, heat production may increase to 60 times above resting values. Such animals do not continue to run, unlike humans, if their central temperature reaches a certain level. The distance over which animals can pursue prey is limited only by the rise in body temperature which is dependent on the weight and speed of the predator. Humans, on the other hand, continue physical work in spite of high body temperature and risk serious consequences. Therefore, careful monitoring of ambient conditions, hydration, acclimatization, and conditioning of athletes is imperative to avoid disasters due to overheating.

F. Heat Illness

Four sports-related conditions in which body temperature is elevated include heat stroke, heat hyperpyrexia, anhidrotic heat exhaustion, and acute anhidrotic heat exhaustion. Heat stroke is associated with high body temperature, impaired consciousness, delirium, and convulsions. Heat hyperpyrexia is a condition in which body temperature is above 41°C, but the other features of heat stroke are not present. This occurs in well-trained and heat-acclimated subjects during marathon competition. Anhidrotic heat exhaustion or absence of sweating because of sweat gland abnormalities causes abnormally high body temperatures and is always associated with mild infection and a hot and humid environment. The presence of a mild upper respiratory tract infection, even in well-trained and heat-acclimated athletes, should be an indication to ban them from serious competition because of this danger. In this setting, the first symptom of infection may be a failure of sweating, inappropriate for the hot ambient temperatures. The fever accompanying such infection may not be heralded by the usual chill and rigor, but rather by dry, hot skin. The subject may notice sudden absence of sweating, headache, anorexia, confusion, and mild ataxia with exertion. Prompt cooling and cessation of physical activity are imperative. Sweating usually returns in a day or two with recovery from the infection.

G. Heat Stroke

Rectal temperatures of 41–43°C associated with disturbed consciousness are classified under this heading. Mortality from heat stroke ranges from 50 to 70%. The situation is not limited to athletic events, but can occur during excessive summer heat and even in individuals performing accustomed physical labor. Preventive measures, in general, include education of those at risk. Athletes should avoid excessive heat loads by limiting physical activity, particularly if they are not heat acclimatized. Hydration and adequate, but not excessive, salt intake during physical work are important. Heat stroke is not confined to healthy young athletes or military recruits in training, but occurs also in the elderly during heat waves. A variety of drugs, including phenothiazines, anticholinergics, sedatives, and diuretics predispose to excessive heat storage by interfering with heat dissipation.

1. SYMPTOMS AND SIGNS OF HEAT STROKE

Heat stroke is a medical emergency and delay in diagnosis and treatment results in irreversible damage or death. It should be suspected in persons whose mental state changes during heat stress. Diagnostic criteria include, but are not limited to, high environmental temperature and humidity, high rectal temperature, and sometimes, though not always hot, dry skin. Cardiovascular and central nervous system abnormalities progress to clouded consciousness and circulatory collapse.

In heat stroke associated with exercise, the changes in cardiovascular function are those that usually occur during adaptation to heat with exercise. There is, therefore, increased heart rate and cardiac output and decreased systemic vascular resistance. Effector organs respond appropriately to increase heat dissipation. The hemodynamic changes of impending heat stroke in persons in whom exercise results in excessive circulatory loads are indistinguishable from those in well-acclimatized endurance athletes during long competition. In contrast, however, elderly subjects suffering from heat stroke unaccompanied by exertion have a decreased cardiac output, an increased peripheral resistance, and striking skin dryness.

Hypovolemia is invariable in heat stroke associated with exercise and also in disease-related heat stroke. Administration of large amounts of intravenous fluid does not, even in the elderly, seem to result in pulmonary circulatory overload, perhaps because of an inappropriately low cardiac output in such individuals.

Hyperventilation occurs with extreme heat and in heat stroke respiratory alkalosis is the rule. Because of the hypovolemia and hypotension, the increased metabolic demands of the tissues generated by the high temperature cannot be met and lactic acidosis also occurs in those not actively exercising at the time of the collapse. Blood gas values must be adjusted for the elevated body temperature so that the patient's true metabolic state can be appropriately assessed and treated. Hypokalemia, hypocalcemia, and hypophosphatemia are common. Rhabdomyolysis can occur in exercise-induced heat stroke, but is uncommon in patients with hyperthermia not associated with exertion. Hypoglycemia is a feature of exertion-induced heat stroke, but hyperglycemia is the rule in the elderly with non-exercise-associated heat stroke.

Patients with heat stroke may lose consciousness or have a feeling of impending doom, headache, dizziness, confusion, and weakness. Rarely, euphoria precedes coma and agitated delirium may make it difficult to convince patients to withdraw from competition. If high body temperature has not persisted too long, cooling produces prompt return to consciousness. If the patient, however, remains unconscious for 24 hours or more and seizures occur, recovery is rarely complete and varying degrees of neurological deficit persist after the acute phase of the illness. The cerebellum is particularly vulnerable and cerebellar deficits may be permanent.

Physical examination shows a rapid pulse and wide pulse pressure. The electrocardiogram may have S-T segment depression and T wave changes often with supraventricular tachycardia. Eventually the cardiac output falls. Survival depends on an increase in cardiac output to meet the excessive circulatory demands. Blood flow is high in skin and muscles (a result of decreased vascular resistance), particularly in patients who were exercising prior to the heat stroke. Splanchnic blood flow, on the other hand, is reduced. Even when body temperature is restored to normal, the cardiac output remains high and the peripheral resistance low for hours, a condition similar to that seen after trauma or during severe infections. Myocardial injury and increased pulmonary vascular resistance may result in heart failure. Petechiae and often large hemorrhages occur together with consumptive coagulopathy. This has been attributed to heat-induced endothelial damage, which has been identified on electromicroscopy. Dehydration and electrolyte imablance tend to be severe in sports-associated cases, particularly in marathon runners. Therefore, acute renal tubular necrosis is relatively common (10–35% of cases) and is compounded by direct heat injury to renal tubules, circulating blood pigments, and reduced renal blood flow. Liver damage may be manifest by jaundice and, histologically, central lobular necrosis with extensive bile stasis. These findings are prominent in biopsies from gold miners who have had heat stroke. In such subjects, extreme heat exposure, severe exertion, and dehydration are usually present. Sometimes the reduced splanchnic blood flow is sufficient to cause intestinal mucosal ischemia and transient malabsorption problems after recovery.

2. TREATMENT OF HEAT STROKE

The two important aspects of treatment are cooling and support of vital functions. Clothing should be removed and the patient placed in an ice cold bath or cooling blanket. In the field, substitution of wet clothing and increased air circulation, together with shading from the sun, may be all that is available. Recent evidence from study of heat stroke victims during the pilgrimages to Mecca shows that water at skin temperature sprayed on the naked body together with increased air movement are more efficient than many other methods of cooling. The reason for this is probably that water at skin temperature does not cause cutaneous vasoconstriction and therefore does not impede heat transfer from the core to the surface. Massage of the extremities also promotes cooling because it combats cutaneous circulatory stasis. When the body temperature is near normal, cooling maneuvers should be stopped. Reflex shivering may be initiated by a precipitous drop in core temperature and should be counteracted by phenothiazines.

Support of vital functions includes correction of dehydration, hypovolemia, and acid–base disturbances to ensure adequate cardiac output and prevent cardiac failure. Fourteen hundred milliliters (or more if needed) of intravenous fluids may be given in the first hour. Urine output should be monitored and mannitol given if needed to promote adequate diuresis. If digitalis is required for congestive heart failure, one should keep in mind that respiratory alkalosis may predispose to digitalis toxicity. β-Adrenergic stimulation with isoproterenol may increase cardiac output. α-Adrenergic stimulation decreases skin perfusion and impedes heat exchange and is contraindicated in this setting. Oxygen may be helpful, though hypoxemia and shunting of blood through the lungs are not common. Disseminated intravascular coagulation should be treated with heparin (7500 units every 4 hours). If coma persists in spite of a normal body temperature and renal function, cerebral edema is almost surely present and use of dehydrating agents is indicated. Anticonvulsants should be used for seizure control. Most patients recover within a few hours if cooling and hydration are accomplished promptly and are maintained.

3. MARATHONS AND HEAT STROKE

The death of a competitor during a marathon race generates a great deal of publicity. Some deaths have been attributed erroneously to acute myocardial ischemia, when, in fact, they resulted from heat stroke. The explosive increase in marathon participation by older individuals, some of whom are inadequately prepared, makes these occurrences likely to be frequent. Therefore, the climatic and situational factors that contribute to heat stroke even in relatively cool ambient conditions must be kept in mind. These factors are

1. High running speed, particularly at the beginning of the race when large amounts of blood are shunted away from the skin and other organs to contracting muscles.
2. Higher body temperature, which normally accompanies strenuous muscular activity and leads to sweating.
3. High environmental temperatures, particularly when humidity is also high.
4. Windless conditions that decrease evaporative heat loss. In such a situation, there is further decrease in skin blood flow (therefore reduction in heat transfer) in order to maintain cardiac output for sustained muscular activity.
5. Normally high sweat rates contribute to dehydration.
6. Dehydration prevents maintenance of the cardiac output; skin blood flow falls further in order to provide adequate blood supply to the muscles.
7. Inadequate prerace acclimatization and hydration.

A vicious cycle is initiated by the falling cardiac output, decreased heat transfer from core to the surface, and increased sweating rates, all of which promote heat storage. Once the runner is dehydrated, progressive and rapid rise in body temperature results in collapse. The clouding of consciousness, ataxia, decreased sweat rate, and competitor's inability to gauge the seriousness of the situation places a great burden on the medical attendant to control an inexorably progressive situation, which leads to disaster if competition is not stopped.

H. Heat Stress and the Exercising Child

Exercising children do not adapt to high climatic heat as effectively as adults (5) because of greater surface area/mass ratio than adults which induces greater heat transfer between the environment and the body. Children produce more metabolic heat per mass unit than adults when walking or running and sweating capacity is not as great in children as in adults. The capacity to convey heat by blood from the body core to the skin is also reduced in the exercising child. These characteristics do not interfere with the exercising child's ability to dissipate heat in a neutral or mildly warm climate. However, when air temperature exceeds skin temperature, children have less tolerance to physical activity than do adults. The greater the temperature gradient between the air and the skin, the greater the effect on the child.

The rate of heat acclimatization to exercise is slower in children than in adults (5). Therefore, a child needs more exposure to the new climate to sufficiently acclimatize.

Children frequently do not drink enough liquids to replenish fluid loss during prolonged exercise and may become severely dehydrated (6) with the consequence of excessive increase in body temperature.

Obesity, febrile illness, cystic fibrosis, gastrointestinal infection, diabetes insipidus, diabetes mellitus, chronic heart failure, caloric malnutrition, anorexia nervosa, sweating insufficiency syndrome, and mental deficiency pose potentially greater risks of heat stress to children with these problems (10).

The Committee on Sports Medicine of the American Academy of Pediatrics (10) recommends that intensity of activities that last 30 minutes or more be reduced whenever relative humidity and air temperature are above critical levels. Exercise intensity and duration should be increased gradually over 10–14 days to accomplish heat acclimatization at the beginning of a strenuous exercise program or after traveling to a warmer climate. The child should be fully hydrated prior to prolonged physical activity, and should drink periodically (150 ml of cold tap water each 30 minutes for a child weighing 40 kg) during the activity. Clothing should be lightweight and limited to one layer of absorbent material to facilitate sweat evaporation.

I.   Hypothermia

Rectal temperature below 30.2°C is often associated with clouded consciousness, restless stupor, slurred speech, ataxia, and occasional involuntary movements. On examination, pallor, cyanosis, sometimes edema of the face, and slow cerebration with a croaky voice are reminiscent of hypothyroidism. The body is characteristically cold, but the cold is not confined to the extremities. It also extends to covered portions including axillae and groin. Pupils may be dilated or pinpoint and react sluggishly to light. Generalized rigidity and neck stiffness may be present without shivering. If shivering occurs just after prolonged physical activity such as endurance races, hypothermia is imminent. Athletic competition and other events may be held in relatively cold environments with scantily dressed participants. Occasionally in mountain races, sudden worsening of the weather, increasing winds, and wet clothing make the risk of hypothermia, often associated with fatal outcome, unpredictable. Hypothermia may occur in persons exposed to relatively mild temperatures. If prolonged exertion, dehydration, and relative lack of caloric intake are factors, hypoglycemia may be superimposed on the other stresses. It is important to recognize deterioration in judgment and failure of physical strength as early signs of hypothermia so that appropriate steps can be taken to avoid disaster. Heaters are provided in the dressing facilities at the finish of some of the better known marathons even when the race is run in heat. Runners stand with blankets in front of the hot air, shivering, and on the brink of hypothermia at the end of the race. Tendon reflexes are diminished and plantar responses are extensor in the hypothermic subjects, but revert to normal with rewarming. It is important to look for hypotension, compensatory tachycardia, slow atrial fibrillation, and gangrene of the toes during evacuation of victims. Respirations are slow and sighing characteristically, but may be Cheyne Stoke's, particularly if the victims of hypothermia are at altitude. When respiration is depressed, hypoxia and acidosis are also present. Abdominal distention and decreased peristalsis may indicate pancreatitis. Bowel sounds are absent and sometimes gastric dilatation with vomiting occur. Massive hepatic necrosis is a rare complication of hypothermia. Renal blood flow decreases and creatinine clearance is reduced. Despite diminished glomerular filtration, diuresis occurs because of decreased secretion of antidiuretic hormone and reduced responsiveness of renal tubular cells to this hormone. Eventually, however, dehydration and continued fall in renal blood flow cause oliguria. Renal failure from acute tubular necrosis may occur and severe muscle necrosis with myoglobinuria can further compromise renal function.

Accidental hypothermia out of doors, and sometimes in the elderly in their homes, may be a complication of drug ingestion, including alcohol, which intereferes with thermoregulation and accelerates heat loss. Though alcohol is often used for treating hypothermia, it may, in fact, only reduce discomfort and anxiety of cold exposed subjects. Studies of its effect on thermoregulation are controversial; some showed no difference in heat loss in those taking alcohol compared to control exposed subjects, and others even showed decreased heat loss after alcohol ingestion. In other studies of alcohol in induced hypothermia, hypoglycemia, which can further reduce core temperature and interfere with hepatic detoxification of alcohol, was also found. Moreover, when alcohol was given to subjects prior to experimental immersion in cold water, central body temperature declined faster, recovery of normal temperature after removal from the water was delayed, and shivering was considerably decreased. Nevertheless, in subjects ingesting alcohol with lower core temperature and decreased shivering, cold was perceived less and the environment was judged warmer than in controls. Alcohol intake during or after prolonged physical activity, particularly in cold weather, is dangerous. It may accelerate the fall in central body temperature and decrease awareness of impending serious complications. In addition, alcohol potentiates exercise-induced cutaneous vasodilatation and increases heat loss from the extremities. Moreover, alcohol ingestion after a marathon may be responsible for the occasional syncope of finishers because of cutaneous vasodilatation in addition to maximal dilatation of blood vessels at the end of the race. Systemic blood pressure falls precipitously in this situation.

Preexisting disease may be masked by hypothermia and nervous system lesions may not be appreciated because of the general depression in nervous system function. Elevated enzymes from pressure necrosis of muscles in the unconscious patient together with electrocardiographic changes that occur in both hypothermia and myocardial infarction make the diagnosis of myocardial ischemia difficult. Last, but not least, it must be stressed that the diagnosis of brain death is impossible during hypothermia. Patients may be deeply comatose with absent reflexes and the pupils can be fixed and dilated. Respirations may hardly be detectable; bradycardia and severe hypotension plus marked slowing and flattening of the electroencephalogram do not rule out complete recovery. Thus, the hypothermia-related disturbances of function may recover fully even though clinical examination and previous experience suggests the contrary.

1. THE DIAGNOSIS OF HYPOTHERMIA

The diagnosis of hypothermia depends on accurate measurement of body temperature, which is normally different in various parts of the body. For example, skin temperature of the extremities fluctuates with changes in environmental temperature. In accidental hypothermia, extremity temperature may be much lower than temperature in other body parts because of vasoconstriction. Hypothermia is only dangerous if core temperatures are low; hence, reasonable estimates of central body temperature are necessary. These may be obtained from external auditory meatus or rectum. If the central temperature is 32°C or below, and the individual is otherwise healthy, he may be actively rewarmed in hot water. In the field, success depends on availability of warming equipment. Vests covering the upper abdomen and chest containing tubing that allows hot water to circulate around the upper body work well. Surrounding the victim with warm nonhypothermic bodies in a sleeping bag is also effective. Complications must be treated. Blood gases, routine blood, urine, and liver function should be studied in those who do not recover rapidly with rewarming. If sophisticated equipment is available, rewarming through inhalation of humidified, warm oxygen can give gratifying results.

2. FROSTBITE

High winds and cold temperatures are associated with an increased risk of frostbite. The exposed body parts and distal extremities are most likely to be affected because vasoconstriction occurs in these areas in response to normal thermoregulatory drive. Furthermore, hand contact with cold or rapidly evaporating fluids (gasoline) may precipitate frostbite. Tissue freezing produces the damage, and if rewarming is not prompt, serious injury results. Early mild frostbite often leads to numbness of the fingertips and paresthesias, which persist for several weeks and recover. This has been attributed to damaged digital nerve endings. Serious frostbite and hypothermia often go together. Rewarming in a warm water bath (40–43°C) with care to protect the cold-injured extremity from mechanical trauma is indicated. Infections may also complicate recovery. Often, Raynaud's phenomenon persists for years in frostbitten digits.

Prevention of frostbite and hypothermia by appropriate education, layered clothing that can be easily taken off and zipped up again, and the use of woolen headgear is important (heat loss through the scalp is great because of copious blood supply particularly during exercise). The chill factor of high wind may produce cold urethritis associated with temporary incontinence, particularly in runners. This can be avoided by use of windproof undergarments now widely available.

Subjects on the brink of hypothermia or frostbite often have the so-called "cold muscle syndrome" characterized by weakness, stiffness, and clumsiness from impaired muscle excitation–contraction coupling. Both muscle action potentials and contraction times are prolonged. This may be evident when individuals have trouble removing their clothing because of impaired function of hands and fingers.

In patients with neuromuscular disease, hypothermia can further impair function. Examples are those with hypocalemic and hypercalemic periodic paralysis, paramyotonia congenita, and myotonic dystrophy. Such individuals learn early to avoid cold exposure.

IV. ALTITUDE, PERFORMANCE, AND NERVOUS SYSTEM ACTIVITY

Humans are increasingly participating in physical activity at altitudes at which they formerly sojourned for only short periods of time. Permanent inhabitants do exist between 1500 and 4600 m, but considerable populations live and work at altitudes of about 3000 m (10,000 ft). Very few venture much beyond 5500 m (18,000 ft) and even fewer perform physical tasks at such altitudes. It is beyond the scope of this section to discuss the adaptive mechanisms that occur in those who acclimatize to varying altitudes, but the commonest manifestation of maladapted sojourners is acute mountain sickness (AMS) and, occasionally, high altitude pulmonary edema (HAPE).

The important clinical manifestations of AMS are severe, often pounding headache, nausea, dimmed vision, restlessness, palpitation, anorexia, sleeplessness, and anxiety. Rapid ascent increases the chances of developing AMS and may be associated with HAPE in a minority of sojourners. This condition occurs in a setting of increased thoracic intravascular volume and consequent extravascular fluid accumulation, especially in the peribronchial spaces, and lung edema. If HAPE is present, there is almost always also increased vascular permeability in other tissues. This may manifest itself as retinopathy, increased intraocular pressure, and cerebral and peripheral edema. Hypoxia is the underlying cause of these complications, but low barometric pressure may also be important. The delay in onset of symptoms after arrival in the hypoxic environment suggests that secondary or tertiary factors are the actual triggers of altitude illness. Fluid retention occurs in all individuals on altitude exposure, along with increased sodium excretion. Those with altitude illness retain relatively more sodium than those who are not affected by the problem. The cause of the fluid retention in this situation is not known.

A. Cerebral Edema

One part of altitude illness is cerebral edema. Although this is a complication of altitude exposure, it is usually seen at rather high altitudes and in those who are unacclimatized. The manifestations of altitude cerebral edema are the same as those of cerebral edema elsewhere and include retinal hemorrhages, papilledema, clouded consciousness, confusions, and, eventually, coma. Nevertheless, judging from logs of Himalayan expeditions of acclimatized mountaineers, mental function sufficient to record at least meteorologic data is adequate at altitudes up to 8500 m. And, experimentally, at altitudes of up to 5500 m, no measurable impairment of cerebral metabolism has been found.

B. Treatment and Prevention of Altitude Illness

The oral use of acetazolamide for 2 or 3 days prior to ascent is protective against AMS and perhaps against HAPE. Treatment requires oxygen administration and, most importantly, immediate evacuation to lower altitudes. The use of diuretics, morphine, or other drugs once AMS or HAPE is present is not effective. AMS alone may be treated symptomatically with aspirin, cold fluids, and carbohydrate-containing food which alleviates the condition until acclimatization occurs. HAPE and cerebral edema, however, should not be managed at altitude and evacuation is essential. Endurance training may provide some protection from altitude illness, but good evidence for this is not available. Moreover, once a person has had HAPE, it is likely to recur on reexposure to appropriate altitude. Anecdotal evidence suggests that well-acclimatized persons not suffering from mountain sickness experience personality changes that may affect the success or failure of an expedition.

Studies of neuropsychological effects of high altitude indicate similarities between mountaineers, sojourners, and those who are mildly intoxicated with alcohol. Increased vigilance manifests itself as difficulty in sleeping rather than in performance tests. Electroencephalograms recorded at 5500 m may show arousal patterns and decreased mean α frequency. Occasionally, the normal suppression of α rhythm with eye opening did not occur, and electroencephalographic signs of sleep were present in individuals who had their eyes open. Subjects were easily aroused from deep sleep and they experienced multiple arousals during an all-night EEG recording at altitudes of 4300 m. Visual and somatosensory evoked responses showed either no change, lengthening, or shortening of latencies. It is clear, however, that brain function and the EEG are altered at altitude. Other recognized effects include somnolence, withdrawal, inattention, lethargy, fatigue, frequent desire to sleep, but inability to fall asleep, and, occasionally, drowsiness. Psychomotor skills and decision making are variably affected in different individuals by altitude exposure. The intellectual changes associated with high altitude are similar to the impairment and slowing of mental function of advancing age. Perseveration, difficulty with calculations, faulty judgment, and unpredictable emotional outbursts have been reported. Unimpaired judgment is often critical to survival and success of mountaineering expeditions. Nevertheless, comparatively little change occurs in testing situations in the ability to perform skillful tasks at altitudes below 5500 m.

In the visual system light sensitivity is impaired, acuity is decreased, and critical flicker fusion (dependent on the metabolic rate of retinal ganglion cells) also becomes impaired at 3000–3500 m and above. Intraocular pressure increases, particularly with exercise at altitude, but has never reached pathological levels in those in whom it has been measured. Decreased central visual acuity, attributed to retinal arteriolar hemorrhage, and hypoxia of ganglion cells may occur at altitudes of 5500 m or greater. Previous high altitude exposure to about 5000 m even though the subject is no longer altitude acclimated seems to protect against visual disturbances and, particularly, against retinal hemorrhages upon reexposure. Recovery from retinal hemorrhages, except for those that involve the macula, is usually complete. Scotomata from macular hemorrhage may persist indefinitely though the rest of the visual impairment recovers completely.

Incoordination occurs at about 5500 m and subjects are unsteady on standing and are unable to stand on one leg or with eyes closed. Truncal ataxia may be so severe that support during motion is required. This usually improves with cessation of physical activity and disappears when lower altitudes are reached. Drop attacks may occur and tetraplegia to the extent that subjects were only able to communicate by facial grimacing and with the aid of neck muscles has been reported. Tendon reflexes decrease in amplitude above 4500 m, and increase again at about 6100 m and above. This has been attributed to cerebral and brainstem hypoxia.

In general, the sensory system is not affected by altitude exposure, except in those who, in addition to altitude, also suffer from cold injury which affects limb sensation.

C. Exercise at High Altitude

Adaptation to altitude increases capacity to perform muscular work, but capacity is still less than at sea level for a given individual. Not only is oxygen less available to muscles, but vital capacity also decreases. Transient efforts lasting no more than a few minutes may, in fact, be enhanced at altitude because of decreased air resistance. However, athletic events requiring more than a few minutes for completion are considerably altered by altitude and performance is worse. This applies also to acclimatized athletes though acclimatization and training at high altitude may improve performance significantly for endurance events (3).

When altitude illness is present, subjects should not participate in athletic events because muscular work accentuates the hypoxia. Surprisingly, oxygen consumption for a given amount of work at high altitude is proportionately greater than at lower elevations. This is mainly due to oxygen debt. Efficiency of muscle contraction is reduced, and cardiopulmonary recovery is prolonged. Acclimatization improves oxygen delivery to the tissues by its effect on hematocrit, tissue capillary density, and 2,3-diphosphoglycerate, and this might be further improved by training at altitude. Three weeks or longer of altitude training is required before full physiological adjustment can be expected and maximum potentials for a given altitude are attained. Performance is always worse in any individual athlete at altitude if effort duration is more than a few minutes. The methods of training at altitude to achieve optimum and speedy acclimatization have not been fully investigated. Those athletes not suffering from mountain sickness can engage in athletic activity at maximum effort without harm. Speed and short-duration efforts might be emphasized in order to build power and coordination because of prolonged recovery periods at higher altitude.

Some diseases of the nervous system may be influenced by altitude sojourn. If properly treated, epilepsy, hypertension, and diabetes mellitus seem not to interfere with physical activity at altitude. No one is certain how many patients with epilepsy are climbers, and accidents during climbs have not been attributed to seizures. Some anticonvulsants protect the central nervous system from ischemic or hypoxic damage. Whether they are also protective against the ill effects of high altitude is not certain. Cerebrovascular and heart disease can be aggravated by hypoxia superimposed on an already compromised circulation; however, serious accidents have not been reported from altitude exposure of these patients. Even well-controlled myasthenia gravis and multiple sclerosis in remission may be affected adversely by altitude exposure and weakness, ataxia, and spasticity may be aggravated or brought on by the patient's traveling to elevations above 3000 m.

Tolerance to alcohol and sedative drugs is decreased at high altitude. This may be related to the similarity of effects of altitude and alcohol on central nervous system function. The effects of sedative drugs might be compounded by their respiratory depression in a setting of hypoxia. Migraine may be precipitated by altitude exposure. Nonneurological conditions influenced by high altitude include sickle cell disease in which crises leading to vascular occulsion of splenic infarct may occur at altitudes of about 2300 m or above. There is also increased propensity to cold injury, particularly associated with decreased judgment and the psychological stress of altitude exposure.

The eyes and exposed skin should be protected from ultraviolet radiation, which is increased by the thin atmosphere and reflections from snow, and when combined with hypoxia, may severely injure these organs (14).

Decompression sickness and other diving-related diseases are discussed in detail in Chapter 18.

V. SPORTS AND THE PERIPHERAL NERVOUS SYSTEM

Almost all peripheral nerve injuries are due to compression or direct trauma and are usually traceable to excessive, unaccustomed activity either in organized sports or recreational pursuits. The improper use of and inadequate protective gear also have a role. Those who oppose physical activity often suggest, after reviewing nerve injuries, that it would be safer to face a television screen sitting in an easy chair rather than to expose such important structures to often serious damage. But, watching television sports is not without its dangers. Ulnar and radial neuropathies can occur and these might, as in all pressure mononeuropathies, be aggravated by the concomitant excessive use of alcohol.

To localize lesions in the peripheral nervous system, it is necessary to know the anatomy of peripheral nerves and their relationship to bony prominences, tendons, and muscle tunnels. This is beyond the scope of the present section and the reader is referred to appropriate texts. Only those syndromes associated with recreational, athletic, or competitive activities, their symptoms, signs, and prognoses will be covered here. The pathogenesis, which in most cases is compression, excessive traction, or direct trauma, will be briefly touched on.

A. Plexus and Nerve Root Problems

''Burners'' or ''stingers'' are common complaints of football players and are due to injuries of the upper trunk of the brachial plexus or upper cervical roots. A sharp, burning pain in the shoulder radiating sometimes down the lateral arm and forearm to the thumb occurs soon after a blow to the head or neck. The pain and dysesthesia may last seconds and occasionally are associated with momentary weakness. This syndrome also occurs after a hockey stick blow to the shoulder which may cause long-lasting brachial plexus injury. Burners and stingers are occasional complaints of wrestlers after head and shoulders are twisted in opposite directions or after a fall on the shoulder with the head turned to the opposite side. Weakness may persist for some days after the pain and numbness have gone.

Trap shooting and big game hunting with powerful rifles can cause firearm recoil palsies probably due to entrapment of the upper trunk of the brachial plexus when the clavicle is forced backward onto the underlying scalenus muscle. The thoracic outlet syndrome (scalenus anticus syndrome) or supraclavicular discomfort and transient tingling in the fourth and fifth digits has been reported in competitive swimmers. Eventually, severe numbness and aching improved after section of the anterior scalenus muscle. The symptoms in swimmers tend to occur on the side opposite that to which the head is turned in order to breathe. Intervertebral disc herniation and osteoarthritis of the lumbosacral spine may be associated with radiculopathies in some long-distance runners who have an exaggerated lumbar lordosis or an overly long stride with excessive hip extension. L 3-4, L 4-5, or L 5-S1 are the usual roots involved. These symptoms may be treated with reduction in the activity which led to them. Often stretching, muscle-strengthening exercises, icing, and diathermy together lead to speedy resolution of the problem unless intervertebral disc herniation or severe osteoarthritis with root pressure precludes recovery. These problems should be evaluated surgically.

B. Symptoms Referable to the Shoulder Girdle and Upper Extremity

Throwing movements with the arm across the chest and twisting may stretch the suprascapular nerve in its notch and pain and weakness result. The pain is deep in the posterior aspect of the shoulder and arm abduction and external rotation are weakened. Long-standing cases may have atrophy of the supra- and infra-scapular muscles evidenced by unusual prominence of the spinous process of the scapula. This occurs in baseball and during relay races when runners stretch to pass the baton to the next runner. Isolated suprascapular nerve palsies may also occur with falls on the shoulder when the head is stretched to the opposite side. In these falls the brunt of the mechanical trauma is on the brachial plexus itself. This occurs in horseback riding, motorsports, polo, skiing, and, occasionally, football. Partial injury to the suprascapular nerve may occur with acromioclavicular separations and the resulting pain erroneously attributed to the shoulder. Electrophysiological tests can confirm nerve injury, but worsening of pain by deep pressure on the suprascapular notch or relief of the pain with local anesthetic block of the supra-scapular nerve are helpful diagnostic maneuvers (15).

C. The Long Thoracic Nerve

The long thoracic nerve has no cutaneous sensory function. Therefore, symptoms of injury are entirely confined to weakness. Excessive contraction of the scalenus muscle, forced abduction of the shoulder beyond 90°, blows to the neck or shoulder, and downward traction on the shoulder can damage the nerve. Pain and weakness are usual symptoms. The pain involves the neck in the region of the scalenus muscle and often radiates to the shoulder, axilla, or the lateral chest. The serratus anterior muscle is weak, manifest by impaired ability to elevate the arm or to push forward. Attempts to do this cause winging of the scapula.

Activities associated with injury to the long thoracic nerve include punching bag training, vigorous swinging at golf balls, and excessive and violent contraction of the scalenus medius muscle during swimming and playing tennis. Poorly padded heavy backpacks or improper distribution of pack weight during prolonged hikes may injure the long thoracic nerve. "Pack palsy" is usually seen in relatively untrained young people who carry packs for long periods of time at the beginning of the backpacking season. Occasionally, discus throwers stretch their long thoracic nerve and similar injuries have been reported in football and basketball players.

D. Musculocutaneous and Axillary Nerve Injuries

Axillary nerve injuries usually result from its compression against the lateral aspect of the humerus. Occasionally, direct pressure in the axilla, stretching from posterior dislocation of the shoulder or downward displacement of a dislocated shoulder, or severe direct trauma to the anterior shoulder causes axillary nerve injuries. Deltoid weakness and numbness, tingling, and occasionally referred pain in the sensory distribution of the axillary nerve (skin overlying the deltoid) occur. Deltoid atrophy gives a square or boxlike appearance to the shoulder on the affected side. Sometimes, in old injuries, compensatory hypertrophy of the supraspinatus muscle may be found.

Musculocutaneous nerve injury causes atrophy of the anterior aspect of the upper arm and occasionally compensatory hypertrophy of the brachioradialis muscle.

Contact sports are the usual cause of axillary and musculocutaneous nerve injuries, which can be confirmed by electromyographic studies.

E. The Anterior Interosseus and Median Nerves

The commonest site for median nerve injury is in the carpal tunnel and there the symptoms of mild compression are pain and, occasionally, numbness. Weakness in the muscles innervated by the median nerve in the hand (abductor pollicis brevis, mainly) occurs in the more severe injuries. Damage to the median nerve in the carpal tunnel is usually caused by force applied to the palm, repetitive wrist movement such as in racquet ball and occasionally catching baseballs with a poorly padded glove. It is sometimes seen in weight lifters and individuals who do many pushups applying direct pressure on the median nerve. Pressure from handlebars on the median nerve is occasionally seen in bicyclists who do not wear the protective, padded bicycle gloves. Repetitive pronation can injure the median nerve at the pronator teres muscles, and anterior interosseus damage may result from compression during muscle contraction, sometimes seen in tennis players and weight lifters. Clinically, this injury is characterized by the "pinch sign," i.e., it is impossible to make a perfect circle with the thumb and index finger because of inability to flex the thumb and the distal interphalangeal joint of the forefinger.

A traumatic neuroma resulting from bowling (bowler's thumb) gives rise to pain and hyperesthesia on the medial aspect of the thumb. This is due to repeated pressure of the bowling ball on the base of the thumb. Surgical exploration usually shows subcutaneous scarring, and neurolysis perhaps with a change in bowling technique is curative.

F. Ulnar Nerve

Sports injuries to the ulnar nerve usually occur at the elbow or in the palm. Bicycle and motorcycle riding injuries to the motor branch of the ulnar nerve in the palm are common and have been known to exist for many years. If the deep motor branch in the palm is involved, weakness and atrophy of the intrinsic hand muscles without sensory deficits are usually present. Loss of strength in the lumbrical muscles in the fourth and fifth digits causes the characteristic flexion posture of these digits ("main en griffe"). When there is loss of adductor power in the thumb, the thumb flexion on attempting to hold a paper between the index finger and the thumb is characteristic (Froment's sign). In bicycle riders, the neuropathy may affect sensory and motor parts of the ulnar nerve seen in racing cyclists with a prolonged and tight grasp of the handlebar and pressure on the palms. Karate practitioners and weight lifters also occasionally have ulnar nerve injuries either in the hand or at the elbow. Pitching baseballs can traumatize the ulnar nerve at the elbow, causing pain and numbness in the hand typical of ulnar mononeuropathy. Oarsmen and Nordic skiers may compress the ulnar nerve in the hand by gripping skipole or oar and, occasionally, the flexor carpi ulnaris tension injures the nerve at the elbow. Electromyographic and nerve conduction studies confirm the site of the injury.

G. Radial and Posterior Interosseus Nerves

Sudden triceps contraction can damage the radial nerve in the arm. Elbow extension against weights and the throwing movement may also cause this injury. When the posterior interosseus nerve is damaged, the brachioradialis strength is preserved and wrist extension is only partially possible. Pronation and supination can injure the posterior interosseus nerve as it runs through the supinator muscle. Activities associated with this injury include swimming, Frisbee throwing, hitting a tennis ball backhand, and, occasionally, throwing numerous snowballs.

Occasionally, the supraclavicular nerve passes through the clavicle on its way to innervate the skin on the anterior and midportion of the shoulder. Such normal variants may be more easily injured by compression or stretch during contact sports. The symptoms are pain and numbness of the anterior shoulder and midportion of the clavicle. Electrical studies can successfully detect the site of the injury.

H. The Sciatic Nerve and Its Branches

Injuries to the sciatic nerve can occur by pressure in the region of the ischial tuberosity often also called unicyclists sciatica or "Bozo's syndrome." Such injuries are also seen after horseback riding. The peroneal nerve branch of the sciatic can be compressed as it winds around the lateral aspect of the neck of the fibula and clinically this is manifest by foot drop. Stretch lesions due to twisting of the ankle or occasionally from knee dislocations can also injure the peroneal nerve. This occurs in contact sports (rarely during the twirling of a Hula Hoop) if the athlete is somehow predisposed to peripheral nerve disease because of a metabolic disturbance (latent diabetes or covert alcoholism). Peroneal palsy may occur quite easily with relatively minor ankle sprains or pressure directly on the nerve. The traction on the nerve during the ankle sprain or while the peroneus longus muscle is tensed with direct pressure on the nerve is the commonest cause of this palsy. Occasionally, a stretch may cause an intraneural hematoma, which results in delayed recovery or permanent damage after an ankle sprain. Taping the ankle tightly after a sprain may also injure the nerve and lead to foot drop. Compression of the deep peroneal nerve from tight ski boots can produce sensory symptoms between the first and second toe and pain over the dorsum of the foot or lower tibia when the nerve is compressed by a high boot. Persistent numbness between the first and second toes and weakness of toe dorsiflexion may result from prolonged compression by ski boots and interfere with athletic performance.

The posterior tibial nerve is rarely injured except in the tarsal tunnel which gives rise to burning dysesthesia of the sole of the foot. It can occur with horseback riding or prolonged squatting or when the shoes are too tightly laced during a hike. Heel pain in joggers can also be due to repeated trauma to the medial plantar nerve or from extra pressure from the use of orthotics. Reeducation is sometimes helpful. The runner should be instructed to strike the lateral (normal) aspect of the heel first on ground contact. Occasionally, tight ski boots also cause numbness in the back and sole of the foot by compression of the calcaneal and sural nerves.

The superficial femoral artery may become thrombosed in Hunter's canal in skiers and joggers from repeated compression by the surrounding hypertrophied muscles. Symptoms of this rare occurrence, hypesthesia or numbness of the great toe, simulate those of deep peroneal nerve compression.

Genitofemoral nerve injury by direct trauma to the groin produces pain during walking or hip hyperextension. This is sometimes seen in long-distance bicycle riders on unaccustomed hard seats. A femoral sensory neuropathy has been reported after heavy weight lifting and a combined femoral and sciatic sensory-motor neuropathy occurred following situps and "legovers." Paresthesias may occur on the medial aspect of the knee after injuries to the infrapatellar branch of the saphenous nerve, a branch of the femoral nerve. This symptom frequently occurs after meniscectomies and can be mistaken for knee joint pathology.

Meralgia paresthetica from lateral femoral cutaneous nerve injury is an affliction of gymnasts and also individuals who hike for prolonged periods, particularly those in whom the nerve passes through the inguinal ligament or is acutely angled across it, both normal anatomic variants. Occasionally, direct pressure by packbelts cause burning paresthesias and impaired sensation in the upper lateral aspect of the thigh (area of supply of the lateral femoral cutaneous nerve).

The pudendal nerve is occasionally directly compressed during bicycling causing penile insensitivity. With frostbite, the sensory abnormalities of the penis may be prolonged, perhaps because of cold damage to the pudendal nerve.

I. Exercise and Peripheral Neuropathies

Peripheral nerve disease usually caused by metabolic or toxic disorders affects the longest nerve foremost and most severely. Such neuropathic disorders are well known and many are complicated by severe autonomic nervous system dysfunction often manifest by abnormalities in temperature regulation (impairment of sweating) and postural hypotension. Such disabilities preclude prolonged physical exercise. Postural hypotension, in particular, requires appropriate management for rehabilitation. One way of achieving this without pharmacotherapy is by habituation. This eventually allows adequate cerebral perfusion in the face of gravitationally induced falls in systemic blood pressure. For patients with orthostatic hypotension conditioning can be achieved in two ways. Patients may sleep in a propped-up position, with an increase in the angle of incline as tolerance permits. Alternatively, one can place the patient on a tilt table and gradually increase the angle of tilt with blood pressure monitoring, keeping the head up for 5 minutes at a time and the blood pressure at a level that just prevents syncope. Gradually the angle and duration of headup tilt is increased until the patient can maintain adequate perfusion in the upright position for some time (2).

Patients with so-called pressure-sensitive neuropathy should not squat or do deep knee bends, which may, even though pressure on nerves is minimal, cause transient increase in symptoms.

In acute affections of the peripheral nervous system, for example, in the

Landry–Guillain–Barre syndrome, exercise should be avoided until clinical recovery is evident. These admonitions stem from the well-documented earlier studies of poliomyelitis victims whose paralysis was much more pronounced in muscles that had been exercised prior to the onset of clinical weakness.

J. Musculoskeletal Injuries and Complaints Sometimes Referred to Neurologists

In this section, we will not deal with muscle contusion, tears, low back muscle spasm, impingement syndromes, the so-called down leg and knee syndromes, plantar fasciitis, shin splints, and stress fractures, undoubtedly the more common complaints of participating athletes, but hardly within the purview of neurologists. Muscle aches and cramps are normal accompaniments of exercise, pregnancy, dehydration, salt depletion, and the like. However, cramps may also signal the presence of myopathic disorders related to thyroid dysfunction, uremia, electrolyte abnormalities, such as hypomagnesemia, intermittent claudication of the legs, spinal cord, or cauda equina, and amyotrophic lateral sclerosis. Those conditions attributed to relative muscle ischemia in tight compartments (though there may be other causes of the compartment syndromes) will also not be considered here.

1. DISEASES OF MUSCLES PRESENTING WITH MUSCLE PAIN AND FATIGUE IN SPORTS PARTICIPANTS

Excessive fatigue or weakness of the extremities during exercise may be the result of primary muscle disease. Though these are uncommon, they should be considered because of the relative ease of proper management and, in most cases, the possibility that affected persons may continue to participate in sports.

Disease affecting muscles as part of a generalized disorder is commoner than primary myopathies. Fatigue, painful cramps, and weakness are the hallmarks of these conditions and include inflammatory myopathies such as dermatomyositis, polymyositis, polymyalgia rheumatica, hypocalemic myopathy often drug induced, alcoholic myopathy, and muscle affection by certain drugs including clofibrate, amphetamine, lithium, tolbutamide, and other toxic agents. Myopathies may also accompany metabolic bone disease. Predominantly proximal weakness occurs in primary and secondary hyperparathyroidism, in hypophosphatemia, in dysfunction of the renal tubules, and in chronic anticonvulsant intoxication. It is unlikely that patients with these disorders participate in or desire to start athletic endeavors.

2. MYOPHOSPHORYLASE AND PHOSPHOFRUCTOKINASE DEFICIENCIES

Myophosphorylase and phosphofructokinase deficiencies are rare disorders presenting in childhood with attacks of stiffness, pain, and cramps brought on by moderate exercise and relieved by rest. Shortening and hardening of muscles occurs. The cramps may disappear within a minute after exercise or may persist for several hours after experimentally prolonged ischemic exercise. Creatine kinase is not greatly increased and characteristically cramps are not present at rest. Lactate increases very little during exercise and the muscles depend on oxidation of free fatty acids for fuel. Therefore, artificially manipulating free fatty acid levels in these subjects prolongs their exercise tolerance, as is also seen after low-level warmup exercise. The failure of lactate release is diagnostic of the condition and muscle biopsy is usually not necessary.

3. CARNITINE PALMITYL TRANSFERASE DEFICIENCIES

Carnitine palmityl transferase deficiencies are rare muscle disorders of children and teenagers characterized by attacks of cramps, weakness, and myoglobinuria following exercise. The symptoms are facilitated by fasting or ingestion of high fat diets. In these patients, the enzyme defect interferes with oxidation of long-chain fatty acids which results in postexertional muscle pain that may persist for several days. Marked elevation of creatine kinase occurs. Such patients usually have only three or four attacks per year, and between attacks, their exercise tolerance is normal. Rare attacks of weakness and pain occur independently of exercise. If examined soon after an attack or while still somewhat symptomatic, slight proximal or generalized muscle weakness may be associated with diffuse muscle aches. Otherwise clinical and electromyographic examinations during symptom-free periods are normal. These patients do not develop ketosis during fasting. Muscle biopsy at the height of symptoms shows lipid accumulation between myofibrils, but may be normal when the patient is asymptomatic. Definitive diagnosis is made by demonstrating deficient enzyme activity.

4. MYOADENYLATE (AMP) DEAMINASE DEFICIENCY

Some patients, but not all, with AMP deaminase deficiency have exercise related cramps, stiffness, and weakness. Symptoms usually begin in the second or third decade and cramping, if it occurs, is induced by moderate exercise of the calves. It is also present in hands, forearms, and shoulders. Between attacks, the patients may be normal clinically or may have mild weakness. Symptoms of AMP deaminase deficiency are not as pronounced as those of myophosphorylase or carnitine palmityl transferase deficiency. AMP deaminase deficiency and gout have been reported in a subject with exercise-induced cramps, suggesting that disordered purine metabolism may have something to do with exercise intolerance, but the nature of this relationship is not clear. Specific therapy is not available for this condition. The diagnosis depends on demonstration of low levels of muscle AMP deaminase or failure to show increased venous ammonia after ischemic forearm exercise (13).

Muscle enzyme levels in athletes should be interpreted carefully. Serum creatine kinase is increased particularly after competition and for some days thereafter. This has been attributed to increased muscle membrane permeability, but proof for this is lacking. Fatigued or recovering muscle membrane attributed to inadequate oxygen supply has been implicated, but this occurs even in highly trained athletes after relatively minor exertion. Moreover, ultrastructural studies of muscles in athletes do not show tissue damage. The degree of exertion and training of the athlete affects the serum level of creatine kinase and other muscle enzymes after vigorous exercise. Even in the same individual, if untrained muscles are exercised, creatine kinase is higher than when the well-trained musculature is subjected to similar exertion. If one examines creatine kinase levels in athletes at rest, it is necessary to demand abstention from training for at least 10 days before resting levels are expected.

Creatine kinase MB isoenzyme (CK-MB) correlates with serum myoglobin and it has been suggested that it is a sensitive biochemical marker for exertional rhabdomyolysis. This same isoenzyme is also a sensitive and specific marker for myocardial injury. Male marathon runners during training and after competition showed CK-MB elevation to levels seen after myocardial necrosis. However, myocardial scanning with Tc-99m-pyrophosphate showed no evidence of infarct. These findings are consistent with, but do not prove, the idea that enzyme leakage from skeletal muscle, including the CK-MB isoenzyme fraction, occurs, and that at least in highly trained marathon runners with elevated isoenzyme, there was no clinical or radiographic evidence of myocardial necrosis.

5. NONDYSTROPHIC MYOTONIAS

A number of individuals suffering from primary myotonias including myotonia congenita, paramyotonia congenita, and Isaac's syndrome (stiffness, cramps, and continuous muscle fiber activity sometimes associated with hyperhidrosis) may be helped by advice to facilitate exercise. Myotonia and stiffness are usually worse during the first voluntary movements and improve with repeated effort. Therefore, continuous low-level activity prior to athletic participation facilitates muscle relaxation. Rest should be avoided. Extended warmups of low intensity, particularly if carried out in a warm environment, are also useful. Warmth alone lessens stiffness and myotonia. In patients with the true myotonias, increasing the oral quinine dose in the morning before competition and high carbohydrate intake facilitate prolonged physical activity and decrease myotonia. The high carbohydrate meal improves exercise capacity because it decreases plasma potassium and its deleterious effect on myotonia. The carbohydrate meal-induced insulin release allows glucose and potassium to enter the muscle and decreases myotonia.

K. Epilepsy and Physical Activity

Participation in sports resulting in head injuries may occasionally cause epilepsy. Conversely, however, the commonest problem is to decide whether patients with seizures should participate in athletic activities after the first or subsequent convulsions and whether the type of athletic endeavor should restricted. No good evidence is available for or against athletic participation of patients with fits. Most of the following is conjectural based on inadequate data and is subject to controversy.

Active participation in athletics was largely confined to children and young people until recently; hence, most of the evidence for or against athletic participation in epileptics is based on subjects in this age group. Nevertheless, many physicians will now be confronted with older epileptics and the problem of determining the effect of athletics on their symptoms. Even less factual and reliable information is available for these patients.

The Committee on Medical Aspects of Sports of the American Medical Association (9) has vacillated in its recommendations on participation of epileptics in contact or collision sports. The latest recommendations "give legal support to doctors who do not discourage epileptic patients from participating in contact sports." Nevertheless, many physicians feel that epileptics should be excluded from contact sports, gymnastic, and other athletic activities. In other parts of the world, a lenient attitude toward children with seizures is the rule (Japan) and it seems that a good case can be made for a similar attitude in this country. Epilepsy is a common disorder. About 75% of the approximately 2 million epileptics in this country have seizures before the age of 18. Of these, some 277,000 young people with epilepsy are of school age and thus might be required to participate in school sports.

A number of outstanding athletic achievements have been attained by epileptics. One epileptic young woman ran 2000 miles from Minneapolis–St. Paul to Washington, D.C., and an epileptic man, whose seizures were well controlled with phenytoin, was a member of a successful Mt. McKinley mountaineering expedition. Anecdotally, there are athletic geniuses with epilepsy who have contributed to major professional sporting events. Nevertheless, parents and physicians generally are overprotective of epileptics and thus may thwart some gifted individuals from reaching their full athletic potential.

The possible preventive effects of exercise on seizures has been reported anecdotally since antiquity, and the United States Department of Health, Education, and Welfare's Commission for the Control of Epilepsy and its Consequences has stated, "Physical activity appears to play a role in seizure prevention." Moreover, epileptologists have noted that fits seem to occur preferentially when the patient is sleeping, resting, or just idle. Rarely is a fit documented during athletic activities. Studies on patients with epilepsy who were in the German Air Force and in Israel during the Second World War showed that seizures were rare during intense physical activity. Thus, it has been suggested that exercise prevents convulsions, but no good studies exist to support this opinion. Proposals have been made for possible mechanisms of beneficial effects of exercise on seizures. Electroencephalographic evidence indicates that stimulation inducing mental activity, arousal, increased concentration, alertness, and enjoyment of tasks may protect against seizures. Thus, epileptiform discharges in the EEG are much more frequent when the patient is inactive than when he is alert. It is, therefore, implicated that during sports, particularly during competition, the vigilance and concentration required may influence seizures beneficially. It is also known that sometimes fits can be inhibited in certain patients by sensory stimuli and similar stimuli in other patients may, infact, precipitate seizures. Exercise-induced metabolic changes may have a salutary effect on seizures. Lactic acidosis during exercise has been associated with normalization of the EEG. Acidosis may reduce neuronal irritability by increasing the putative inhibitory neurotransmitter, γ-aminobutyric acid in the brain. Other studies, however, have not indicated that increased lactic acid levels inhibit central abnormal nervous system electrogenesis. Some suggest on the basis of EEG activity during recovery after exercise that physical activity, in fact, predisposes to seizures and that the higher the acidity and base excess during recovery from exercise, the greater the epileptiform activity. Unanimity of opinion does not exist about the origin of beneficial effects of exercise on seizure frequency. Exertion-induced biochemical changes and their relationship to EEG activity need further study.

The literature supporting physical activity as protective against seizures is more voluminous than that which proposes the opposite view. Hyperventilation, a known activator of absence or complex partial seizures, is an example, but the role of exercise-induced hyperpnea in precipitating such attacks is not clear. Hyperventilation with exercise depends on the type of athletic event, physical condition, and age. Children are more susceptible to hyperventilation-induced seizures than are adults. The rate and mechanics of breathing change with improved exercise tolerance so training becomes important. Despite these caveats, the literature on hyperventilation-induced seizures with exercise is anecdotal. Epileptics should be warned against hyperventilation prior to diving to allow longer submergence (12). Drowning deaths have occurred in healthy swimmers using these techniques and hyperventilation might, of course, precipitate seizures under water in epileptics. Because of the hyperoxic environment, emotional and other stresses associated with scuba diving, and the high likelihood of drowning secondary to a seizure deep underwater, this sport activity is not recommended for epileptics. Increased ventilation associated with rapid ascent to higher altitudes rather than slow acclimatization might increase seizure risk. This is particularly applicable to skiers who fly from lower altitudes to resorts at 10,000 or 12,000 ft. There is no definitive information, however, that shows that such practices are associated with other than altitude illness. Fatigue, associated with physical activity, sleep deprivation, and sometimes jet lag are precipitants of convulsions. These alter the physiological balance and may occasionally induce seizures in nonepileptics. The definitive risk of these conditions to epileptics has not been assessed.

Known activators of seizures in certain epileptics include visual and auditory stimuli and movement. Fits have occurred for the first time during athletic events when movement was the inducer. This must be rare. Reflex epilepsy is most common in the first decade of life and only occasionally occurs after the age of ten. Persons in this age group are hardly likely to embark on a physical training program. The risk of movement-induced seizures in athletic events is minimal.

Stress of any sort may precipitate seizures in epileptics who are otherwise well controlled. The stress of athletic competition, however, is not definitively associated with increased seizure activity even in well-known epileptic athletes. The idea that collision and perhaps associated head trauma during sports may aggravate existing epilepsy has no scientific basis. Epileptics may sustain head injury and have a seizure immediately after the impact; however, this may occur in those without epilepsy (7).

Fits during sporting events is a nebulous, poorly documented area. Absence seizures, which may be more suceptible to physiological and biochemical changes associated with athletic competition and training, may occasionally occur during such activity, but the number of patients so far reported is small.

The mortality and morbidity in epileptics are a matter of controversy. About 7% die from accidents and 5% of the deaths are attributed to injuries sustained during a fit. Most of these are bathtub drownings. The risk of an epileptic child drowning while swimming in the sea or pool is less than one in 400 epileptic child years. This fourfold increased risk can be reduced by instruction and supervision. Other sports-related injuries and fatalities have not been attributed to seizures so it has been suggested that children with epilepsy be allowed to participate normally in school and camp physical education programs. Nevertheless, those who have seizures that are not preceded by an aura are at greater risk than those who have a warning of the impending fit and can, therefore, protect themselves from injury. Even brief loss of tone, balance, or arrest of movement during climbing or skiing may result in serious accidents. The frequently reported sudden death syndrome in epileptics has not been associated with sporting activities. Withdrawal of medication from children whose seizures are well controlled may pose a problem and become more urgent in athletically active persons because of the possible unfavorable influence of anticonvulsants on physical performance. In general, the seizure relapse rate with varying follow-up periods of 2–20 years is between 8 and 24%. Those who have been seizure-free on anticonvulsants usually remain so after anticonvulsant withdrawal.

Single seizures are not uncommon and often pose a difficult problem. Should young people who have had a single fit continue in athletics? Single seizures occurred in 18 per 100,000 persons, ages 5 to 24 years in one study. Two-thirds of these had more fits after varying periods of time, but most recurred within 2 years. So-called single fits may result from infection, toxic or metabolic cause, or trauma. Sleep deprivation, fatigue, excessive exertion, and emotional stress may also predispose to single seizures. An obvious precipitating cause for a single fit is not present in many patients. A single fit immediately after head trauma is of no prognostic significance. An example of this is Ingemar Johansson, former heavyweight world champion boxer who convulsed immediately after being knocked out by Floyd Patterson in the 1950s. It is interesting that Johansson has recently finished a marathon in around four hours. The knockout-associated seizure has not prevented him from attaining reasonable physical fitness after his years as world heavyweight champion during which he must have sustained many other serious head injuries.

The question of subsequent athletic activity in children with febrile convulsions is often raised. Should they participate in fitness programs and team sports? The incidence of epilepsy after one febrile seizure is around 2%. If a family history of non-fever-related seizures exists, the patient is abnormal neurologically or the initial seizure is complex, the percentage of subsequent epilepsy is higher. Forty-two percent of children who develop subsequent seizures unassociated with fever do so within 1 year of the first febrile convulsion, and 94% do so within 5 years of the fever-associated fit. Each seizure patient requires individual assessment of the psychological and physical risks and benefits of athletic participation.

Seizures within the first week after head injury usually signify intracranial pathology and increased risk for posttraumatic epilepsy (approximately 19% for patients over 16 years of age). In children, even minor head injuries not associated with loss of consciousness, amnesia, depressed skull fracture, or intracranial hematoma are likely to be followed by late epilepsy with an incidence similar to that of severe head injuries if a fit occurs in the first week after injury. Forty to 50% of patients who develop posttraumatic epilepsy do so within 6 months, 70% by 1 year, and 80% by 2 years after the head injury. Therefore, most individuals who go 2 years without a seizure are unlikely to develop posttraumatic fits (7).

L.   Rehabilitation of the Neurologically Handicapped through Sports

Handicapped individuals have unique biomechanical requirements for performance of certain sports. Wheelchair Ping-Pong is quite different from the ordinary variety. On the other hand, the biomechanics of wheelchair archery are not significantly different from that of the traditional sport.

Recreational activities and athletic competition are now available for paraplegics, amputees, and poliomyelitis patients, and special Olympics have been organized for the physically and mentally handicapped. Evaluation of weakness and spasticity plus analysis of force velocities, motion, and electromyographic kinesiology in the neurologically handicapped help one to advise particular physical activities most suited for a patient. It is important to recognize the functional rather than the purely diagnostic category of the neurological deficit. For example, spasticity is not enough, but should include description of the speed of muscle activation, the delay between intent and actual movement, and the tension and strength of a particular limb. In addition, delay in relaxation may occur and influence athletic activity. Mirror movements and overflow of purposeful activity to other limbs in cerebral palsy patients should be assessed as well as control of respiratory muscles. Moreover, visual tracking, often impaired in patients with extrapyramidal lesions, can affect sports that require accurate visual coordination.

Some patients with nervous system disorders have concomitant myocardial involvement. Examples of this are Friedrich's ataxia and some muscular dystrophies. This is important because endurance training in some nonprogressive muscular dystrophies improves exercise tolerance including the usefulness of minimally or noninvolved muscles and, therefore, overall function of the patient.

Exercise testing of patients with neurological disorders prior to assignment to certain sports or training must be modified for each patient. For example, bicycle ergometer or treadmill testing, usually employed in assessments of nonhandicapped individuals, would not be appropriate for some neurologically impaired persons. Finally, the psychological aspects of sports and training must be considered since self-respect and satisfaction are derived from participation in athletics. Some believe that the psychological advantages of competition or athletic activity to the neurologically handicapped far outweigh risks inherent in such pursuits. Therefore, leniency should rule the advice given to patients (8).

1. WHEELCHAIR SPORTS

Paraplegics can participate in basketball, tennis, sprint distances and slalom involving maneuvering of wheelchairs around obstacles and ramps, weight lifting, archery, table tennis, javelin, bowling, and shot put from a wheelchair. International competitor's standards exist for many of these sports and though originally developed for posttraumatic spinal cord problems, paraplegics with other lesions are now included. Classification systems allow patients with roughly equal handicaps to compete against each other. In international competition, ten different divisions ensure fair competition based on individual function.

Wheelchairs are modified for competition, some so sophisticated that they are of no use except for athletics. One of the largest competitive events is the wheelchair division of the marathon in which participants are usually sent off some time before the actual start of the footrace. The opportunity to compete in athletic events undoubtedly gives a tremendous psychological boost to paraplegics.

Amputees are equally capable of athletic participation appropriate to their handicap. The role of the nervous system in adaptation of skills after limb amputation is best illustrated by the Hungarian, Karoly Takacs, who ranked among the top pistol shooters in the world when he participated in the 1936

Olympic Games. In 1938, his right arm was accidentally amputated midway between the elbow and wrist. He then retrained his nervous system, including his eye, to shoot the pistol with his left hand. He later became world pistol shot champion in 1939, a year after the amputation and won gold medals at the Olympic Games in London in 1948 and in Helsinki in 1952. He again participated in his fourth world competition at the Olympic Games in Australia in 1956.

2.   CEREBRAL PALSY AND SPORTS

The clinical manifestations of cerebral palsy are related to timing, sequencing, and isolation of various movements. Motor performance is distorted and movements overflow to other parts of the body. Stress magnifies spasticity, athetosis, and ataxia, and the competition even in handicapped categories is usually too much for affected children. Nevertheless, they do participate in adaptive ball games in which special balls travel slower than normally weighted ones. Occasionally cerebral palsied children participate in volleyball. Motor handicapped children swim freestyle and competition is against the patient's own previous performance rather than other individuals. Consideration similar to that of motor deficits must also be given to affected respiratory muscles. Endurance events much beyond 400 m are usually beyond the capacity of the spastics. Activities that require agility and rapid movements are not for cerebral palsied persons.

3.   PHYSICAL ACTIVITY FOR THE BLIND

Blind persons can participate in many athletic events either with a guide or with devices that emit auditory signals. If children participate in sports, though blind, they develop more self-reliance and security in moving about in the environment alone.

International and national sports organizations for the handicapped are available for advice to those who wish to train in one or other sports discipline. Sports for the mentally retarded are best explored through the Special Olympics Program established by the Joseph P. Kennedy, Jr., Foundation. The United States Olympic Program has a committee devoted to sports for the handicapped which promotes national and international competition for the disabled. Other organizations deal with sports for the deaf, blind, or paraplegic. The neurologically handicapped should be encouraged to participate in athletics without feeling it necessary to compete.

M.   Sports and Headache

"One should be able to recognize those who have headaches from gymnastic exercises or running or walking or hunting or any other unseasonable labor or from immoderate venery." So wrote Hippocrates. Many exercise-related symptoms, including headache, have appeared with the mushrooming of participant sports in this country (4). Previously, exercise-induced headaches were worthy of reporting. Now this is a frequent complaint though definitive figures on its incidence are not available. Acute headache associated with exercise, straining, coughing, sneezing, laughing, or stooping can be a symptom of life-threatening intracranial disorders, or may result from poorly understood benign cause. Exertional headache must be distinguished from the more common aggravation by exercise of an established headache. This is particularly true of vascular headaches of the migrainous type which often increase in severity with physical exertion. An exception is cluster headache, which may be alleviated by short-term exercise. Premenstrual symptoms, including headache, improve in some instances with endurance training placing such activity into the therapeutic armamentarium for this condition. So-called benign exertional headache is commoner in men than in women and is more frequent in older individuals. Organic lesions associated with exertional headache are rare but include Arnold–Chiari deformities, platybasia, basilar impression, chronic and subacute subdural hematoma, hemangioendothelioma, and parietal gliomas. In such conditions, the type of exercise is not specific, but the severity of the headache is related to the degree of effort. Headache onset in a particular site is not characteristic of a specific lesion, but in exertional headache unassociated with organic intracranial disease, the pain may be bilateral, frontal, occipital, or generalized. Benign exertional headache is usually abrupt in onset, often severe, may be sharp, stabbing, or lancinating and lasts for minutes and may outlast the exercise for a time. The etiology of "benign exertional" headache in nonathletes is obscure. Scalp tenderness is not present and the pain is not influenced by pressure on the scalp or extracranial vessels. In a large series of brain tumors, the associated headaches were only rarely exertional. Similarly, in subdural hematomas, exertional headache is rare.

The treatment of exertional headache associated with recognizable pathology is that of the primary problem. Benign exertional headache unassociated with intracranial lesions in nonathletes has been treated with sedatives, analgesics, and ergot preparations alone or combined without much success. In nonathletes with benign exertional headache, 75 mg/day of indomethacin is occasionally helpful.

Rare brain tumors associated with exertional headache are sometimes also characterized by headache induced by changes in position or precipiated by effort. This rarely occurs, but characteristically, in intermittent obstruction of CSF pathways in the third or fourth ventricle usually by colloid cysts. This type of headache is frontal or fronto-occipital and can be bilateral or unilateral. The headache is sometimes relieved by sudden changes in position opposite to that which triggered it. Vomiting may be present at the height of the pain and visual disturbances, clouded sensorium, tinnitus, and impaired alertness, often intermittent, have been reported.

Significant hemorrhage into previously unrecognized brain tumors has been reported in two joggers. These may have been related to the rise in blood pressure (proportional to physical fitness) during the first few minutes of exercise and to the fragility of blood vessels within the tumor.

1. EFFORT MIGRAINE

Migrainous attacks after athletic effort of any kind can occur, but tend to be more frequent at high altitude, which in itself is a migraine trigger. During Olympic competitions in Mexico City (elevation: 4375 m), effort migraine was frequent and recurrent in some athletes with repeated competition. Many effort migraine attacks have only part of the syndrome, scotomata, which usually occur immediately after exertion. Hyperventilation, nausea, and then severe pulsatile retro-orbital, unilateral pain, indistinguishable from ophthalmic migraine, may occur. This is rare in well-trained athletes. It is more common in poorly trained individuals and in this setting may be precipitated by dehydration, excessive heat load, hypoglycemia, and unaccustomed altitude. The pain is intense and throbbing and may be occipital or frontal. Focal neurological deficits other than scotomata are not seen, though threatening intracranial disorders are often feared. Headaches of this type are generally benign and are not apt to recur with repeated exertion provided physical fitness improves and other precipitating factors are avoided.

Occasionally would-be athletes, inexperienced and untrained, have exertional headache at low levels of activity. Such people complain of occipital, throbbing headache accompanied by nausea. Focal neurological symptoms or signs are not present, and the pain is aggravated by increasing effort and neck movement. Such pain may persist for hours after cessation of exertion. Support of the neck muscles and analgesics taken before exertion prevent attacks.

Ischemic muscular exercise can be associated with excruciating headaches. This has been reported in patients with occlusion of the aorta below the origin of renal vessels and also in subjects who performed treadmill exercise with circulation to the legs experimentally occluded. With ischemic work, blood pressure rises to levels comparable to those found during hypertensive crises, and the height of the blood pressure is related to the degree of ischemia. The reflex increase in blood pressure presumably causes the headache.

Paroxysmal neurogenic hypertension in quadriplegics is accompanied by elevated plasma catecholamines. However, norepinephrine levels achieved by infusion must be 21 times higher than those in quadriplegics in order to raise the blood pressure to similar heights. Therefore, the plasma norepinephrine per se is probably not the cause of neurogenic hypertension and headache in paraplegics or in those performing ischemic exercise. The pathogenetic importance of catecholamines in the headache associated with physical activity (which increases plasma catecholamines), in autonomic hyperreflexia, or in coital headache has not been assessed.

2. HEADACHE AT ALTITUDE

Mountain sickness is an acute disorder, which includes, among other things, headache. It occurs in unacclimatized individuals above an altitude of 2600 m. It is more frequent when ascent is rapid and is characterized by throbbing usually generalized head pain, though it may be predominantly frontal. The headache is aggravated by exertion, coughing, straining, or sudden jolts to the head, and also by lying down. It may be transiently improved by ingestion of cold fluids. Because subjects are anorectic, it is necessary to force food and carbohydrate intake. Carbohydrates may protect against altitude headache whereas other foods tend to increase the pain. The cause of altitude headache is not completely understood, but it does not seem to be an immediate hypoxic effect since it takes 6–9 hours after arrival at altitude before it develops. Severe mountain sickness headache may precede serious manifestations of altitude-induced cerebral edema, usually a complication of rapid, very high altitude exposure seen mainly in mountaineers. The pathogenesis of high altitude cerebral edema is not fully explained, but intracranial pressure rises with ascent and papilledema and retinal hemorrhages occur. Shifts of fluid from extracellular to intracellular compartments and reduced plasma volume may all play a part. Altitude illness including altitude headache may be prevented by acclimatization, that is, a 2- to 4-day stay at intermediate altitudes (1200–1300 m) and gradual ascent to higher levels. Supplemental oxygen is useful, particularly during sleep. Descent to lower elevations abolishes mountain sickness headache. Hypnotic drugs and similar medications should be avoided because they depress respiration. Acetazolamide can prevent or diminish the symptoms of acute altitude exposure and is best taken before ascent. Though the effect of the drug is transient, it gives enough respite for physiological compensation and thus allows acclimatization. Furosemide has also been reported to be useful and ergotamine tartrate may relieve pulsatile headache at high altitudes.

3. DIVING HEADACHES

Skip breathing, common in recreational and some professional dives, is said to cause headache. Many experienced divers do not suffer from the headache even though they continue to skip breathe. Those who do get headaches are thought to have it on the basis of increased CO_2 levels and increased sensitivity of cerebral arteries to vasodilatation by CO_2. Moreover, exercise at depth may further raise the CO_2 level because of faster production and decreased respiratory excretion from the slower ventilatory rate. Nevertheless, the commonest cause of headache associated with diving is sinus pain. The cold and, perhaps, allergies may cause mucous membrane swelling and block sinus drainage. The pressure within the sinuses can no longer be equalized with environmental pressure and pain results.

If the teeth contain gas pockets, diving can precipitate toothache. Muscle contraction headache can develop from gripping the mouthpiece tightly with the teeth. A similar headache occurs in luge because of the prolonged and strong contraction of neck and jaw muscles during competition and training. This is said to be markedly improved by use of a biteplate.

Scotomas and headache developed in some volunteers in hyperbaric chambers, but most who had these symptoms were known migraineurs. Decreased platelet counts and increased platelet clumping has been documented after depth diving. It is possible that neurological accompaniments of migraine are initiated by platelet-related events, which have been implicated in the aura of migraine at any elevation. Platelet clumping releases vasoactive substances, which may trigger a migraine attack.

Exercise may also induce headaches in patients with pheochromocytoma. In a relatively large number of patients with proved pheochromocytomas, only a few had exertion-related headaches. Most of them experienced episodic headache not clearly associated with exercise.

4. HEAD TRAUMA AND MIGRAINE

Athletes who subject their heads to frequent trauma as part of their sport may suffer from migraine. Soccer players and occasionally boxers develop migrainous attacks after heading the ball or taking a blow on the head. These attacks of classic migraine with tunnel or blurred vision or ill-defined gaps in the visual fields occur within a few minutes of the injury. Football players also develop migraine in relation to head injury and occasional migraineurs have been found among rugby players and wrestlers. Sometimes, sensory and motor symptoms, visual deficits combined with somnolence and occasionally speech problems and confusion, accompany sport-induced posttraumatic migraine. Oral ergotamine before a game prevented headache in some sufferers, but protection was not complete.

5. JOGGER'S HEADACHE

Runners and joggers often complain of ill-defined head pain, but the pathogenesis of this is not clear. Hypothetically, the exercise-associated increased secretion of endogenous opioids and the accompanying opioid-induced gastric stasis might trigger headache by stimulation of the gastric branch of the vagus nerve which also contains a meningeal branch. This, in turn, might cause vasodilatation of meningeal vessels and give rise to headache.

Effort-associated rupture of intracranial aneurysms occurs. This, however, is rare during physical activity associated with athletics, though its possibility is uppermost in the minds of physicians and knowledgeable subjects. Similarly, initial rupture of arteriovenous malformations must be extremely rare during athletic events. Though it is said that many of the symptoms of migraine can be mimicked by arteriovenous malformations, particularly if they are situated in the posterior parts of the hemispheres. Nevertheless, exertion, whether athletic or otherwise, that raises systemic blood pressure is contraindicated in persons with known aneurysms or arteriovenous malformations until the vascular abnormality is corrected.

N. Stroke and Transient Ischemic Attacks, Multiple Sclerosis, and Degenerative Central Nervous System Diseases

Patients with completed strokes and progressive central nervous system disease have completed marathons and ultramarathons. In general, however, those with transient ischemic attacks (TIA) should not exercise since TIAs may result from emboli to the cerebral circulation and exercise might increase this risk.

Patients with multiple sclerosis in remission have participated in games and even in endurance training. Increased environmental and body temperatures may, however, aggravate existing symptoms or bring on new ones. Clearly those patients who are sensitive to heat should not participate in activities that tend to raise body temperature. Many multiple sclerosis patients with stable disease find that exercise improves strength and dexterity of affected parts, and these persons can participate or even compete within the limits of their disability.

O. Exercise-Induced Syncope

Syncope results from global cerebral ischemia due to failure of cerebral perfusion. Perfusion failure and syncope in athletes during or at the end of an athletic event are usually related to either hyperthermia with the previously discussed mechanism of drop in cardiac output, or occurs with alcohol intake after prolonged exertion. During prolonged exercise, blood vessels to the muscles are maximally dilated and those to the skin are maximally constricted. Alcohol ingestion causes vasodilatation of skin vessels (direct vasodilator effect). Cutaneous vasodilatation while blood vessels to muscles are still dilated compromises cardiac output to the extent that it is no longer sufficient to perfuse the brain and syncope results.

The treatment of syncope is directed at the cause. If the patient is hyperthermic, volume replacement and cooling, discussed previously, are appropriate. If syncope is associated with alcohol consumption, horizontal positioning for a time allows cardiac output to maintain brain perfusion.

P. Exercise and Endorphins

Evidence exists that movement induces endogenous opioids secretion, particularly β-endorphin and β-lipotropin, and recent studies indicate that endurance training enhances the movement-induced secretion of these substances. On the other hand, transcendental meditation, which does not involve rhythmic movements, but is associated with tranquility or heightened awareness similar to that experienced during prolonged athletic performance, does not change endogenous opioid levels. Secretion of these substances varies with the length of the endurance event, and with very prolonged physical activity, endorphin levels decrease even though work output remains the same. For example, during long runs in the Himalayas, endorphins were markedly increased during the first 3 or 4 days of the expedition. Subsequently, despite similar terrain and miles per day, endorphin levels of the runners returned to base line. Additionally, studies of participants in a yearly mountain race showed that the percentage increase of β-endorphin at the end of the race, though still statistically significantly higher than before the race, decreased in a significant manner in the same individuals and race in a subsequent year. Whether this progressive and significant decrease in the secretion of movement-induced β-endorphin in highly trained endurance athletes signifies decreasing stress of the race with continued training or a feedback inhibition remains unknown.

Though changes in endogenous opioids with exercise have been seized on by behaviorists as explaining the anecdotally reported effects of endurance training on mood, this link has not been satisfactorily established and remains highly problematic. β-Endorphins are significantly elevated in the circulation for only a short time after termination of exercise making it unlikely that they are responsible for exercise-related mood and behavior changes. Central nervous system opioids, on the other hand, affect mood and behavior, but the relationship of these to exercise is unknown. Circulating opioid levels may not reflect brain levels or indicate opioid receptor function. At present, the evidence from animal and other studies does not indicate that endurance training affects central neuropeptide levels or receptor function (1).

REFERENCES

1. Appenzeller, O. (1981). What makes us run? *N. Engl. J. Med.* **305,** 578–580.
2. Appenzeller, O. (1982). "The Autonomic Nervous System: An Introduction to Basic and Clinical Concepts," 3rd ed. Elsevier North-Holland Biomedical Press, Amsterdam.
3. Appenzeller, O., and Atkinson, R., eds. (1981). "Sports Medicine: Fitness·Training·Injuries." Urban & Schwarzenberg, Baltimore, Maryland.
4. Atkinson, R., and Appenzeller, O. (1981). Headache in sports. *Semin. Neurol.* **1,** 334–344.
5. Bar-Or, O. (1980). Climate and the exercising child—a review. *Int. J. Sports Med.* **1,** 53–65.
6. Bar-Or, O. *et al.* (1980). Voluntary hypohydration in 10- to 12-year-old boys. *J. Appl. Physiol.* **48,** 104–108.
7. Bennett, D. R. (1981). Sports and epilepsy: To play or not to play. *Semin. Neurol.* **1,** 345–357.
8. Challenor, Y. B. (1981). Exercise and the handicapped child. *Semin. Neurol.* **1,** 358–364.

9. Committee on the Medical Aspects of Sports of the American Medical Association (1979). "Medical Evaluation of the Athlete: A Guide." AMA, Chicago, Illinois.

10. Committee on Sports Medicine, American Academy of Pediatrics (1982). Climatic heat stress and the exercising child. *Pediatrics* **69,** 808–809.

11. Greenhouse, A. H. (1981). The relation of physical activity to disorders of neurologic function. *Semin. Neurol.* **1,** 237–241.

12. Greer, H. D. (1981). Neurologic casualties in diving. *Semin. Neurol.* **1,** 263–274.

13. Moxley, R. T., III (1981). Muscle and "muscle-like" complaints associated with sports: Potential out-patient problems for the neurologist. *Semin. Neurol.* **1,** 324–333.

14. Petajan, J. H. (1981). The effects of high altitude on the nervous system and athletic performance. *Semin. Neurol.* **1,** 253–262.

15. Weber, L. E. (1981). Sport injuries at the peripheral nerve, plexus, and nerve root levels. *Semin. Neurol.* **1,** 291–300.

CHAPTER **11**

Cardiovascular Disorders and Exercise

ALFRED A. BOVE
*Cardiovascular Division
and Department of
Physiology
Mayo Foundation
Rochester, Minnesota*

229

Exercise Medicine: Physiological Principles
and Clinical Applications

I. BASIC PRINCIPLES

In years past, a common approach to the patient with cardiac disease was to discourage exercise and thus commit the patient to life-long sedentary behavior which often resulted in permanent physiological and psychological impairment. Because of a lack of understanding of the cardiovascular adaptation to exercise, many physicians in the earlier part of the twentieth century were not willing to advise indivuals with heart disease to participate in limited amounts of exercise. Rather, the advice generally was given to follow a program of total inactivity to avoid undue stress to the heart (1). This concept is still advocated for treatment of severe cardiomyopathies (2,3), but over the past 20 to 30 years, changing concepts of the cardiovascular responses to exercise have allowed physiologists and physicians dealing with heart disease patients to develop an approach to the patient with cardiovascular disease which includes some degree of physical activity tailored to the patient's needs and capacity. These newer concepts have allowed a more liberal approach to children with heart disease, and many children previously considered to be incapable of strenuous exercise are able to lead normal lives with participation in all types of exercise. This change in the approach to patients with heart disease is based on physiological studies that have provided a better understanding of the responses of the cardiovascular system and the heart to exercise.

Since physical exercise requires increased mechanical activity of skeletal muscle, and since skeletal muscle requires increased oxygen and fuel to produce increased activity, the heart and circulation are affected by all levels of exercise. The cardiovascular system normally demonstrates an immediate response to exercise (5,6). This response includes local alterations in blood flow and vascular resistance which evoke reflexes that stimulate the heart to provide an increased cardiac output. Because of this inevitable challenge to the cardiovascular system by exercise, patients with cardiac disorders often first manifest symptoms with exercise.

From the cardiovascular standpoint, exercise is anything that raises the resting oxygen consumption above basal levels. Thus, climbing a flight of stairs, walking at a comfortable but reasonable pace, and lifting small or heavy objects, are all sensed by the heart and cardiovascular system as forms of exercise and require an increased output (7). Since, exercise is an important component of normal activity for survival (8) (i.e., for obtaining food and defending against natural enemies), all mammals are equipped with a reserve system that allows for performance at higher than resting levels of physical activity without producing injury or damage to organ or tissue systems. The principle that most tissues and organs contain a functional reserve is well accepted and applies also to the heart (7, 8). Thus, the heart at rest is working at a small percentage of its maximal capacity, and measurement of maximal cardiac performance may be necessary to accurately assess the extent of heart disease in a given patient. Reduction of the maximal capacity of the heart and circulation occurs early in heart disease and may be undetected for long periods of time unless the patient or physician tests the reserve and finds it diminished, or cardiac impairment progresses to the point where the loss of reserve is significant enough to affect resting cardiac performance.

Early work by Master (9) and subsequent studies by Bruce (10,11), Ellestad (12), Naughton (13), and others (14,15) have pointed out the need to measure cardiovascular reserve when assessing an individual with heart disease. Based on this principle, exercise stress testing has become a useful clinical means of assessing cardiovascular reserve. Although exercise testing is often used to detect coronary disease, its application in testing for cardiac reserve is also important and useful (10–12). With the addition of measurements of left ventricular performance during exercise using radionuclide techniques (16,17), it is now possible to assess overall physical performance during exercise and measure specific alterations in the heart which will identify abnormal cardiovascular responses to exercise (18,19).

In dealing with patients with heart disease, it is important to understand the relationships among external physical exercise or work, myocardial work, myocardial oxygen consumption, and blood flow to the myocardium. Understanding these relationships will provide the basis for assessing the performance of an individual with heart disease in an exercise environment.

II. CARDIAC WORK, OXYGEN CONSUMPTION, AND BLOOD FLOW

It is generally accepted that the heart does not markedly increase its extraction of oxygen as its work demands increase. Usually only a small increase in oxygen extraction occurs (e.g., from 10 to 12 ml of oxygen per 100 ml of blood) whereas large increases in myocardial blood flow provide the increased oxygen needs when myocardial work load increase (20) (Fig. 1).

Work on the physiology of the coronary arteries by Wiggers and co-workers in 1935–1940 (21) and later by Sarnoff *et al.* (22) demonstrated the relationship of blood flow to cardiac work. It was found that increased cardiac work could arise from increases in arterial pressure with little change in the amount of blood flow passing through the heart (pressure work), or by increases in blood flow with almost constant pressure (volume work). It is possible to have types of exercise which will produce either primarily pressure work on the heart or primarily volume work on the heart. For example, isometric exercises associated with heavy lifting raises the arterial blood pressure and causes an increase pressure load on the heart, whereas the work associated with aerobic exercise such as

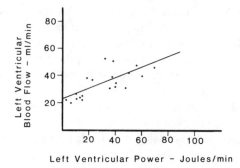

Fig. 1.   Blood flow–power relationships in the heart.

running causes an increase flow demand on the heart and results in a volume load on the heart. The studies of Sarnoff *et al.* (22) demonstrated that a pressure work load is more demanding in terms of myocardial oxygen consumption than an equivalent volume work load. It is important to remember this difference when prescribing exercise programs for individuals with impaired myocardial oxygen supply.

Work by Gregg and co-workers (23,24) detailed the relationships among cardiac contraction, oxygen consumption, and myocardial blood flow. From these studies it has become evident that the myocardium depends on increasing blood flow to supply oxygen demands; when flow restrictions occur, for example, in the presence of coronary stenosis, the myocardium cannot obtain adequate oxygen by increasing oxygen extraction. A recent study in dogs by Bache (25) demonstrated endocardial blood flow deficits that occur during exercise in the presence of coronary narrowing.

In addition to the overall blood flow response to exercise, it is also important to have some understanding of the distribution of blood flow in the myocardium. Recent investigations, taking advantage of the flow distribution measurements provided by radioactive microspheres, have demonstrated that blood flow distribution in the myocardium is not uniform at rest or during increase work loads. Normally the endocardium requires more blood flow, a finding that fits with the concept that the stress in the endocardial layers of the myocardium is greater than in the epicardium (26,27). Thus, on the average, endocardial fibers produce greater amounts of work and demand somewhat greater amounts of blood flow. Normal endocardial–epicardial blood flow ratios are often 1.2–1.4 (27), suggesting that flow to the endocardium is normally greatest at rest and during exercise. Factors in the myocardium and in the coronary artery distribution system may act to product a maldistribution of blood in the myocardium, and this flow maldistribution must be considered when evaluating patients with underlying heart disease for exercise. Chronic pressure or volume overload-induced hypertrophy of the myocardium, coronary artery disease, and congenital heart disease all may affect myocardial oxygen consumption, myocardial blood flow, and blood flow distribution to the myocardium. Better understanding of the these blood flow principles will aid significantly in assessing the expected results of an exercise exposure in an individual that has a cardiac disorder.

III. CORONARY ARTERY DISEASE

Coronary artery disease is the most highly prevalent, life-threatening disease in the United States. It affects 2 million people per year with new onset of the disease, and 500,000 people per year die from coronary artery disease (28). From the physiological standpoint, the basic abnormality of coronary disease is partial or complete obstruction of the epicardial coronary arteries, which are the main conductance vessels for transmitting blood from the aorta to the myocardial microcirculation. Complete or partial occulsion of one or more coronary arteries limits the blood flow that can be delivered to the myocardium, and in the presence of increased myocardial demand or in the presence of additional coronary vasoconstriction, myocardium becomes ischemic. If ischemia is prolonged or severe enough, there will be death of myocardial cells, i.e., myocardial infarction. Exercise has been well established as an important component of the treatment of patients with coronary artery disease (29) as a rehabilitation measure after myocardial infarction, angina pectoris, or cardiac surgery; in the prevention of coronary disease in asymptomatic patients (30–32); and in patients not suspected of having such disease as a means for reducing known coronary risk factors. The basic principle that should guide the physician in caring for patients with coronary disease who wish to exercise is that exercise prescriptions must be tailored to each individual in such a way that myocardial ischemia is prevented during exercise. This principle can be applied to nearly all patients with coronary disease except those with acute myocardial infarction or unstable angina pectoris. Even patients with moderate to severe left ventricular failure may be provided with low-level exercise programs to match their markedly reduced exercise tolerance.

Coronary stenosis limits the blood flow that can pass through the stenosed artery (33). The total resistance to flow in the coronary artery includes the resistance of the peripheral vascular bed plus the resistance of the stenosis (34). As long as the stenosis is mild, flow can be controlled by the resistance of peripheral vascular bed and normal coronary blood flow response to the increased work load of exercise will occur. When a stenosis becomes significant (greater than 50% reduction in cross-sectional area), resistance of the stenosis at high flow rates becomes significant and will limit the ability of the peripheral coronary circulation to control flow (35). As the stenosis becomes more severe, its resistance becomes a significant component of the total resistance to flow, and ultimately a stenosis that causes 85–90% narrowing is the dominant factor controlling flow through the coronary artery (36). When stenosis produces 90% narrowing, peripheral vascular regulation has little or no effect on altering blood flow under states of increased demand. In this situation, the maximal possible flow through the coronary artery may be adequate only to supply the myocardial demands at rest. Any amount of exercise above resting then will induce myocardial ischemia. It is evident from the stenosis versus flow characteristics of the coronary artery shown in Fig. 2 that resting studies used to detect the presence of myocardial ischemia may not reveal a severe underlying stenosis. In the presence of coronary stenosis it may be necessary to stress the myocardium to demonstrate the imbalance between myocardial flow capability and myocardial oxygen demand. There are several approaches to detecting these flow abnormalities clinically, and it is also possible through cardiac catheterization to outline the specific anatomic abnormality of the coronary vessel. Use of invasive and noninvasive tests for exercise evaluation of coronary patients will be discussed below.

There are several consequences of the induced imbalance between myocardial oxygen supply and demand during exercise-induced increases in cardiac work. Angina pectoris or serious ventricular arrhythmias may occur; the ischemic myocardium may develop an acute local or global reduction in contractile capability. The signs and symptoms that accompany this latter response include onset of a third heart sound with exercise, development of marked dyspnea on exertion, development of bibasilar rales shortly following exercise, fall in blood pressure with exercise, and early fatigue. Reduced contractile performance and possible

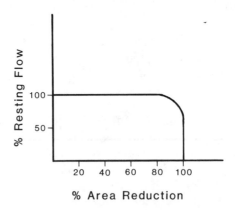

Fig. 2. Coronary flow versus degree of stenosis.

increases in diastolic stiffness induced by ischemia may combine to produce congestive heart failure during exercise. Coronary disease of this severity generally requires a thorough evaluation prior to development of an exercise therapy program, and often patients will require alteration of life-style, cessation of cigarette smoking, and drug therapy for stablization prior to instituting an exercise rehabilitation program.

An important component of coronary disease which has been recently reiterated is the presence in some patients of coronary vasomotion that produces instability of coronary stenoses under external stimuli such as emotional stress and possibly catecholamine release (36). Coronary vasomotion of this type can produce signs and symptoms of unstable angina. Several studies (37,38) have suggested that coronary vasomotion or coronary spasm may be induced by exercise in some patients who will demonstrate sudden onset of myocardial ischemia postexercise with S-T elevation, chest pain, and other indices of severe myocardial ischemia. These patients require treatment that differs from patients with anatomically fixed stenoses. Nitrates and calcium blocking drugs may be needed to control coronary vasomotion (39) prior to induction into an exercise rehabilitation program. Alterations in coronary arterial tone which result in changing severity of coronary stenosis may be detected by a history of spontaneous onset of angina pectoris at rest and sudden onset of angina shortly after exercise rather than a slow progressive onset of angina associated with exercise. Occasionally, 24-hour or long-term electrocardiographic monitoring with an appropriate search for alterations in S-T segment may be needed to find periodic episodes of asymptomatic ischemia. Maseri and co-workers (40) have demonstrated that patients who have a vasotonic component to their myocardial ischemia may show ischemia changes in the electrocardiogram in the absence of symptoms. When this type of response is thought to be present, clear documentation of the response must be obtained prior to developing an exercise program since the periodic ischemic episodes may coincide with exercise exposures.

The clinical consequences of coronary artery disease have been known for several centuries, and include the classic description of angina by Heberden in 1768 (41). In developing an exercise program for patients with known coronary disease, an initial effort should be made to instruct the patients on symptoms of myocardial ischemia. A discussion of pain symptoms should include chest pain or tightness, and information about nonthoracic pain such as arm and neck pain should also be provided so that the patient will not disregard important variants of anginal pain. In addition, significant ventricular arrhythmias may occur during exercise as a sole indicator of ischemia. Thus subjects undergoing exercise programs with coronary disease should be instructed on detection of arrhythmias either by pulse count or by perceiving the abnormal rhythm in the chest. Patients with dizziness or syncope following exercise who have coronary disease should be prevented from exercising until adequate rhythm monitoring can be obtained and serious ventricular arrhythmias can be ruled out as a cause of their syncope or lightheadedness. Changes in exercise tolerance may also occur when ischemic heart disease is severe enough to cause the ventricle to develop heart failure under the increased load state of exercise. In this case careful evaluation of the patient's exercise tolerance on a periodic basis with efforts to detect changes should provide information on the possible development of heart failure due to ischemic heart disease. The most troublesome patient with coronary disease is the patient who has no symptoms or arrhythmias but who develops marked ischemia detected only by electrocardiogram or by 24-hour ECG monitoring during exercise (not all patients with exercise ECG abnormalities have coronary disease, however). These patients require careful evaluation of exercise capacity to provide an exercise prescription or exercise guideline that prevents exercise intensities that induce myocardial ischemia. Patients with asymptomatic ischemia may be at greater risk for sudden death since they developed no premonitory symptoms when severe myocardial ischemia is occurring.

IV. EXERCISE PROGRAMS FOR PATIENTS WITH CORONARY DISEASE

A variety of programs have reported beneficial responses to exercise programs in coronary patients (29,30). These programs may be formal, providing frequent supervised exercise sessions often with continuous cardiac monitoring by telemetry, or they may be informal, with initial evaluation of the cardiac patient followed by description of a program to be followed without supervision. The benefits accrued from cardiac rehabilitation programs are difficult to define. There is ample physiological evidence that an exercise program improves the cardiovascular response to work (42,43); however, this response is due in large part to improved efficiency of skeletal muscle (44). It is not presently clear whether the moderate exercise programs provided to the cardiac patient are sufficient to provide this type of improved skeletal muscle performance. A study by Ehsani et al. (45) suggests that some benefit can be gained in poorly conditioned cardiac patients. Less easy to document it is the subjective response to exercise training. Supervisors of exercise programs and many subjects in exercise programs claim that an improved feeling of well-being and better outlook concerning their physical capacity and health image are important benefits of an exercise program (46). Similar responses are claimed by normal subjects who undertake regular exercise programs.

Present exercise rehabilitation programs for cardiac patients usually follow a well-established protocol (see Chapter 19). This protocol includes initial submaximal exercise testing to define the patients exercise capacity, exercise prescription based on the results of the exercise test, and then entrance of the patient into a supervised exercise program in which the exercise prescription is applied to the daily activities for the patient. These programs are generally designed to provide exercise work loads less than 70% of maximal, and may provide even lower work loads, depending on the general health status of the patient. In supervised programs, the exercise can be walking, slow jogging, or stationary bicycle exercise. Swimming can also be used; however, special care must be taken to prevent the individual interested in using swimming as an exercise for rehabilitation from becoming exposed to sudden plunges into cold water. Thermal changes of this type can induce reflex vasoconstriction, tachycardia, and a rise in blood pressure (47). These changes induce an increase in myocardial oxygen demand and may result in myocardial ischemia.

In most cardiac rehabilitation programs, three phases of activity can be defined. Phase 1 is provided to the patient during the early postmyocardial infarction period. This activity consists of minimal exercise either in bed or at the bedside even while the patient is in the Coronary Care Unit. It can include brief periods of sitting erect, simple arm activities that are necessary for self-care, and even passive range of motion activities provided by a physical therapist. These activities are usually increased during the hospitalization with the rate of progression judged by the patient's daily response. Ideally, during this early period each time the exercise activity is provided, heart rate, cardiac rhythm, and blood pressure should be recorded before and after the exposure to be certain that no adverse hemodynamic responses occur from this mild level of activity.

When the cardiac patient becomes ambulatory, Phase 1 activities can include walking, mild stretching exercises, and, near the completion of the hospital stay, possible use of stairs. Upon discharge from the hospital following acute myocardial infarction, most patients should be exercist tested at submaximal levels to determine their current exercise capacity, and to search for serious cardiac problems that might develop with the mild exercise necessary for normal activity outside the hospital. This early postinfarction submaximal exercise test can be used to describe the exercise needed to commence the next phase of cardiac rehabilitation. Phase 2 of rehabilitation is undertaken in the subsequent early weeks postmyocardial infarction and can last 8–12 weeks. The goal of this period is to restore the patient to a normal activity, including return to a normal working environment, reversal of any detraining effects that may have occurred during hospitalization, and education concerning cardiac risk factors and the role of exercise and other modalities useful for reducing further cardiac risk. Exercise activities in Phase 2 include walking on a treadmill, in a gymnasium, or outside, possibly alternating with activity on a stationary bicycle, mild calisthenics, and stretching exercises. The target heart rate used for the exercise prescription in Phase 2 is determined from the early postinfarction treadmill exercise test, and this exercise prescription is generally designed to maintain a work level below

70% achieved maximal, a value commonly lower than the normal age related expected maximal in the early postinfarction period. Exercise activities during Phase 2 are commonly supervised and may include on-line cardiac rhythm and rate telemetry. Phase 2 programs can also be used for patients recovering from cardiac surgery.

Phase 3 cardiac rehabilitation usually commences about 3 months following myocardial infarction or cardiac surgery. This phase is instituted by a treadmill exercise stress test that is done in an effort to achieve near maximal stress exposure. At that time, the exercise test should achieve 85–90% of maximal heart rate based on the assumption that after 3 months the patient is capable of full activity. An exercise prescription based on this test then is designed to stress the patient to 70% of his age related maximum, and the prescribed program may not involve supervision. During Phase 3, the patient may fulfill the exercise prescription by undertaking exercise activities that can be done at home. It is also possible to continue a patient desiring Phase 3 rehabilitation in a supervised program. Patients with known or suspected problems related to exercise should be in a supervised Phase 3 program.

The exercise test plays an important role in designing the exercise activity for Phase 2 and Phase 3 cardiac rehabilitation. It is difficult to properly prescribe an exercise program for a cardiac patient without first simulating the exercise exposure in the controlled environment available during an exercise test. The electrocardiogram and blood pressure should be monitored and the patient observed throughout the test for symptoms such as severe dyspnea, chest pain or tightness, palpitation, lightheadedness, or weakness. By integrating the clinical observations during exercise with the information provided by electrocardiogram and the recording of blood pressure, it is possible to assess a patient's capacity for physical activity. Patients with ischemic changes at low levels of exercise should have a further diagnostic study to determine the nature of their coronary disease, and patients who demonstrate serious ventricular arrhythmias should be treated prior to instituting an exercise program. A variety of clinical limitations to exercise can be detected by a standard submaximal exercise test where the patient is not severely stressed, but is stressed to levels that simulate normal daily activities (48). Three months after infarction when the patient is to return to full activity, a stress test is again indicated to determine the ability for the patient to return to full activity related to employment or recreation.

It is important to note that the exercise stress test in these applications is not considered to be a diagnostic study but rather a procedure for determining physical capacity and on which to base continuing therapy. It is quite possible that patients with known coronary disease may not demonstrate ischemic changes on the exercise electrocardiogram; conversly, it is possible for patients with no significant coronary obstruction to demonstrate a positive exercise stress test. Since in the coronary patient the diagnosis of coronary disease in general has already been made, one should not consider the exercise test in this application as a diagnostic procedure. Criticism of exercise testing because of a high frequency of false-positive studies in some populations is not pertinent to the application described above. Although the use of nuclear scanning techniques with exercise enhances the diagnostic accuracy of exercise tests (49,50), they are not needed to institute an exercise program for most patients with known coronary disease. However, in cases where there are electrocardiographic abnormalities that preclude observations for ischemia, such as left bundle branch block, the addition of a blood flow scan to the exercise test will often provide the information needed to determine if local ischemia is present. The abnormal S-T segments present at rest in left bundle branch block mask the ischemic changes that would commonly be found during exercise. In some instances gated blood pool scanning is useful when a patient is suspected of having congestive heart failure as part of his or her coronary disease. In these cases it is of importance to assess the performance of the left ventricle under an exercise load. Since the gated blood pool scan can provide a noninvasive estimate of left ventricular end diastolic volume, stroke volume, and ejection fraction, which correlate well with angiographic measurements (51), it is useful to obtain information of this type during exercise to determine whether a patient demonstrates progressive left ventricular failure during exercise. It is evident from numerous studies that a reduced ejection fraction can be found in many patient with coronary disease during exercise (49). This finding suggests that there is myocardial failure due to inadequate myocardial oxygen supply under exercise load. These patients may appear to have normal left ventricular function during a resting study. Often a revision of drug therapy can be made to minimize the degradation in ventricular performance during exercise and the response to drug therapy and exercise can be followed by the noninvasive assessment of ventricular performance provided by the gated blood pool technique.

It should be emphasized that nuclear studies are not necessary for developing an exercise program in most cardiac patients.

V. CARDIOVASCULAR DRUGS AND EXERCISE

Because patients referred for cardiac rehabilitation programs are often taking a variety of cardiac and blood pressure medications, it is necessary to understand the response of patients taking such medications to exercise.

Patients on large doses of antihypertensive medication may have significant inhibition of normal control mechanisms of the vascular system and may have poor exercise tolerance. Medications that inhibit blood pressure rise during exercise may result in exertional syncope. Because of these effects, these patients require careful attention to early signs and symptoms of inadequate blood pressure response during exercise and are best handled in a supervised program with frequent observations of blood pressure and on-line telemetry of heart rate.

Patients taking drugs that produce β-adrenergic blockade may also have unique problems with exercise. These patients have significant inhibition of heart response to exercise; therefore, measurement of heart rate does not provide the index of exercise work load which is generally found in the patients who have normal autonomic responsiveness (52,53). Because of this difference, one must carefully observe these patients for subjective signs of exercise level using perceived exercise scores (54). When stress testing a patient on β-blockade, a relative maximum heart rate can be achieved by comparing the perceived exercise score with the heart rate when the patient has significant fatigue. Once this maximum heart rate is determined, the usual rules for exercise prescription can be followed; however, if a calculated heart rate is exceptionally low for a training work load, some adjustment upward can be made so that the patient will have appropriate exercise in the program.

There is some suggestion that adrenergic blockade will inhibit maximum exercise performance, and although exercise programs are generally designed to avoid maximum performance and provide submaximal exercise exposures, it is important to advise individuals who wish to compete in athletic activities that their maximum capacity may be inhibited by β-blockade.

Although diagnostic stress testing should be done in the absence of β-blockade, when developing exercise prescription for a patient on these medications it is necessary to test exercise capacity in the presence of a full therapeutic regimen. In this way an exercise program can be designed to fit the drugs that the patient is taking. Normally if a patient has a change in the dose of cardiovascular medication especially β-blockers, the patient should have a repeat exercise stress test to determine the heart rate response so that a new exercise prescription can be provided in the presence of the new drug dose.

Patients on nitrate medications for coronary disease generally have no specific problems related with nitrates. It is desirable that the patient not take nitrates immediately prior to exercise because of their blood pressure lowering effect. However, in some patients with angina, the ingestion of nitrates immediately prior to exercise will enhance exercise tolerance. Judgment concerning the taking of nitrate medications prior to exercise should be made for each patient individually.

VI. EXERCISE IN PATIENTS WITH CHRONIC HEART FAILURE

A. Cardiovascular Response to Exercise in Congestive Heart Failure

Many patients with chronic congestive heart failure seek to improve their capacity for physical activity so that they can perform normal activities associated with employment or daily existence. To fulfill this goal, patients with heart failure can be entered into exercise rehabilitation programs. To date, evidence suggests that the advantage gained by exercise training is primarily in the alteration in the adaptation of skeletal muscle to exercise (44). This alteration allows skeletal muscle to extract more oxygen per unit of blood flowing through the muscle, therefore requiring less blood flow for a given external work load and thereby reducing the cardiac output. For the same reason, systemic blood pressure may be lower and blood pressure control may be enhanced during exercise (see Chapter 14). Although these responses are not direct cardiac effects, they tend to unload the heart during exercise so that myocardial oxygen demand and myocardial work are reduced for a given work load. Presently, there are few data to suggest that significant alterations in myocardial performance or in blood flow delivery to the myocardium occur in response to exercise (55,56). Several studies on collateral circulation during exercise done in experimental animals, however, have shown that exercise does enhance the distribution of collateral blood flow in regions distal to coronary stenoses (57,58).

In patients with congestive heart failure, the basic principle of first exercise testing to determine work capacity and heart rate response should be adhered to. In this case, however, heart rate response should be only one of the variables used to determine exercise capacity. In the presence of heart failure the heart rate response will be exaggerated so that extremely high heart rates will be achieved at low work loads. This response indicates that myocardial performance is reduced and an excess catecholamine response occurs during exercise in attempt to enhance cardiac output (59). Observation of the blood pressure, the patient's state of respiration, and general status during exercise are also important and will determine an end point for exercise testing and exercise prescription. Commonly with exercise, a patient with heart failure will develop increased left ventricular end diastolic pressure and pulmonary congestion, manifested as excess dyspnea. Examination at this time will reveal an increased intensity or the presence of a third heart sound. The object of an exercise program in the patient with congestive heart failure is to provide an exercise exposure that does not induce pulmonary congestion but that provides the patient with improved capacity of their skeletal muscle by training. Determining an optimal level of exercise is often difficult and the assessment of the patient's progress may require frequent stress test reevaluation to provide the best exercise prescription for these patients. The evaluation of left ventricular performance available from an exercise nuclear study is useful in determining a patient's response to exercise. Marked decline in ejection fraction associated with exercise should be avoided, and an exercise prescription should be designed to take advantage of the fact that exercise ejection fraction may remain stable at low exercise levels and will fall with higher levels of exercise.

Also of importance in considering an exercise program for the patient with congestive heart failure is the interaction of various heart failure medications with exercise. Many patients with congestive heart failure are being treated with digitalis derivatives, diuretics, and blood pressure lowering drugs for reducing afterload on the left ventricle. The considerations for blood pressure lowering medications are those mentioned previously for patients being treated for hypertension (see Chapter 14). These agents block autonomic responses to exercise, and may cause hypotension during exercise. Patients taking digitalis generally have no problem with exercise. It is important to note that digitalis can cause S-T segment alterations in the stress test which appear as ischemic changes but are not necessarily related to coronary artery disease. Patients on digitalis for atrial fibrillation may have inhibition of heart rate response because of the arterioventricular block induced by the drug. In this case as in the case of β-blockade the heart rate response cannot be used as a reliable indicator of the intensity of exercise and a perceived exertion score (54), plus observation of the patient for dyspnea, alterations of blood pressure, or third heart sound are more useful than heart rate alone in this setting. Patients on diuretics generally do not have significant interaction of these drugs with exercise. In the case of excess diuretic effect, with decreased circulating blood volume, patients may develop reduced exercise tolerance, low cardiac output, and hypotension during exercise. Potassium depletion induced by diuretics can also produce muscle weakness. Patients exercising in hot environments may also experience excess fluid loss when taking diuretics. Thus, patients taking diuretics should be cautioned to maintain adequate fluid intake before, during, and after exercise in warm environments.

B. Signs and Symptoms of Heart Failure Induced by Exercise

When designing an exercise program for patients with congestive heart failure, it is helpful to advise the patient about symptoms that will provide clues to inadequate circulatory response to exercise. In addition, exercise supervisors should be trained to watch for signs associated with inappropriate exercise response. Heart rate alone may be an unreliable indicator of exercise work level in these patients either because of drugs that interfere with the heart rate response or because abnormal electrocardiographic findings may prevent the observation of ischemic changes of the electrocardiogram. Lung congestion will induce dyspnea when significant elevation of left ventricular diastolic pressure occurs (60). Thus, warning the patient that excess dyspnea should be avoided and instructing exercise supervisors to observe patients for severe dyspnea should help prevent exercise at levels that cause significant pulmonary congestion.

Many patients with cardiomyopathy and congestive heart failure develop chest pain that may be associated with a relatively inadequate blood flow occurring with dilation of the heart and increased oxygen demand during periods of increased venous return (61,62). In addition, chest sensations interpreted as pain are often related by patients who have arrhythmias during exercise. Dealing with nonanginal chest pain in patients with heart failure is often difficult. It is sometimes helpful to allow the patient to exercise with minimal amounts of chest discomfort as long as ischemia and cardiac arrhythmias can be reasonably ruled out as causes. The nonspecific chest pains induced by exercise may inhibit the training response because of an attempt to maintain an exercise level which produces no chest discomfort.

Patients with congestive heart failure may develop syncope with exercise because of inability to generate an appropriate cardiac output, vasodilation of skeletal muscle, and lowering of blood pressure (63). This response will be aggrevated by the presence of medications that inhibit autonomic response such as those used for afterload reduction or hypertension. Careful monitoring of blood pressure during the initial exercise test and periodic evaluation of blood pressure during exercise training in patients with heart failure will provide information on the threshold for safe exercise. Many times, exercise levels must be kept quite low in the patient with heart failure.

C. Development of an Exercise Program for the Patient with Congestive Heart Failure

To design an exercise program for a patient with congestive heart failure, the basic principles of exercise rehabilitation should be followed (see Chapter 19). Evaluation should include an exercise test with heart rate and blood pressure measurements, and a careful assessment of the patient's general response to exercise including pattern of breathing, onset of dyspnea, skin color, and mental state. Stress tests for patients with heart failure are generally done at lower levels, and exercise prescriptions may be of quite low intensity compared to that given to a relatively asymptomatic patient following coronary bypass surgery, for example. For patients who have abnormal electrocardiograms that mask ischemic changes the addition of a nuclear study with exercise can be useful. The information obtained from a single exercise nuclear test can be used both to understand the cardiac resonse exercise in terms of ejection fraction and diastolic size, and the electrocardiographic correlates of this finding. An exercise prescription can be designed from the work load achieved during the nuclear study so that one test can provide all the information necessary to prescribe the program. Patients should be maintained on their usual medications when tested. However, patients on vasodepressor agents should be observed for alterations of blood pressure which would suggest inadequate vasomotor control and the possibility of syncope. Patients with arrhythmias should be maintained on antiarrhythmic drugs and observation of cardiac rhythm during exercise should be emphasized. In patients with cardiac arrhythmias and congestive heart failure good communication among the physicians providing treatment is needed to arrive at an appropriate antiarrhythmic regimen properly adjusted to fit the patients' exercise program.

VII. VALVULAR AND CONGENITAL HEART DISEASE

With patients that have valvular heart disease or some form of congenital heart disease, two questions must be addressed: first, one must question what increased physical activity will do to the overload state that is present on the heart as a result of the valvular or congenital lesion. Second, one must question the overall circulatory response to exercise in the presence of the lesion. The presence of an abnormality per se is not a contraindication to exercise. However, the consequences of exercise on either the myocardium or on the ability of the heart to supply the necessary blood flow must be considered.

A. Pathophysiological Principles

In considering the pathophysiology of the various lesions one should be cognizant of the myocardial consequences of the lesions. Overload lesions of the heart can be classed as either pressure or volume overload types (64). Pressure overload lesions include the concentric left ventricular hypertrophy that results from aortic stenosis (65), whereas volume overload of the left ventricle can occur from aortic or mitral regurgitation (66,67) or in the right ventricle from atrial-septal defect (68). The response of the myocardium to these overload states is different depending on whether the overload is a pressure or volume type. Indeed, the myocardium appears to adapt specifically to handle the type of load imposed on it.

In either type of hypertrophy the increased muscle mass that occurs in response to chronic overload demands an increased myocardial blood flow (69). Thus, the blood flow to either the pressure or volume overloaded hypertrophied heart is increased above normal resting levels. It is presently unclear whether maximum blood flow remains the same or is limited by a relative undergrowth of the vascular bed in relationship to the amount of contracting muscle tissue. Experimental evidence suggests that in pressure overload hypertrophy there is a reduction in the capillary to myocardial cell volume ratio, thus leaving the myocardium with the inability to adequately perfuse all areas of heart muscle under high load states (70). Because of this relative underperfusion, it is likely that zones of ischemia may occur in severe pressure overload hypertrophy. The subendocardial ischemia found on the exercise ECG in aortic stenosis and chronic hypertension with hypertrophy is one example of an abnormal flow distribution in hypertrophied myocardium. The flow and capillary to cell ratio in chronic volume overload hypertrophy is less well documented. Some evidence does suggest that there is, like the changes found in pressure overload hypertrophy, a reduction in the capillary to cell volume ratio suggesting that regions of the volume overloaded heart may also be underperfused under states where flow demands are high (71).

In all instances it is reasonable to assume that the first areas to be rendered ischemic during increased exercise in hypertrophied hearts will be the subendocardial zones of the myocardium. This occurs for several reasons: first, the forces in the subendocardial layers of the myocardium are higher, thus requiring somewhat greater oxygen demand from the cells of the endocardial regions; second, the resistance vessel of the subendocardium are most distant from the supplying arteries which reside in the epicardium. Early hypertrophy, which may even be undetected by electrocardiogram, can be associated with evidence of subendocardial ischemia as detected by exercise stress testing for example (72). Fortunately, the changes induced in the endocardium by maldistribution of blood flow under exercise loads is often detected by the exercise stress test, which can be used to evaluate the presence or absence of subendocardial ischemia in patients who have volume or pressure overloads due to acquired or congenital heart disease. Although there are specific exceptions (see below), it is possible to provide an exercise prescription for patients with congenital or valvular heart disease. Here again, the basic principle of simulating the exercise exposure in the controlled environment of the exercise stress test with electrocardiographic and blood pressure monitoring should be followed. This information is then used to determine the individual patient's capacity for exercise. By approaching the patient with valvular or congenital heart disease in this manner, it is possible to achieve a level of exercise below that which would induce ischemia of the myocardium or produce excess overload.

B. Circulatory Considerations

Certain specific circulatory abnormalities which are present in acquired valvular and congenital heart disease need special consideration when involving patients in exercise programs. Patients with circulatory obstruction such as aortic stenosis, mitral stenosis, aortic coarctation, or pulmonic stenosis may have limitations to exercise because of the resistance to forward flow and inadequate cardiac output that may occur because of the narrowed segment of the circulation. When an imbalance occurs between peripheral circulatory demand and cardiac output, blood pressure will fall and the patient will develop syncope. Indeed, this mechanism may be one of the causes for sudden death in patients with aortic stenosis. Although it is generally not advised to perform exercise stress tests in patients with significant obstructing lesions, these patients must perform some level of exercise in their daily activity. Because it is useful to document the exercise tolerance of individuals with obstructive circulatory lesions, carefully controlled submaximal exercise testing may be done to assess a patient's capacity for exercise. When conducting an exercise stress test in such a patient, it is important to monitor not only heart rate and electrocardiogram, but also blood pressure. The test should be done with a knowledgeable physician present and with careful continuous observation of the patient in addition to measurement of heart rate and blood pressure. Moderate degrees of stenosis (e.g., aortic valve area of 1.5 cm or greater) need not contraindicate low levels of exercise. However, patients with even moderate degrees of valvular stenosis or other obstruction in the central circulation which inhibit the normal cardiac output rise with exercise should not participate in competitive sports (73). The environment of the competitive athlete is such that the immediate demands of the sporting event may force the individual to exceed his normal exercise capacity and syncope or sudden death may occur.

In lesions that produce volume overload on the heart a major consideration is whether exercise causes a significant dilation of the left or right ventricle during submaximal exercise. Because the response of the ventricular volume to exercise in the presence of a shunt lesion is of importance, assessment of exercise capacity in patients with regurgitant lesions or shunts should be done using a technique that provides an estimate of left ventricular volume during exercise. The gated radionuclide scan fills this purpose well. Patients with regurgitant or shunt lesions are generally less likely to develop syncope or severe hypotension with exercise, but are more likely to develop pulmonary congestion and evidence of severe dyspnea. With this response, the patient often can judge what his or her exercise limits are. This is often not the case in the patient with obstructive lesions of the circulation. Thus, an exercise prescription for patients with regurgitant or shunt lesions should be determined in the usual fashion with an exercise test and an examination of capacity considering all variables measured. This author has seen teenagers with minor ventricular septal defects and no evidence of cardiac loading participating in competitive sports such as basketball and track with no adverse effects and with excellent athletic performance records.

Considerations mentioned above apply both to valvular regurgitation and to shunt lesions such as atrial and ventricular septal defect. In patients with minimal or no symptoms who have either atrial or ventricular septal defects, if pressures in the central circulation are normal, the shunt will be directed from left to right and no arterial desaturation occurs. Any patient with a right to left shunt and arterial hypoxemia will normally have severely limited exercise capacity (74), and although exercise programs can be prescribed to these patients, these will of necessity be very low level activity programs and should be provided with caution and with clear instructions to the patient concerning the nature of the cardiovascular problem and the need for limitations to exercise.

An interesting and uncommon problem associated with scuba diving with atrial or ventricular septal defects is the risk of paradoxical embolism of gas bubbles which occur in the venous circulation during decompression (75). Since intra-atrial and intraventricular shunts can be bidirectional at different phases of the cardiac cycle (76), presence of an atrial or ventricular septal defect is a contraindication to approval of individuals for diving. Because scuba diving is currently a popular sport, it is possible that individuals with asymptomatic atrial or ventricular septal defects may seek medical consultation requesting permission and medical clearance for recreational or commercial diving. These individuals should be advised against this activity. The consequence of arterial gas embolism induced from transport of gas from the peripheral veins to the left heart is cerebral gas embolism with significant neurological deficit (77).

In isometric exercises such as weight lifting, aortic and mitral regurgitation can become more severe with larger amounts of blood flowing in a reverse direction during the rise in blood pressure induced by the weight lifting maneuvers. Thus, patients with valvular regurgitation should be cautioned against severe degrees of isometric exercise.

VIII. CARDIAC ARRHYTHMIAS

Patients with or without heart disease may develop a variety of arrhythmias during exercise. The importance of the arrhythmia varies depending on the type and on the patient's history. It is important to thoroughly understand the patient's arrhythmia, the events which evoke it, and the consequences of the arrhythmia. Many arrhythmias need not be treated, whereas others demand treatment for safe exercise activity.

A. Supraventricular Arrhythmias

Premature atrial beats, supraventricular tachycardia, and atrial fibrillation may occur associated with exercise and produce symptoms of lightheadedness or frank syncope (78). Supraventricular tachycardia and atrial fibrillation in the young adult population may often be associated with a normal heart (79); however, in the presence of these arrhythmias, one should carefully evaluate the individual to rule out mitral stenosis, hyperthyroidism, and hypertension. Rarely, pulmonary emboli may produce atrial arrhythmias in this asymptomatic population, and this diagnosis should also be considered. Generally, premature atrial contractions are of no consequence and are found frequently in normal persons who exercise and even in well-trained athletes. Treatment of these supraventricular arrhythmias should follow standard lines including the drugs that would normally be used for therapy. In normal individuals, therapy for the arrhythmia may produce more troublesome symptoms than the arrhythmia itself. Thus, care in selection of both therapy and the patient requiring therapy is necessary. After ruling out significant cardiac disease or systemic illness such as hyperthyroidism or hypertension, one should evaluate the patient for ingestion of cardiac excitatory agents such as caffeine (coffee, cola drinks, and various combination over-the-counter analgesics), catecholamine-like drugs such as those found in anti-allergy medications, alcohol, and nicotine. It is probably helpful in these patients also to evaluate the psychic or emotional stress in the patient's environment since excess stress appears to be related to an increased frequency of supraventricular arrhythmias.

B. Ventricular Arrhythmias

Ventricular arrhythmias manifest as isolated premature ventricular contractions may be found in normal individuals in the absence of heart disease, and these should be assessed for their behavior during exercise (see below). Normally, premature contractions which demonstrate a multifocal pattern, R on T phenomenon, or frequent coupling of sequential premature beats should be considered as serious, and therapy should be provided. In patients who present for exercise advice and are found to have serious ventricular arrhythmias, a thorough cardiac evaluation should be performed prior to prescribing exercise or permitting the patient to exercise, since arrhythmias of this type may often result from cardiac disease and may be made worse by exercise. Antiarrhythmic therapy can take several approaches: β blockade alone may often be sufficient whereas in other cases combination antiarrhythmic drugs may be necessary to provide adequate control for the arrhythmias. Because of the known increased mortality of patients with coronary disease who manifest serious ventricular arrhythmias (80), it is important to understand the behavior of these arrhythmias during exercise and to provide appropriate therapy when necessary. Because an important complication of exercise is worsening of ventricular arrhythmias (81) it is of utmost importance to achieve adequate control of the ventricular arrhythmias prior to prescribing exercise.

C. Vagotonic Arrhythmias

Exercise training is known to augment vagal tone and induce a resting bradycardia with a relative slowing of heart rate at all exercise work loads compared to the untrained state (43). Often vagal tone may be so high that resting heart rates in the 30s and 40s are present. These are normally well tolerated because of the appropriately increased stroke volume, and normally, athletes do not show significant symptoms because of the bradycardia. Occasionally, a bradycardia induced by exercise in an athlete may result in a lowering of cardiac output to the point where symptoms are evident, and in this case the bradycardia must be treated following usual clinical guidelines. Therapy can include vagal blocking agents, sympathomemetic drugs, reversal of the training state to a less-trained state, and rarely the insertion of a permanent cardiac pacemaker. Increased vagal tone may be manifest by alterations in conduction of the A-V node as well. Occasionally, because distribution of vagal innervation is dominant at the A-V node, a Wenkebach type of conduction abnormality may be noted at rest in well-trained individuals who do not have other significant cardiac disease. This rhythm will wax and wane with respiration, and normally disappears with moderate amounts of exercise. Bradycardias and A-V nodal conduction changes induced by training will disappear with exercise in every case; and if this response is not noted, one should suspect anatomic abnormalities of the conduction system which may require specific therapy (82).

IX. CONDUCTION ABNORMALITIES

Patients with conduction system abnormalities normally demonstrate evidence of cardiac disease as the cause of these abnormalities. Congenital heart disease, certain valvular heart diseases (aortic stenosis with valvular and A-V ring calcification), cardiomyopathy, and coronary heart disease all may be associated with chronic conduction system abnormalities. Children with congenital complete heart block may have no limitations to exercise because of the significant increase in stroke volume which compensates for the inability of heart rate to increase with exercise (78). Most patients with acquired complete heart block, however, are limited in their exercise capacity because of inability to increase cardiac output. Patients with acquired complete heart block should be treated along standard clinical lines, and most commonly a permanent pacemaker is implanted to provide adequate cardiac output and heart rate. Other degrees of heart block must be treated according to the underlying disease process that produces them. Indications for permanent implanted pacemakers should not be based on the need to exercise, but rather on standard clinical indications, such as the expectation for sudden bradycardia, and on the underlying disease process.

X. PREEXCITATION SYNDROMES

Patients with short P-R intervals, with and without QRS abnormalities may develop rapid tachycardia at rest or during exercise (83,84). However, many patients with short P-R intervals are asymptomatic and this finding on the electrocardiogram is not in itself a contraindication to exercise. Patients who develop rapid tachycardia during exercise should be evaluated for the presence of the preexcitation syndrome; if recurrent paroxysmal or exercise induced tachycardia is a significant symptoms, then appropriate diagnostic and therapeutic procedures should be followed. Exercise induced syncope may be induced by tachyarrhythmias, and evaluation of the electrocardiogram during exercise will aid in this diagnosis. Tachycardias associated with a prolonged Q-T interval should also be considered (85).

XI.   ASSESSMENT OF ARRHYTHMIAS AND CONDUCTION SYSTEM ABNORMALITIES

Patients with suspected arrhythmias or conduction system abnormalities induced by exercise should be evaluated clinically to predict whether they will develop significant rhythm or conduction system abnormalities during exercise. The basic principle in assessing these rhythm and conduction disturbances is to simulate the exercise load in a controlled environment with continuous electrocardiographic monitoring and clinical observation. This approach can be achieved either with standard stress testing and continuous ECG monitoring or with the 24-hour electrocardiographic recording used while the patient conducts his normal daily activities, including exercise. Arrhythmias induced by exercise can be detected during treadmill exercise tests, and the behavior of premature ventricular beats during exercise can be observed. Premature ventricular beats that become more frequent with exercise or which are associated with hypotension should be controlled prior to instituting an exercise program. Often isolated premature ventricular beats will disappear with exercise as the heart rate rises and supresses the ectopic focus. In most cases, patients who override their premature ventricular beats with exercise and show no evidence of recurrence or more frequent premature ventricular beats following exercise can exercise without significant concern. Premature ventricular beats may become more frequent immediately postexercise when a suppressed ventricular ectopic focus may become manifest and produce a serious arrhythmia. The development or progression of serious ventricular arrhythmias either during or after exercise is a contraindication to further exercise until the arrhythmia is controlled. Evaluation of ventricular arrhythmias obtained from 24-hour ECG recordings also provides information upon which to base treatment (86).

It is also helpful in patients being treated for arrhythmias who are undertaking exercise programs to instruct the patient on self-detection of arrhythmias. Patients can be informed of the pulse pattern associated with premature beats and can be taught to count the frequency of premature beats from the peripheral pulse. Patients trained to detect their own arrhythmias can provide an early warning of changes in cardiac rhythm.

Patients who have permanent implanted pacemakers with fixed rates will be limited by a fixed heart rate during exercise, and these patients should be cautioned to maintain low levels of exercise so that cardiac output will be allowed to adjust appropriately to the exercise. Newer atrioventricular sequential pacemakers may provide a better adjustment to exercise in patients with complete heart block who have normally functioning sinus nodes and atria. These pacemakers sense the atrial stimulus and provide an atrioventricular sequential stimulation so that heart rate can respond to autonomic regulation. As these pacemakers become more available patients who received them will be able to withstand more significant degrees of exercise because their heart rate will respond appropriately to the exercise load.

XII. CARDIAC SURGERY

A. Coronary Bypass Surgery

Patients with successful coronary bypass surgery who wish to exercise need not be denied this activity. The basic principles of testing for capacity and providing an exercise program that stresses the patient to 60–70% capacity can still be followed. Early exercise prescriptions for these patients (2–3 weeks postsurgery) can be provided to assist the patient in recovering from surgery. These patients should be approached in a manner similar to the postmyocardial infarction patient. At 6–8 days postoperatively the patient can have a submaximal stress test to assess low level exercise capacity and a low level exercise prescription can be provided. At 10–12 weeks the patient should return for a more vigorous stress test that tests for maximal capacity. Based on this stress test an exercise prescription should be provided to allow the patient to exercise indefinitely and improve physical conditioning over long periods of time. Some postcardiac surgical patients will retain an ischemic S-T segment response with exercise; however, this response usually occurs at a higher work load than found prior to surgery. Evidence of continued ischemia on a postoperative exercise stress test suggests that complete myocardial revascularization has not been achieved. This situation may result from the diffuse nature of coronary disease present in some patients, from closure of a bypass graft or new disease. Although some myocardial ischemia may still be present following coronary bypass surgery, exercise capacity is usually improved. The fundamental approach of assessing exercise capacity and then providing an exercise prescription of 65–70% of capacity can still be followed.

Our experience with cardiac surgery patients in the early postoperative period indicates that these patients tend to have higher heart rates than nonsurgical cardiac patients. Because of this finding of higher heart rates in the postoperative period extending for 3–4 weeks, exercise prescriptions should be provided with slightly higher heart rate limits (15–20% higher) than comparable prescriptions for nonsurgical patients. Patients who have recovered long term from surgery have been known to run competitive races including marathons (26.2 miles) and to participate in strenuous sports to a degree that one would consider their performance normal. With adequate revascularization this level of physical activity is possible. Based on the patient's coronary anatomy and the completeness of the coronary revascularization it is likely that some patients will return to vigorous sports and other athletic activities.

B. Valvular Surgery

Prosthetic cardiac valves create two important problems. First is the inability of the prothetic valve poppet to undergo motions as rapidly as the natural valves when a rapid heart rate occurs. This limitation of the prosthetic heart valve occurs because the valve poppet has finite mass and artificial valve orifices are narrower than the natural orifice of the valve. Thus, in high output states, there may be a significant gradient across the valve, and with high heart rates, the valve poppet may not open and close completely, thus aggravating the gradient or producing significant valve regurgitation. Because of these limitations, patients who have prosthetic cardiac valves should be provided with low level exercise programs that maintain maximal heart rates no greater than 120–130 per minute. The use of center opening valves, including heterograft valves with tissue leaflets that open with larger orificies and have less mass, provides the possibility for greater cardiac output and, therefore, greater exercise capacity. Patients with heterograft valves can be provided with more vigorous exercise prescriptions after an initial 2- to 3-month recovery period from surgery.

The second consideration in patients with prosthetic cardiac valves is anti-coagulation. Because exercise often results in minor trauma to various parts of the body, patients on chronic anticoagulation should be warned to avoid exercise situations that can produce blunt trauma, injury, or bruising. Heterograft valves provide a significant advantage in this regard since patients with heterograft aortic valves can be followed without anticoagulation after an initial period for recovery from surgery (87). Patients with heterograft mitral valves often are maintained on anticoagulation.

Patients recovered from cardiac surgery for either valvular, coronary, or congenital heart surgery can enter exercise programs with certain limitations. The approach to the patient depends on reproducing an exercise environment under controlled conditions where heart rate, electrocardiogram, blood pressure, and the general status of the patient can be observed carefully by the physician. Even though many patients who have had cardiac surgery have significant limitations, their daily lives will require some level of exercise. By appropriate testing, an exercise prescription can be provided for these individuals which will allow them to maintain optimal physical conditioning for the status of their heart and the surgical procedure that was performed.

ACKNOWLEDGMENTS

The author is grateful to R. Vlietstra and R. Squires, Mayo Clinic, for their thoughtful reviews.

REFERENCES

1. Wenger, N. K. (1981). In hospital rehabilitation after myocardial infarction. *In* "Physical Conditioning and Cardiovascular Rehabilitation" (L. S. Cohen, M. B. Mock, and I. Ringquist, eds.), pp. 139–144. Wiley, New York.
2. Abelmann, W. H. (1978). Treatment of congestive cardiomyopathy. *Postgrad. Med. J.* **54**, 477.
3. Burch, G. F., and DePasquale, N. P. (1970). Recognition and prevention of cardiomyopathy. *Circulation* **42**, A-47.
4. Stone, H. L. (1977). Cardiac function and exercise training in conscious dogs. *J. Appl. Physiol.* **42**, 824–832.
5. Nadel, E. R. (1980). Circulatory and thermal regulations during exercise. *Fed. Proc., Fed. Am. Soc. Exp. Biol.* **39**, 1491–1497.
6. Åstrand, P.-O., Cuddy, T. E., Saltin, B., and Stenberg, J. (1964). Cardiac output during submaximal and maximal work. *J. Appl. Physiol.* **19**, 268–274.
7. Mitchell, J. H. (1980). Regulation in physiological systems during exercise. *Fed. Proc. Fed. Am. Soc. Exp. Biol.* **39**, 1479–1480.
8. Folkow, B. (1971). Role of sympathetic nervous system. *In* "Coronary Heart Disease and Physical Fitness" (O. A. Larson and R. O. Malmborg, eds.), pp. 68–73. Univ. Park Press, Baltimore, Maryland.
9. Master, A. M. (1950). The two-step electrocardiogram: a test for coronary insufficiency. *Ann. Int. Med.* **32**, 842–863.
10. Bruce, R. A., and McDonough, J. R. (1969). Stress testing in screening for cardiovascular disease. *Bull. N. Y. Acad. Med.* [2] **45**, 1288–1305.
11. Bruce, R. A., and Hornsten, T. R. (1969). Exercise stress testing in evaluation of patients with ischemic heart disease. *Prog. Cardiovasc. Dis.* **11**, 371–391.
12. Ellestad, M. H., and Wan, M. K. C. (1975). Predictive implications of stress testing. *Circulation* **51**, 363–369.
13. Naughton, J. P., and Haider, R. (1973). Methods of exercise testing. *In* "Exercise Testing and Exercise Training in Coronary Heart Disease" (J. P. Naughton and H. K. Hellerstein, eds.), pp. 79–91. Academic Press, New York.
14. Redwood, D. R., and Epstein, S. E. (1972). Uses and limitations of stress testing in the evaluation of ischemic heart disease. *Circulation* **46**, 1115–1131.
15. Mattingly, T. W. (1962). The postexercise electrocardiogram. *Am. J. Cardiol.* **9**, 395–409.
16. Mann, D. L., Mackler, P. T., and Bove, A. A. (1981). Reduced left ventricular contractile reserve in aged subjects. *Clin. Res.* **29**, 220A.
17. Rerych, S. K., Scholz, P. M., Sabiston, D. C., and Jones, R. H. (1980). Effects of exercise training on left ventricular function in normal subjects: A longitudinal study by radionuclide angiography. *Am. J. Cardiol.* **45**, 244–252.

18. Zaret, B. L., Strauss, H. S., Hurley, P. J., Natarajan, T. K., and Pitt, B. (1971). A noninvasive scintiphotographic method for detecting regional ventricular dysfunction in man. *N. Engl. J. Med.* **284**, 1165–1170.

19. Strauss, H. W., Zaret, B. L., Hurley, P. J., Natarajan, T. K., and Pitt, B. (1971). A scintiphotographic method of measuring left ventricular ejection fraction in man without cardiac catheterization. *Am. J. Cardiol.* **28**, 575–580.

20. Jorgensen, C. R., Kitamura, K., Gobel, F. L., Taylor, H. L., and Wang, Y. (1972). Hemodynamic correlates of coronary blood flow and myocardial oxygen consumption during vigorous upright exercise in normal humans. *In* "Myocardial Blood Flow in Man" (A. Maseri, ed.), pp. 251–259. Minerva Medica, Torino.

21. Johnson, J. R., and Wiggers, C. J. (1937). The alleged validity of coronary sinus outflow as a criterion of coronary reactions. *Am. J. Physiol.* **118**, 38–51.

22. Sarnoff, S. J., Braunwald, E., and Welch, G. H. (1968). Hemodynamic determinants of oxygen consumption of the heart with special reference to the tension-time index. *Am. J. Physiol.* **192**, 148–156.

23. Gregg, D. E. (1963). Physiology of the coronary circulation. *Circulation* **27**, 1128–1177.

24. Sabiston, D. C., and Gregg, D. E. (1957). Effect of cardiac contraction on coronary blood flow. *Circulation* **15**, 14–20.

25. Bache, R., and Ball (1976). Distribution of myocardial blood flow in the exercising dog with restricted coronary artery inflow. *Circ. Res.* **38**, 60–66.

26. Bove, A. A., McGinnis, A. A., and Spann, J. F. (1979). Ventriculographic correlates of left ventricular oxygen consumption during acute afterload changes in the intact dog. *Fed. Proc. Fed. Am. Soc. Exp. Biol.* **38**, 1267.

27. Buckberg, G. D., Fixler, D. E., Archie, J. P., and Hoffman, J. I. F. (1972). Experimental subendocardial ischemia in dogs with normal coronary arteries. *Circulation*

28. Anonymous (1981). "Heart Facts," pp. 10–11. American Heart Association, Dallas, Texas.

29. Wenger, N. K., Gilbert, C. A., and Skorapa, M. Z. (1971). Cardiac conditioning after myocardial infarction. *Card. Rehab.* **2**, 17–22.

30. Scheuer, J., Greenberg, M. A., and Zohman, L. R. (1978). Exercise training in patients with coronary artery disease. *Mod. Concepts Cardiovasc. Dis.* **47**, 85–90.

31. Fox, S. M., and Paul, O. (1969). Physical activity and coronary heart disease. *Am. J. Cardiol.* **23**, 298–306.

32. Paffenbarger, R. S., Wing, A. L., and Hyde, R. T. (1978). Physical activity as an indicator of heart attack risk in college alumni. *Am. J. Epidemiol.* **108**, 161–175.

33. Santamore, W. P., and Bove, A. A. (1982). Alterations in the severity of coronary stenosis: Effects of intraluminal pressure and proximal coronary vasoconstriction. *In* "Coronary Artery Disease" (W. P. Santamore and A. A. Bove, eds.), pp. 157–172. Urban & Schwarzenberg, Baltimore, Maryland.

34. Gould, K. L., and Kelly, K. O. (1982). Hemodynamics of coronary stenosis. *In* "Coronary Artery Disease" (W. P. Santamore and A. A. Bove, eds.), pp. 173–198. Urban & Schwarzenberg, Baltimore, Maryland.

35. Logan, S. E. (1975). On the fluid mechanics of human coronary stenosis. *IEEE Trans. Biomed. Eng.* **BME-22**, 327–334.

36. Prinzmetal, M., Kennamer, R., Neerliss, R., Wada, T., and Bor, N. (1959). Angina pectoris. I. A variant form of angina pectoris. *Am. J. Med.* **27**, 375–388.

37. Yasue, A. R., Omote, S., Takazawa, A., *et al.* (1979). Circadion variation of exercise capacity in patients with Prinzmetal's variant angina: Role of exercise induced coronary spasm. *Circulation* **59**, 938–948.

38. Specchia, G., DeServi, S., Falcone, C. *et al.* (1979). Coronary arterial spasm as a cause of exercise induced ST segment elevation in patients with variant angina. *Circulation* **59**, 948–954.

39. Pepine, C. J., Feldman, R. L., and Conti, C. R. (1982). Diagnosis and treatment of coronary spasm. In "Coronary Artery Disease" (W. P. Santamore and A. A. Bove, eds.), pp. 233–246. Urban & Schwarzenberg, Baltimore, Maryland.

40. Maseri, A., Mimmo, R., Cherchia, S. et al. (1975). Coronary artery spasm as a cause of acute myocardial ischemia in man. Chest 68, 625–633.

41. White, P. D. (1970). The evolution of our knowledge of the heart and its diseases. In "The Heart" (J. W. Hurst and R. B. Logue, eds.), 2nd ed., pp. 3–4. McGraw-Hill, New York.

42. Clausen, J. P. (1976). Circulatory adjustments to dynamic exercise and effects of physical training in normal subjects and in patients with coronary artery disease. Prog. Cardiovasc. Dis. 18, 459–495.

43. Scheuer, J., and Tipton, C. M. (1977). Csrdiovascular adaptations to physical training. Annu. Rev. Physiol. 39, 221–251.

44. Hollosy, J. O., and Booth, F. W. (1976). Biochemical adaptations to endurance exercise in muscle. Annu. Rev. Physiol. 38, 273–291.

45. Ehsani, A. A., Heath, G. W., Hagberg, J. M., Sobel, B. E., and Holloszy, J. O. (1981). Effect of 12 month intense exercise training on ischemic ST depression in patients with coronary artery disease. Circulation 64, 1116–1124.

46. Naughton, J., Bruhn, J. G., and Lategola, M. T. (1968). Effect of physical training on physiologic and behavioral characteristics of cardiac patients. Arch. Phys. Med. Rehabil. 49, 131–137.

47. Bove, A. A., Hardenberg, E., and Miles, J. A. (1978). Effect of heart and cold stress on inert gas (^{133}Xe) exchange in the rabbit. Undersea Biomed. Res. 5, 149–158.

48. Brock, L. (1973). Early reconditioning for post-myocardial infarction patients. In "Exercise Testing and Exercise Training in Coronary Heart Disease" (J. P. Naughton and H. K. Hellerstein, eds.), pp. 315–323. Academic Press, New York.

49. Borer, J. S., Barcharach, S. L., Greeen, M V. et al. (1977). Real time radionuclide cineangiography in the noninvasive evaluation of global and regional left ventricular function at rest and during exercise in patients with coronary-artery disease. N. Engl. J. Med. 296, 839.

50. Berger, H. T., Reduto, J. A., Johnstone, D. E. et al. (1979). Global and regional left ventricular response to bicycle exercise in coronary artery disease. Am. J. Med. 66, 13–21.

51. Dennenberg, B. S., Makler, P. T., Bove, A. A., and Spann, J. F. (1981). Normal left ventricular emptying in coronary disease at rest: Analysis by radiographic and equilibrium radionuclide ventriculography. Am. J. Cardiol. 48, 311–315.

52. Lawlor, M. R., Thomas, D. P., Michele, J., Paolone, A. M., and Bove, A. A. (1982). Effect of propranolol on cardiovascular adaptation to endurance training in dogs. Med. Sci. Sports Exercise 14, 123

53. Thomas, D. P., Lawlor, M. R., Michele, J., Paolone, A. M., and Bove, A. A. (1982). Metabolic adaptations to endurance training in dogs: Effects of chronic propranolol therapy. Med. Sci. Sports Exercise 14, 124.

54. Borg, G. A. V. (1973). Perceived exertion: A note on history and methods. Med. Sci. Sports 5, 90–93.

55. Bove, A. A., Hultgren, P. B., Ritzer, T. F., and Carey, R. A. (1979). Myocardial blood flow and hemodynamic responses to exercise training in dogs. J. Appl. Physiol. 46, 571–578.

56. Carey, R. A., Santamore, W. P., and Bove, A. A. (1981). Effects of tachycardia on myocardial blood flow and oxygen consumption in exercise trained dogs. Fed. Proc. Fed. Am. Soc. Exp. Biol. 40, 500.

57. Eckstein, R. W. (1957). Effect of exercise and coronary artery narrowing on coronary collateral circulation. Circ. Res. 5, 230–235.

58. Burt, J. J., and Jackson, R. (1965). The effect of physical exercise on the coronary collateral circulation of dogs. J. Sports Med. 5, 203–206.

59. Chidsey, C. A., Braunwald, E., and Morrow, A. G. (1965). Catecholamine excretion and cardiac stores of norepinephrine in congestive heart failure. *Am. J. Med.* **39**, 442–451.
60. Wasserman, K., and Whipp, B. J. (1975). Exercise physiology in health and disease. *Am. Rev. Respir. Dis.* **112**, 219–248.
61. Weiss, M. B., Ellis, K., Sciacca, R. R., Johnson, L. L., Schmidt, D. H., and Cannon, P. J. (1976). Myocardial blood flow in congestive and hypertrophic cardiomyopathy. *Circulation* **53**, 484–494.
62. Pasternac, A., Noble, J., Streulens, Y., Elie, R., Henschke, C., and Bourassa, M. G. (1982). Pathyophysiology of chest pain in patients with cardiomyopathies and normal coronary arteries. *Circulation* **65**, 778–788.
63. Zelis, R., Longhurst, J., Capone, R. J., Lee, G., and Mason, D. T. (1976). Peripheral circulatory control mechanisms in congestive heart failure. *In* ''Congestive Heart Failure'' (D. T. Mason, ed.), pp. 129–142. Dunn-Donnelley Co., New York.
64. Rushmer, R. F. (1961). ''Cardiovascular Dynamics,'' pp. 444–448. Saunders, Philadelphia, Pennsylvania.
65. Spann, J. F., Bove, A. A., Natarajan, G., and Kreulen, T. H. (1980). Ventricular pump performance, pump function, and compensatory mechanisms in patients with aortic stenosis. *Circulation* **62**, 576–582.
66. Osbakken, M. D., Bove, A. A., and Spann, J. F. (1981). Left ventricular regional wall motion and velocity of shortening in chronic mitral and aortic regurgitation in man. *Am. J. Cardiol.* **47**, 1005–1009.
67. Osbakken, M. D., Bove, A. A., and Spann, J. F. (1981). Left ventricular function in chronic aortic regurgitation with reference to end-systolic pressure, volume and stress relations. *Am. J. Cardiol.* **47**, 193–198.
68. Natrajan, G., Bove, A. A., Coulson, R. L., Carey, R. A., and Spann, J. F. (1979). Increased passive stiffness of short term pressure overload hypertrophied myocardium in cat. *Am. J. Physiol.* **237**, 4676–4680.
69. Hultgren, P. B., and Bove, A. A. (1981). Myocardial blood flow and mewchanics in volume overload-induced left ventricular hypertrophy in dogs. *Cardiovasc. Res.* **15**, 522–528.
70. Breisch, E. A., Houser, S. R., Carey, R. A., Spann, J. F., and Bove, A. A. (1981). Myocardial blood flow and capillary density in chronic pressure overload of the feline left ventricle. *Cardiovasc. Res.* **14**, 469–475.
71. Thomas, D. P., Phillips, S. J., Spann, J. F., and Bove, A. A. (1981). Myocardial blood flow and capillary density in experimental volume overload. *Fed. Proc. Fed. Am. Soc. Exp. Biol.* **40**, 445.
72. Wroblewski, E. M., Pearl, F. J., Hammer, W. J., and Bove, A. A. (1982). False positive stress tests due to undetected left ventricular hypertrophy. *Am. J. Epidemiol.* **115**, 412–417.
73. Starek, P. J. K. (1982). Athletic performance in children with cardiovascular problems. *Phys. Sports Med.* **10**, 78–89.
74. Epstein, S. E., Beiser, G. D., Goldstein, R. E. *et al.* (1973). Hemodynamic abnormalities in response to mild and intense upright exercise following operative correction of atrial septal defect on tetralogy of fallot. *Circulation* **47**, 1065–1075.
75. Bove, A. A. (1982). The basis for drug therapy in decompression sickness. *Undersea Biomed. Res.* (in press).
76. Myizawa, K., Smith, H. C., Wood, E. H., and Bove, A. A. (1973). Roentgen video densitometric determination of left to right shunts in experimental ventricular septal defect. *Am. J. Cardiol.* **31**, 627–634.
77. Bove, A. A., Clark, J. M., Simon, A. J., and Lambertsen, C. J. (1982). Successful therapy of cerebral air embolism with hyperbaric oxygen at 2.8 ATA. *Undersea Biomed. Res.* **9**, 75–80.

78. McIntosh, H. D., and Morris, J. J. (1968). The hemodynamic consequences of arrhythmias. *Prog. Cardiovasc. Dis.* **8,** 330–363.
79. Bigger, T. J. (1980). Management of arrhythmias. *In* "Heart Disease" (E. Braunwald, ed.), p. 733. Saunders, Philadelphia, Pennsylvania.
80. Chiang, B. N., Perlmon, L. V., Ostrander, L. D. *et al.* (1969). Relationship of premature systoles to coronary heart disease and sudden death in the Tecumsch epidemiologic study. *Ann. Intern. Med.* **70,** 1159–1166.
81. Lown, B., Kosowsky, B., and Whiting, R. (1969). Exposure of electrical instability in coronary artery disease by exercise stress. *Circulation* **40,** Suppl. 3, 136.
82. Ahlborg, B., Atterhog, J., Ekelund, L., and Ericcson, G. (1977). The significance of AV block I in asymptomatic young men. *Acta Med. Scand.* **201,** 377–380.
83. Wolff, L., Parkinson, J., and White, P. D. (1930). Bundle branch block with short P-R interval in healthy young people prove to paroxysmal tachycardia. *Am. Heart J.* **5,** 685.
84. Lown, B., Ganong, W. F., and Levine, S. A. (1952). The syndrome of short P-R interval, normal QRS complex and paroxysmal heart action. *Circulation* **5,** 695.
85. Vincent, G. M., Abiloskov, J. A., annd Burgess, M. T. (1974). Q-T interval syndromes. *Prog. Cardiovasc. Dis.* **16,** 523–530.
86. Ryan, M., Lown, B., and Horn, H. (1975). Comparison of ventricular ectopic activity during 24 hour monitoring and exercise testing in patients with coronary heart disease. *N. Engl. J. Med.* **292,** 224–229.
87. Levinson, G. E. (1981). Aortic stenosis. *In* "Vavular Heart Disease" (J. E. Dalen and J. S. Alpert, eds.), pp. 171–230. Little, Brown, Boston, Massachusetts.

CHAPTER 12

Pulmonary Disorders
and Exercise

DANIEL C. DUPONT and ALLAN P. FREEDMAN

Division of Pulmonary Diseases
Hahnemann University School of Medicine
Philadelphia, Pennsylvania

The normal ventilatory response to exercise was presented in Chapter 3. The purpose of this chapter is to review the limitation imposed on exercise by various pulmonary disorders, the methods used for assessing impairment, and therapeutic modalities available. Before proceeding further, it is appropriate to comment from the standpoint of a chest physician on the performance of the clinical exercise test.

I. THE CLINICAL EXERCISE TEST

This will serve as an overview of the fundamentals of exercise studies. For a more detailed discussion of pulmonary exercise assessment, several comprehensive references are suggested (1–4).

259

Exercise Medicine: Physiological Principles
and Clinical Applications

The purpose of clinical exercise testing is to evaluate objectively an individual's physical work capacity and factors that limit it. There are several specific goals:

1. To determine whether effort tolerance is normal or abnormal.
2. To determine what disease process is suggested by the pattern of abnormality.
3. To quantitate impairment.
4. To monitor improvement after various interventions.
5. In some situations, to induce a particular symptom or sign that may be diagnostic.

In an exercise test, muscular work is performed, a variety of measurements are obtained, and a data base is formulated from which conclusions can be drawn. Work rates observed in the laboratory setting correlate with ability to perform various tasks at work or at home. By using a unit of power based on the resting metabolic oxygen requirement (the MET—equivalent to 3.5 ml of oxygen per kilogram per minute), exercise capacity can be translated into ability to carry out routine daily and occupational activities. Table I lists some common activities and their energy requirements expressed as METs. Muscular work is performed in the laboratory by simple reproducible activities such as walking, stair climbing, or cycling. Quantitation of effort is best accomplished in the laboratory with a graded treadmill or cycle ergometer.

TABLE I

Energy Cost (in METS[a]) of Some Common Activities

Activity	METS	Activity	METS
Supine rest	1.0	Showering	3.5
Sitting	1.0	Golf (walking)	4.0–8.0
Standing	1.0	Dancing	4.0–8.0
Eating	1.0	Walking downstairs	4.5
Dressing	2.0	Swimming	5.0–8.0
Washing	2.0	Walking (3.5 km/hour)	5.5
Driving car	2.0	Walking uphill	5.5–10.0
Light housework	2.0–3.5	Climbing 1 flight of stairs	6.0–9.0
Golf (power cart)	2.0–4.0	Tennis	6.0–9.0
Bowling	2.0–4.0	Handball	8.0–12.0
Commode use	3.0	Racquetball	8.0–12.0
Walking (2.5 km/hour)	3.0	Jogging 12 min/km	9.0
Conditioning exercises	3.0–8.0	Jumping rope	9.0–12.0
Cycling	3.0–8.0	Jogging 6 min/km	16.0

[a] MET = resting oxygen consumption in a sitting position (approximately 3.5 ml/kg/minute or 1.0 kcal/kg/hour).

Work is usually performed in one of two fashions: a progressive exercise test, where the amount of muscular effort is gradually increased in a stepwise fashion, or a steady-state protocol, where a given level of work is quickly attained and thereafter maintained for the duration of the study. In any case, exercise is not continued past a targeted end point, usually a heart rate 85% of a predicted maximum, or until symptoms occur. These symptoms may reproduce the problem that prompted the study, such as wheezing, chest discomfort, fatigue, or severe dyspnea. A fall in blood pressure or evidence of cardiac ischemia on the electrocardiogram are indications to terminate the study.

There are several possible levels of sophistication in data gathering during an exercise study. Determining maximal achievable work allows different exercise studies to be compared and results extrapolated to activities of daily living. A number of physiological parameters can be readily observed including heart rate, respiratory frequency, and electrocardiographic pattern (see Chapter 3). If expired gas is collected, minute ventilation can be determined. With greater sophistication, gas analyzers can measure CO_2 and O_2 tensions in expired gas samples so that oxygen consumption ($\dot{V}CO_2$), carbon dioxide production ($\dot{V}co_2$), ventilatory equivalent ($\dot{V}_E/\dot{V}O_2$), and anaerobic threshhold (AT) can be calculated. If an indwelling arterial catheter is inserted for blood gas determination, then dead space ventilation (V_D/V_T), alveolar–arterial oxygen gradient ($DA-ao_2$) and cardiac output (CO) can be derived. The use of an ear oximiter instead of an arterial sampling catheter allows estimation of hemoglobin saturation and may be quite useful. Comparing the results obtained with predicted normal values will determine the presence and severity of any abnormal response. Several patterns of impairment are recognized in pulmonary disease. Cardiac disease also has distinct patterns of impairment, and characteristic responses have been described for both the anxious, but healthy, subject and for the malingerer (5).

Exercise testing can also be used to assess a patient's response to training and medical intervention. Several studies have demonstrated that improvement with training in both the acute and chronically ill patient may be predicted from initial exercise performance (6–8). Also, clinical exercise testing has been used to evaluate the efficacy and define the optimal duration of various drugs and medical regimens (9). An exercise prescription as well as possible pharmacologic intervention are more appropriate when based on exercise studies. Finally, serial exercise testing provides objective data to monitor the course of a patients illness.

Several caveats are appropriate. There is a broad spectrum of physiological response to muscular work that falls within the range of normal. The variability in individual response to exertion has been referred to as the "fitness continuum" (10). In other words, individuals without a disease process display a range of response in the parameters described depending on the state of fitness of cardiovascular and muscular systems. With physical conditioning, there is an increase in the capillary network and in the myoglobin stores of skeletal muscle. This aspect of physical conditioning, however, is limited to the specific muscle groups involved (11). Finally, there frequently is an increase in blood volume and the total hemoglobin available for oxygen transport. The net result is better oxygen utilization and an increased aerobic capacity. Anaerobic threshold with attendant lactic acidosis occurs at a higher work level and both maximal oxygen consumption and work capacity are greater.

Conversely, with prolonged bedrest and inactivity, blood volume and hemoglobin content are reduced, and both myoglobin stores and capillary network to skeletal muscle diminish. The sedentary extreme of the spectrum manifests a low anaerobic threshhold. Therefore, there is an early rise in minute ventilation relative to oxygen consumption from the excess production of CO_2 that occurs during anaerobic lactate generation.

Many groups have sought to demonstrate training effects in the pulmonary system. However, there are only minor differences between the fit and unfit with respect to pulmonary function. Lung volumes increase somewhat, and ventilatory muscle strength and diffusing capacity may improve (12–15).

II. EXERCISE AND PULMONARY DISEASE

Many pulmonary diseases limit exercise. The most common impairment is obstructive lung disease, which includes emphysema, bronchitis, asthma, and bronchiectasis. Next is restrictive lung disease, which encompasses a large group of disorders involving infiltration of the pulmonary parenchyma and chest wall defects. Restrictive chest wall defects include obesity, chest wall deformities (i.e., kyphoscoliosis), and neuromuscular disorders. Finally, pulmonary circulation can also be compromised and impair exercise tolerance, such as in thromboembolic disease and primary pulmonary hypertension. We will now discuss the pathophysiology of these pulmonary disorders and general guidelines for prescribing exercise in these states.

A. Exercise Limitation in Chronic Obstructive Airways Disease

Prolonged expiratory time is the hallmark of obstructive disease. Airway narrowing, whether from asthmatic bronchospasm, bronchitic mucosal hypertrophy, emphysematous loss of elasticity, or just edema, increases airway resistance. This causes the "lung bellows" response to be suboptimal (16). Frequently, expiration becomes an active phase of breathing and metabolic demand on the respiratory muscles consequently increases. At the same time, lung volumes may be increased from overinflation and gas trapping. The resultant downward displacement of the diaphragm and increase in chest wall diameter often limit the efficiency of respiratory muscle contraction. Thus, the obstructive diseases are characterized by increased work of breathing from elevated airway resistance and decreased muscular efficiency at the same time that increased dead space ventilation necessitates an undue increase in ventilation. The "oxygen cost of breathing" in patients with cardiorespiratory disease has been shown to be substantially greater than normal (17).

Destruction of parenchymal tissue disturbs matching of ventilation and perfusion in lung units. The emphysematous areas that no longer contribute to gas exchange constitute wasted ventilation. This increased dead space wastes ventilatory effort and further increases the work requirements of breathing. On the other hand, blood still flowing through capillary regions that are poorly ventilated due to airways obstruction is not oxygenated well and contributes to venous admixture, lowering arterial P_{O_2}. This has been shown graphically in Chapter 3, Fig. 2.

Obliteration of the lungs' capillary bed reduces the compliance of the pulmonary vascular system and hypoxic vasospasm elevates the pulmonary vascular pressures. As a result, the lung frequently cannot accommodate the pronounced increase in cardiac output produced by exercise, and pulmonary arterial pressure rises.

Ventilation–perfusion imbalance combined with limited capillary reserve may cause severe worsening of hypoxemia during exercise. Oxygen loading of hemoglobin may be even less complete when the returning venous blood arrives more desaturated from the increased tissue extraction of oxygen demanded by exercise. Also, as blood flows faster through the limited capillary bed, diffusion abnormalities may be unmasked because of the decreased time available for gas exchange. These defects result in decreased ability of capillary blood to acquire oxygen and widening of the alveolar–arterial oxygen gradient. These pathophysiological relationships are summarized in Table II.

The individual with predominantly chronic bronchitis can often improve his ventilation–perfusion distribution and oxygenation during exercise (16). Frequently, the V_D/V_T, A-a gradient for oxygen and arterial blood gases will improve during exercise in these patients (18,19). However, airway obstruction

TABLE II

Exercise Limitation in Obstructive Lung Disease

1. Increased work of breathing: inefficient respiratory muscular performance
2. Increased oxygen cost of breathing
3. Ventilation–perfusion mismatch: bronchitis more than emphysema
4. Limited maximum minute ventilation: due to increased expiratory time
5. Decreased red cell capillary transit time: fixed pulmonary capillary volume

limits maximal minute ventilation and higher levels of oxygen consumption often cannot be attained. Thus, there is a mechanical limitation with insufficient "lung bellows" response (16). In classic emphysema, V/Q distribution is near optimal at rest and does not further improve with exercise. Although minute ventilation is limited, there is an additional problem that may predominate. Oxygen content may decrease because insufficient alveolar capillary surface area limits diffusion (16,18). The extent of desaturation in emphysema cannot be accurately predicted from resting data alone and patients usually have a variable mix of emphysema and chronic bronchitis.

B. The Role of Exercise in Obstructive Lung Disease

The evolution of thought on rehabilitation in obstructive airways disease demonstrates the increased awareness of exercise as therapy. In the 1930s and 1940s, when emphysema and chronic bronchitis were comparatively uncommon, rest was the prescribed life-style for the breathless patient. The late 1950s and 1960s witnessed an increase in the prevalence of chronic obstructive airways disease and its attendant disability. Physician visits, hospitalizations, days lost from work, and death from bronchitis and emphysema doubled every 5 years (20). It is still increasing today.

In 1952, Barach and others began commenting on improved life-style and longer survival in COPD patients (21). By 1956, portable supplemental oxygen was used to enhance exercise ability in chronic respiratory insufficiency (22). The approach to the breathing impaired individual underwent a radical change: exercise was to be prescribed not prohibited. Regular exercise in subjects with obstructive lung disease is clearly beneficial; although the mechanisms that produce improvement are poorly understood. Consistent improvement in a particular cardiopulmonary parameter has not been found with exercise training.

Despite methodological differences, many studies have shown that regular exercise programs improve effort tolerance in patients with obstructive airway disease. Furthermore, the use of regular exercise improves the patient's ability to perform activities of daily living such as bathing and self-care (23). Studies of long-term outcome of pulmonary rehabilitation that includes both conventional medical management and exercise training indicate reduced morbidity (as measured by number of hospital days) and mortality (24,25). However, chronic home oxygen therapy was also employed in these studies and the contribution of exercise training cannot be singled out.

Factors proposed to explain this imporvement in exercise capacity include increased efficiency of oxygen utilization (improved aerobic capacity of muscles) and improved neuromuscular coordination of respiratory muscles, exercising muscles, or both (26–30). Psychological factors including increased motivation and patient confidence are also felt to have a role in the observed improvement in exercise tolerance (31,32). Desensitization to dyspnea has been suggested as an explanation for the increased ability to exercise (33,34).

The use of supplemental oxygen in COPD has received equal attention in the literature. The merits of nasal oxygen in subjects hypoxemic at rest are clear. There is immediate correction of hypoxemia as well as long-term amelioration of pulmonary hypertension and cor pulmonale (35–37). Functional status increases and mortality is reduced in direct proportion to the daily period of oxygen use and may aid even those without documented hypoxemia (38). Oxygen therapy has also been found effective in exercise (26,39–44). The present feeling is that although sufficient evidence is lacking to formulate firm recommendations for oxygen therapy during exercise, this modality is beneficial in hypoxemic individuals (45–47).

Exercise therapy in chronic obstructive lung disease may include walking, cycling, or stair climbing. No one modality has been found superior. Exercise may initially be prescribed as an inpatient since supervision is important until tolerance is determined. The program must be safe, sufficient to elicit the desired improvement, and acceptable to the patient. As a final note, breathing training focusing on respiratory muscle endurance (work where minute ventilation is more than half of maximal) is felt by some to augment traditional exercise training (37,48).

The indications for performing an exercise test in COPD have been scrutinized. There is general agreement that in patients with airways obstruction, exercise testing facilitates determination of aerobic capacity, evaluation of concomitant cardiac limitation, and the need for supplemental oxygen (49). Also, exercise testing has been employed to monitor progress and predict potential for improvement (6,7). The development of an exercise program in the breathing impaired will be outlined below.

C. Exercise-Induced Asthma

Until recently, exercise-induced asthma was considered a distinct entity (50,51). Individuals displaying bronchospasm, cough and dyspnea with muscular work were felt to have a specific clinical condition. Many theories were proposed to explain the effect of exercise on the lung in these susceptible individuals including lactic acidosis, excessive lung receptor activity, hyperventilation, and autonomic imbalance. As investigation proceeded, most of these factors were excluded. Today, this condition is felt to be part of the spectrum of conventional asthma, but with a specific triggering mechanism.

It now appears that exercise-induced asthma is not produced directly from muscular exercise, but rather the airway cooling and drying that occur with a high minute ventilation causes bronchospasm in individuals that are asthmatic (52). Most individuals displaying this phenomenon frequently have or will develop the typical asthma syndrome. Although most commonly observed with exercise, bronchospasm can be produced by voluntary hyperventilation even at rest under the proper circumstances. Cold air, especially, greatly enhances this phenomena.

Several points appear relevent to the prevention of exercise induced bronchospasm. First, the magnitude of heat and water loss appear closely related to the development and severity of bronchospasm. Exercise at levels above anaerobic threshold (when minute ventilation rapidly increases) or in cold environments (such as skiing) may predictably initiate bronchospasm. Interestingly, brief bursts of exercise (including warmup activities) may protect a person from bronchospasm during subsequent activity. This is felt by some to be mediated by catecholamines released during the limited strenuous activity. Finally, various medications have been found effective in modifying this condition. In general, inhaled agents with rapid local activity have been found to be most effective. Cromolyn sodium, β-adrenergic agonists, and atropine have all been found to have a role in managing this problem.

For prevention of exercise induced bronchospasm, exercise should include a warmup period, remain submaximal if possible, and should be modified to minimize airway cooling and water loss. Certain activities such as swimming are thus better suited for the asthmatic provoked by exercise. Medications are most effectively employed before exercise and the inhaled route has been found to be best. Inhaled cromolyn sodium or β-adrenergic agonists should be used approximately 15 minutes before activity is initiated. In cases in which unanticipated exercise triggers bronchospasm, inhaled sympathomimetics may terminate the attack. Local measures to minimize heat and moisture loss may also be effective, especially in cold weather. Nasal breathing and local protection such as a scarf over the mouth often are enough to avoid provoking bronchospasm.

D.   Restrictive Lung Disease

There are many pulmonary disorders of varied etiology that are considered restrictive in nature. The more common conditions are listed in Table III. As shown, these can be subdivided into impairments of the pulmonary parenchyma, the chest wall, the neuromuscular system and the pleura. Obesity is a restrictive disorder that will be considered separately.

In general, restrictive lung disease is characterized by a reduction in the number of functioning lung units that can be recruited during deep inspiration. Because of stiffness or reduced compliance in either lung, pleura, or chest wall, a greater change in pressure and, therefore, more inspiratory effort are necessary to deliver a given volume of air. At rest, individuals with restrictive lung disease frequently settle for a subnormal tidal volume with an increased respiratory rate to maintain alveolar ventilation with the minimal effort. When the restrictive

TABLE III

Restrictive Lung Disorders

Parenchymal
    Sarcoidosis
    Diffuse pulmonary fibrosis
    Inhaled inorganic dusts (pneumoconioses), e.g., silicosis
    Inhaled organic dusts (extrinsic allergic alveolitis), e.g., farmer's lung
    Collagen vascular disorders
    Drug-induced lung disease
    Radiation induced lung disease
    Toxic gases
    Carcinoma, especially lymphangitic metastasis
    Lung resection or scarring
Chest wall
    Skeletal, e.g., kyphoscoliosis
    Neuromuscular, e.g., poliomyelitis, diaphragmatic paralysis
    Obesity
    Persistent pain (splinting)
Pleural
    Effusion
    Pneumothorax
    Thickening/fibrosis

defect involves the pulmonary interstitium, j-receptors described in Chapter 3 may be excessively stimulated, leading to an even more shallow and rapid respiratory pattern. If the impairment is severe, the high minute ventilation necessary for gas transfer may be impossible and alveolar hypoventilation and hypercarbia ensue.

There are several reasons for hypoxemia in restrictive disease. Random derangement of alveolar structures frequently causes ventilation–perfusion mismatching as well as reduction in functional lung units. Also, thickening of the alveolar capillary membrane and impairment of gas diffusion, so-called alveolar–capillary block, contributes to exercise hypoxemia. At rest the red blood cell has sufficient contact time with the alveolus, but with exercise the increased cardiac output reduces the contact time between the red cell and the alveolus so that equilibration of gas cannot occur. This disturbance is due more to increased ventilation–perfusion imbalance than to the diffusion defect described (53,54). Evidence indicates that diffusing capacity does not change significantly despite the distortion of the alveolar–capillary interface (54). The hypoxemia and widened A-a gradient for oxygen often occur when resting pulmonary function is normal, making this parameter a sensitive indicator of early or mild disease.

These physiological alterations limit exercise in several ways (Table IV). The altered breathing pattern is less efficient, since with lowered tidal volume, fixed

TABLE IV

Exercise Limitation in Restrictive Lung Disease

Altered lung mechanics: rapid shallow breaths at rest due to reduced lung volumes and stretch receptor activation. Exacerbated with exercise, further increasing dead space ventilation.
Ventilation–perfusion mismatch: due to derangement of alveolar units.
Diffusion impairment: thickening of alveolar capillary membrane, unmasked by increased heart rate when rbc contact time is decreased.
Alveolar hypoventilation: occurs when lung volumes are reduced to the extent that minute ventilation cannot accommodate CO_2 production.

anatomical dead space occupies a greater fraction of ventilation. From this and from reduced thoracic compliance, oxygen consumption at any given work rate increases from increased work of breathing. Maximal breathing capacity is reduced, and at the same time the ventilatory equivalent for oxygen ($\dot{V}_E/\dot{V}O_2$) increases, increasing work of breathing. The ventilation–perfusion mismatching and alveolar capillary block combine to impair gas transfer at high work rates. The alveolar–arterial gradient for oxygen widens and significant hypoxemia may occur.

E. Impairment of the Pulmonary Circulation

Disorders primarily involving the pulmonary vasculature that limit exercise include thromboembolic disease, primary pulmonary hypertension, and vasculitis. Thromboembolic impairment due to multiple recurrent pulmonary emboli is the most common condition of this type. Pulmonary hypertension may arise from any pulmonary impairment causing parenchymal destruction and hypoxemia; in these cases the hypertension is secondary and the major problem is the underlying pulmonary disease. Idiopathic or primary pulmonary hypertension is quite uncommon but tends to affect young women and be progressive. Pulmonary vasculitis of small vessels accompanies collagen vascular disease including lupus erythematosis, rheumatoid vasculitis, and scleroderma.

As the vascular bed is occluded or destroyed, the population of ventilated but nonperfused alveoli increases dead space fraction (V_D/V_T) and necessitates an increase in minute ventilation. Consequently, ventilatory requirement is increased at rest and at all levels of exercise.

With vasculitis, there may additionally be problems with oxygen delivery. Frequently there is random derangement of alveolar units and ventilation– perfusion mismatch occurs. This V/Q mismatch is not corrected with exercise and combines with the reduced vascular bed to cause exercise induced hypoxemia. This is similar to one of the pathophysiological mechanisms of restrictive parenchymal disease. The physiological alterations that occur in pulmonary vascular impairment, particularly thromboembolic disease, are rather specific. The combination of normal lung mechanics with increased dead space ventilation and progressive exercise hypoxemia points to thromboembolic disease until proved otherwise (55).

There is little to be gained with exercise therapy in correction of the basic defect in the pulmonary circulation. Unfortunately, there is no satisfactory therapy for the chronic alterations of recurrent emboli or iodiopathic hypertension, and the diseases often pursue a relentless course. The benefit of exercise in this setting probably occurs with improved peripheral oxygen stores and muscle efficiency discussed below.

F. The Role of Exercise in Restrictive and Pulmonary Vascular Lung Disease

Frequently the impairment of oxygen transfer reflects the extent of disease. For example, studies of exercise capability in patients with sarcoidosis have demonstrated normal alveolar gas exchange on exercise in individuals with disease confined to hilar lymph nodes (56). On the other hand, parenchymal involvement with sarcoidosis, whether inflammatory alveolitis or fibrosis, impairs gas exchange during exercise. Similar observations have been made for other infiltrative lung diseases including pulmonary fibrosis and pneumoconiosis from inhaled dusts (57,58). However, it should be remembered that other factors, such as an obstructive component and limited musculoskeletal mobility, frequently coexist and complicate assessment of work performance (58,59).

In general, impaired muscular effort can be due to defects in both oxygenation and ventilation. Therapy directed at the disease process is the key to restoring exercise capability. Numerous studies have documented improvement in exercise tolerance with effective treatment (60,61). Corticosteroids are employed for many interstitial lung diseases and immunosuppressants are useful in certain parenchymal and vascular disorders. Other conditions are without specific therapy.

Until relatively recently, therapy was directed toward rehabilitation of work capacity only when a neuromuscular component existed. In truth, most individuals with restrictive lung impairment would benefit from increased muscular activity. The improvement in skeletal muscle coordination alone allows a higher level of activity to be achieved. Training effects on respiratory muscles such as have been demonstrated in obstructive lung disease patients may occur, although to a lesser extent (20,26–30). Also, the motivational, emotional, and psychological impact of regular exercise cannot be ignored in these conditions. Finally, supplemental oxygen is beneficial in reducing the severity of exercise-induced hypoxemia and thereby increasing work tolerance.

G. Obesity

Obesity, defined as a 20% increase above optimal body weight, presents some unique problems with relation to work ability. At rest, most obese subjects have relatively rapid shallow respirations (62). In addition to restriction of chest wall motion, there is moderate limitation to diaphragmatic excursion in significant obesity (63). Breathing shallowly at lower lung volumes promotes small airway closure with regional atelectasis and can lead to ventilation/perfusion imbalance. Perhaps due to the altered oxygen uptake (and consequent increase in $\dot{V}_E/\dot{V}O_2$), resting minute ventilation is increased in the overweight. It is also possible that increased stretch receptor activity contributes to the increased minute ventilation.

These abnormalities in resting pulmonary mechanics are compounded by exercise. The ventilation–perfusion relationships, which normally improve with exercise, become more disturbed. This is due to a suboptimal increase in tidal volume (recall that tidal volume can normally increase up to fivefold) with a persistently high dead space fraction. Also, the exercise oxygen requirement increases as body fat content increases (64). The large metabolizing tissue mass produces excess carbon dioxide and further elevates the ventilatory requirement (65). If the physical work capacity is expressed as the maximal oxygen consumption available to mobilize a kilogram of body weight ($\dot{V}O_2$ max/kg), there is as much as a 50% reduction in obese subjects when compared to normal sedentary adults (64). Frequently, this compromised state is considered the lower range of normal in the "fitness continuum" previously discussed. We see that the impairments to pulmonary function in obestiy include reduced ventilatory efficiency and elevated oxygen requirements.

The overweight individual has an increased proportion of "inert body mass," that is, tissue that does not participate in muscular exercise. Mostly fat, this "dead weight" can approach 40–50% of body mass (66). In a large heterogenous group of obese adults, the average increase in ventilatory requirement was 130% (67). In very obese subjects, minute ventilation and oxygen consumption are frequently double that of normal at any given level of work. The work of breathing in overweight subjects is increased due to the altered chest wall configuration from excess fat in the thorax and abdomen. This results in an increase in chest wall resistence to breathing. Naimark and Cherniak estimate that a third of the increase of mechanical work of breathing in obesity is due to increased elastic work of the chest wall (68).

Impaired gas exchange in obesity initially received attention with the description of the "Pickwickian syndrome." This constellation of obesity, hypoventilation, hypoxemia, polycythemia, and cor pulmonale was described in 1955 by Sicker and associates (69). Subsequent investigations focused on alveolar hypoventilation as the primary defect in gas exchange in the obese. In 1960 Said reported the more common occurrence of ventilation–perfusion imbalance when individuals with obesity were studied (70). Subsequently, investigators demonstrated that hyperventilation was the more common alteration in breathing at rest and exercise in the overweight (71,72). Table V summarizes the factors contributing to the limitations to exercise in obesity.

Two additional aspects of exercise in obesity are of interest. Despite the wealth of data on ventilatory function in obesity, there has been no correlation established with fat content, body mass, or excess body weight (72–74). Also, in one study weight loss of as much as 50% of body fat has failed to improve compromised gas exchange and pulmonary mechanics (74).

Despite the lack of correlation between weight loss and improved gas exchange, reduction in body mass is the most important therapeutic goal in obesity. Muscular exercise assumes a dual purpose in this regard. The increased caloric expenditure with muscular exercise may aid in reduction of excessive body fat. Also, the "training effect" in obesity may be to correction of those factors contributing to altered lung mechanics, work efficiency and gas exchange.

H. Occupational Aspects

Although there is a link between lung disease and certain activities such as occupational exposure to organic dusts (e.g., farmers' lung), inorganic compounds (e.g., silica), and chemical agents (e.g., toluenediisocyanate in industry), these do not appear to be directly related to the performance of muscular activity. Rather, these entities are considered occupational pulmonary diseases due to the environment rather than to exercise. Although there is little doubt that muscular activity can be limited with occupational lung disease, there is little to differentiate these problems from the disorders previously described. Specifically, occupational disorders can either cause classical restrictive defects (interstitial lung disease from inhalation of environmental dust) or typical obstructive defects (occupational bronchitis or asthma).

Occupationally related asthma constitutes a recently appreciated group of disorders that may be immunological or nonimmunological in nature. Agents associated with the work environment initiate an adverse response that may include airway irritability or bronchospasm. Although not directly related to exercise or

TABLE V

Exercise Limitation in Obesity

Limitations common for all restrictive lung disorders: see Table IV
Increased ventilatory requirement: due to elevated CO_2 production from increased body mass
Increased oxygen requirement: due to increased weight
Increased mechanical work of breathing: due to chest wall impairment
Obesity–hypoventilation syndrome

its equivalent, this disorder may appear to the patient related to exertional aspects of his job. Exposure to occupational agents such as sulfur dioxide, fluorocarbons, various inert dusts, animal proteins, enzymes, grain and cereal dust, and many small molecular weight inorganic chemicals have been implicated (75). Individuals describing exercise limitation or bronchospasm that appears work related should be carefully questioned regarding inciting factors. Needless to say, the avoidance of any putative factor is the appropriate initial therapy. This may involve a minor change in occupational activity or a major adjustment in work or life style.

I.   Exercise Prescription in Pulmonary Disease

Regardless of the nature or severity of the impairment, exercise may produce an increase in the level of daily physical activity. Optimal benefit is realized when supervised activity is performed as part of a comprehensive program that involves medical management and education as well as psychosocial and vocational rehabilitation (76). When exercise is rationally applied, the individual frequently becomes more self-sufficient.

Exercise, like medication, should be properly prescribed including the form, dose, and frequency. When dealing with a breathing impairment, base line exercise tolerance should be known. An exercise test with determination of "mets" of activity often is necessary. The individual's motivation, personal goals, and psychosocial limitations should also be appreciated. Is the patient physically limited or does the fear of breathlessness impose a mental barrier? Since normal daily activities may truly represent exercise for this group of patients, a supervised program of regular muscular activity must be carefully planned. The general guidelines that follow are modifications of exercise recommendations of the American College of Sports Medicine (77).

Several types of activity are available for exercise training. The initial exercises should stress flexibility and relaxation activities that utilize limb movements, calesthenics, and isometrics. These may also be used as "warm-up exercise" before performing more strenuous activities. Endurance activity intended to increase cardiorespiratory functional status is the next step. This should utilize normal forms of activity such as walking, stair climbing, and light work. In addition to flexibility–relaxation exercise and endurance activity, brief high level (often anaerobic) activity intended to improve strength in particular muscle groups may be used. However, this form of activity is usually less beneficial than the previously described modes.

The second aspect of exercise prescription involves the intensity of activity measured in mets and its duration. Once specific goals are set, low level work is initiated. The intensity and/or duration are then gradually increased until symptoms (usually breathlessness) or a heart rate in excess of 70% of maximum are noted. Activity is then reduced or maintained at this level until further "training effect" is noted.

The rate at which exercise intensity and duration are increased depends on the individual's age, pulmonary status, and motivation. The initial conditioning exercises can usually be steadily increased. Endurance activity can be gradually accelerated based on the individual's symptoms and heart rate. With training, a given level of activity should be achievable at a lower heart rate (training effect) and this should be closely monitored by the subject.

With careful titration of the intensity and duration of activity, the targeted level of activity in mets can be attained. Often, however, the individual must settle for a lesser degree of activity. The optimal level reached should allow for 15 minutes of steady-state exercise without undue fatigue 1 hour later. A final factor is the frequency of exercise work. Initially, when endurance is minimal, frequent brief sessions may be necessary on a daily basis. As functional capacity increases and duration of activity increases, frequency can be reduced to only several times daily. With conditioning, once daily exercise at least three times per week is sufficient to maintain fitness.

The last item in the exercise prescription is consideration of oxygen requirements. Often the breathing impaired individual will have a significant increase in functional capacity with supplemental oxygen. Although there appears to be no consistent improvement in most of the parameters of exercise performance, there is general agreement that exercise tolerance is improved with supplemental oxy-

TABLE VI

Elements of Exercise Prescription

Type
1. Flexibility and relaxation exercises
2. Cardiorespiratory endurance activity
3. Muscular strength activities

Intensity
1. Initially low level: 50% of maximum predicted
2. Increased by 10% every 2 weeks
3. Maximum intensity determined by symptoms and/or heart rate

Duration
1. Initially brief
2. Titrated along with intensity
3. Should approach fifteen minutes of steady state work

Frequency
1. Initially several times daily
2. With training can be reduced to three times a week

Oxygen supplementation
1. Assessed with exercise study
2. Should have $PaO_2 > 55$ mm Hg

gen in those individuals who become hypoxemic on room air. It may be necessary to determine the oxygen requirements of a symptomatic individual by means of exercise testing with measurement of resting and exercise blood gases. A summary of the factors involved in prescribing exercise is provided in Table VI.

REFERENCES

1. Åstrand, P.-O., and Rodahl, K. (1970). "Textbook of Work Physiology," 2nd ed. McGraw-Hill, New York.
2. Jones, N. L., and Campbell, E. J. (1982). "Clinical Exercise Testing," 2nd ed. Saunders, Philadelphia, Pennsylvania.
3. Wasserman, K., and Whipp, B. J. (1975). Exercise physiology in health and disease. *Am. Rev. Respir. Dis.* **112**, 219–249.
4. Spiro, S. (1977). Exercise testing in clinical medicine. *Br. J. Dis. Chest* **71**, 145–72.
5. Wasserman, K., and Whipp, B. J. (1975). Exercise physiology in health and disease. *Am. Rev. Respir. Dis.* **112**, 244–245.
6. Moser, K. M., Bokinsky, G. E., Savage, R. T., Archibald, C. J., and Hausen, P. R. (1980). Results of a comprehensive rehabilitative program. Physiologic and functional effects on patients with chronic obstructive pulmonary disease. *Arch. Intern. Med.* **140**, 1596–1601.
7. Alison, J. A., Samios, R., and Anderson, S. D. (1981). Evaluation of exercise training in patients with chronic airway obstruction. *Phys. Ther.* **61**, 1273–1277.
8. Mungall, I. P., and Hainsworth, R. (1980). An objective assessment of the value of exercise training to patients with chronic obstructive airways disease. *Q. J. Med.* [N. S.] **49**, 77–85.
9. Bierman, C. W., Pierson, W. E., and Shapiro, G. G. (1977). Effect of drugs on exercise-induced bronchospasm. *In* "Muscular Exercise and the Lung" (J. A. Dempsey and C. E. Reed, eds.). Univ. of Wisconsin Press, Madison.
10. Dempsey, J. A., and Rankin, J. (1967). Physiologic adaptation of gas transport systems to muscular work in health and disease. *Am. J. Phys. Med.* **46**, 582–647.
11. Leith, E. D., and Bradly, M. (1976). Ventilatory muscle strength and endurance training. *J. Appl. Physiol.* **41**, 508–516.
12. Åstrand, P.-O., and Rodahl, K. (1970). "Textbook of Work Physiology," 2nd ed., p. 224. McGraw-Hill, New York.
13. Bannister, R. G., Cotes, J. E., Jones, R. S., and Meade, F. (1960). Pulmonary diffusing capacity on exercise in athletes and non-athletic subjects. *J. Physiol. (London)* **152**, 66P.
14. Clausen, J. P. (1977). Effect of physical training on cardiovascular adjustments to exercise in man. *Physiol. Rev.* **57**, 779–815.
15. Åstrand, P.-O., and Rodahl, K. (1970). "Textbook of Work Physiology," 2nd ed., pp. 391–445. McGraw-Hill, New York.
16. Marcus, J. H., McLean, R. L., Duffell, G. M., and Ingram, R. H., Jr. (1970). Exercise performance in relation to pathophysiologic type of chronic obstructive pulmonary disease. *Am. J. Med.* **49**, 14–22.
17. Field, S., Kelly, S. M., and Macklem, P. T. (1982). The oxygen cost of breathing in patients with cardiorespiratory disease. *Am. Rev. Respir. Dis.* **126**, 9–13.
18. Jones, N. L. (1966). Pulmonary gas exchange during exercise in patients with chronic airway obstruction. *Clin. Sci.* **31**, 39–50.
19. Spiro, S. G., Hahn, H. L., Edwards, R. H. T., and Pride, N. B. (1975). An analysis of the physiological strain of submaximal exercise in patients with chronic obstructive bronchitis. *Thorax* **30**, 415–420.

20. Haas, A., and Cardon, H. (1969). Rehabilitation in chronic obstructive pulmonary disease. A five year study of 252 male patients. *Med. Clin. North Am.* **53,** 593–606.
21. Barach, A. L., Bickerman, H. A., and Beck, G. J. (1952). Advances in treatment of nontuberculous pulmonary disease. *Bull. N. Y. Acad. Med.* [2] **28,** 353–359.
22. Cotes, J. E., and Gilson, J. C. (1956). Effect of oxygen on exercise ability in chronic respiratory insufficiency. *Lancet* **1,** 872–876.
23. Unger, K. M., Moser, K. M., and Hansen, P. (1980). Selection of an exercise program for patients with chronic obstructive pulmonary disease. *Heart Lung* **9,** 68–76.
24. Sahn, S. A., Nett, L. M., and Petty, T. L. (1980). Ten-year follow up of a comprehensive rehabilitation program for severe COPD. *Chest* **77,** Suppl., 311–314.
25. Giminez, M., Pham, Q. T., Uffholtz, H., and Sobradillo, V. (1978). Ten years follow up in patients with chronic obstructive lung disease submitted to a program of pulmonary rehabilitation. *J. R. Soc. Med.* **71,** 61–62
26. Petty, T. L., Nett, L. M., Finigan, M. M., Brink, G. A., and Corsello, P. R. (1969). A comprehensive care program for chronic airway obstruction. *Ann. Intern. Med.* **70,** 1109–1120.
27. Paly, P. N., Phillipson, E. A., Masangkay, M., and Sproule, B. J. (1967). The physiologic basis of training patients with emphysema. *Am. Rev. Respir. Dis.* **95,** 944–953.
28. Alpert, J. S., Bass, H., Szucs, M. M., Banas, J. S., Dalen, J. E., and Dexter, L. (1974). Effects of physical training on hemodynamics and pulmonary function at rest and during exercise in patients with chronic obstructive pulmonary disease. *Chest* **66,** 647–651.
29. Nicholas, J. J., Gilbert, R., Gabe, R., and Auchincloss, J. H., Jr. (1970). Evaluation of an exercise therapy program for patients with chronic obstructive pulmonary disease. *Am. Rev. Respir. Dis.* **102,** 1–9.
30. Belman, M. J., and Mittman, C. (1980). Ventilatory muscle training improves exercise capacity in chronic obstructive pulmonary disease patients. *Am. Rev. Respir. Dis.* **121,** 273–280.
31. Chester, E. H., Belman, M. J., Bahler, R. C., Baum, G. L., Schey, G., and Buch, P. (1977). Multidisciplinary treatment of chronic pulmonary insufficiency. 3. The effect of physical training on cardiopulmonary performance in patients with chronic obstructive pulmonary disease. *Chest* **72,** 695–702.
32. McGavin, C. R., Gupta, S. P., Lloyd, E. L., and McHardy, G. J. R. (1977). Physical rehabilitation for the chronic bronchitic: Results of a controlled trial for exercises in the home. *Thorax* **32,** 307–311.
33. Baum, G. L., Agle, D. P., Chester, E. H., Schey, G., Anteola, E., Buch, P., Bahler, R., and Wendt, M. (1973). Multidiscipline treatment of chronic pulmonary insufficiency: Functional status at one-year follow up. *In* "Pulmonary Care" (R. F. Johnston, ed.), pp. 355–362. Grune & Stratton, New York.
34. Bruno, B. H., and Howell, J. B. L. (1969). Disproportionately severe breathlessness in chronic bronchitis. *Q. J. Med.* [N. S.] **38,** 277–293.
35. Petty, T. L., and Finigan, M. M. (1967). The clinical evaluation of prolonged ambulatory oxygen therapy in patients with chronic airway obstruction with hypoxemia. *Ann. Intern. Med.* **66,** 639–650.
36. Neff, T. A., and Petty, T. L. (1970). Long term continuous oxygen therapy in chronic airway obstruction. *Ann. Intern.Med.* **72,** 621–626.
37. Steward, B. N., Hood, C. I., and Block, A. J. (1975). Long term results of continuous oxygen therapy at sea level. *Chest* **68,** 486–492.
38. Nocturnal Oxygen Therapy Trial Group (1980). Continuous or nocturnal oxygen therapy in hypoxemic chronic obstructive lung disease. *Ann. Inter. Med.* **93,** 391–398.
39. Barach, A. L. (1966). Oxygen supported exercise and rehabilitation of patients with chronic obstructive lung disease. *Ann. Allergy* **24,** 51–57.

40. Vyas, M. N., Banister, E. W., Morton, J. W., and Grzybowski, S. (1971). Response to exercise in patients with chronic airway obstruction. II. Effects of breathing 40 per cent oxygen. *Am. Rev. Respir. Dis.* **103**, 401–412.

41. Longo, A. M., Moser, K. M., and Luchsinger, P. C. (1971). The role of oxygen therapy in the rehabilitation of patients with chronic obstructive pulmony disease. *Am. Rev. Respir. Dis.* **103**, 690–697.

42. Stark, R. D., Finnegan, P., and Bishop. J. M. (1972). Daily requirement of oxygen to reverse pulmonary hypertension in patients with chronic bronchitis. *Br. Med. J.* **3**, 724–728.

43. King, A. J., Cooke, N. J., Leitch, A. G., and Flenly, D. C. The effects of 30% oxygen on the respiratory response to treadmill exercise in chronic respiratory failure. *Clin. Sci.* **44**, 151–162.

44. Bradley, B. L., Garner, A. E., Billiu, D., Mestas, J. M., and Forman, J. (1978). Oxygen-assisted exercise in chronic obstructive lung disease. *Am. Rev. Respir. Dis.* **118**, 239–243.

45. Editorial (1981). Oxygen in the home. *Br. Med. J.* **2**, 1909–1910.

46. Block, A. J., Castle, J. R., and Keitt, A. S. (1974). Chronic oxygen therapy. *Chest* 65, 279–288.

47. Baum, G. L. (1975). Exercise tolerance increased by oxygen therapy or psychologic factors? *Chest* **67**, 736–737.

48. Pardy, R. L., Rivington, R. N., Despas, P. J., and Macklem, P. T. (1981). Inspiratory muscle training compared with physiotherapy in patients with chronic airflow limitation. *Am. Rev. Respir. Dis.* **123**, 421–425.

49. Belman, M. J., and Wasserman, K. (1981). Exercise training and testing in patients with chronic obstructive pulmonary disease. *Basics RD* **10** (2).

50. Herxheimer, H. (1946). Hyperventilation asthma. *Lancet* **1**, 83–87.

51. Anderson, S. D., Silverman, M., Konig, P., and Godfrey, S. (1975). Exercise-induced asthma. *Br. J. Dis. Chest* **69**, 1–39.

52. McFadden, E. R., and Ingram, R. H. (1979). Exercise-induced asthma, observations on the initiating stimulus. *N. Engl. J. Med.* **301**, 763–769

53. Wagner, P. D., Dantzker, D. R., Dueck, R., DePolo, J. L., Wasserman, K., and West, J. B. (1976). Distribution of ventilation perfusion ratios in patients with interstitial lung disease. *Chest* **69**, 256–258.

54. Spiro, S. G. (1977). Exercise testing in clinical medicine. *Br. J. Dis. Chest* **71**, 145–172.

55. Wasserman, K., and Whipp, B. J. (1975). Exercise physiology in health and disease. *Am. Rev. Respir. Dis.* **112**, 237–241.

56. Holmgren, A., and Svenborg, N. (1961). Studies on the cardiopulmonary function in sarcoidosis. *Acta Med. Scand., Suppl.* **336**, 1–37.

57. Stanek, V., Widimsky, J., Kasalicky, J., Narratil, M., Daum, S., and Levinsky, L. (1967). The pulmonary gas exchange during exercise in patients with pulmonary fibrosis. *Scand. J. Respir. Dis.* **48**, 11–30.

58. Gabriel, S. K. (1973). Respiratory and circulatory investigations in obstructive and restrictive lung disease. *Acta Med. Scand., Suppl.* **546**, 1–87.

59. Godfrey, S., Bluestone, R., and Higgs, B. E. (1969). Lung function and the response to exercise in systemic sclerosis. *Thorax* **24**, 427–434.

60. Chester, E. H., Fleming, G. M., and Montenegro, H. (1976). Effect of steroid therapy on gas exchange abnormalities in patients with diffuse interstitial lung disease. *Chest* **69**, 269–271.

61. Emirgil, C., Sobol, B. J., and Williams, M. H. (1969). Long-term study of pulmonary sarcoidosis. The effect of steroid therapy as evaluated by pulmonary function studies. *J. Chronic Dis.* **22**, 69–86.

62. Said, S. I. (1960). Abnormalities of pulmonary gas exchange in obesity. *Ann. Intern. Med.* **53**, 1121–1129.

63. Kerr, W. J., and Lagen, J. B. (1936). The postural syndrome related to obesity leading to postural emphysema and cardiorespiratory failure. *Ann. Intern. Med.* **10,** 569.

64. Miller, A. T., and Blyth, C. S. (1955). Influence of body type and body fat content on the metabolic cost of work. *J. Appl. Physiol.* **8,** 139–141.

65. Dempsey, J. A., and Rankin, J. (1967). Physiologic adaptations of gas transport systems to muscular work in health and disease. *Am. J. Phys. Med.* **46,** 618–621.

66. Sharp. J. T., Henry, J. P., Sweeny, S. K., Meadows, W. R., and Pietras, R. J. (1964). The total work of breathing in normal and obese men. *J. Clin. Invest.* **43,** 738–739.

67. Naimarck, A., and Cherniak, R. M. (1960). Compliance of the respiratory system and its components in health and obesity. *J. Appl. Physiol.* **15,** 377–382.

68. Sicker, H. O., Estes, E. H., Kelser, G. A., and McIntosh, H. D. (1955). A cardiopulmonary syndrome associated with extreme obesity. *J. Clin. Invest.* **34,** 916.

69. White, R. I., and Alexander, J. K. (1965). Body oxygen consumption and pulmonary ventilation in obese subjects. *J. Appl. Physiol.* **20,** 197–201.

70. Dempsey, J. A., Reddan, W., Rankin, J., and Balke, B. (1966). Alveolar-arterial gas exchange during muscular work in obesity. *J. Appl. Physiol.* **21,** 1807–1814.

71. Cullen, J. H., and Formel, P. F. (1962). The respiratory defects in extreme obesity. *Am. J. Med.* **32,** 525–531.

72. Dempsey, J. A., Reddan, W., Balke, B., and Rankin, J. (1966). Work capacity determinants and physiologic cost of weight-supported work in obesity. *J. Appl. Physiol.* **21,** 1815–1820.

73. Alexander, J. K., Amad, K. H., and Cole, V. W. (1962). Observations on some clinical features of extreme obesity with particular reference to cardiorespiratory effects. *Am. J. Med.* **32,** 512–524.

74. Cullen, J. H., and Formel, P. F. (1962). The respiratory defects in extreme obesity. *Am. J. Med.* **32,** 525–531.

75. Salvaggio, J. E. (1982). Overview of occupational immunologic lung disease. *J. Allergy Clin. Immunol.* **70,** 5–10.

76. Hodgkin, J. E., Balchum, O. J., Kass, I., Glaser, E. M., Miller, W. F., Haas, A., Shaw, D. B., Kimbal, P., and Petty, T. L. (1975). Chronic obstructive airway disease, current concepts in diagnosis and comprehensive care. *JAMA, J. Am. Med. Assoc.* **232,** 1243–1260.

77. Sinclair, J. D. (1978). Exercise in pulmonary disease. *In* "Therapeutic Exercise" (J. V. Basmajian, ed.), pp. 565–590. Williams & Wilkins, Baltimore, Maryland.

78. American College of Sports Medicine (1980). "Guidelines for Graded Exercise Testing and Exercise Prescription," 2nd ed. Lea & Febiger, Philadelphia, Pennsylvania.

CHAPTER 13

Gastrointestinal Disorders and Exercise

STANLEY H. LORBER

Department of Medicine
Temple University Medical
School
Philadelphia, Pennsylvania

Exercise Medicine: Physiological Principles
and Clinical Applications

The gastrointestinal tract has not been one of the chief beneficiaries of investigative interest related to exercise. As one reads through monographs, texts, etc., on this subject, one recognizes quickly the paucity of information related to hard data versus the abundance of opinions derived from anecdotal experiences. In this chapter we shall attempt to differentiate the objective and subjective types of information available.

I. PHYSIOLOGY: EXERCISE AND GASTROINTESTINAL FUNCTION

A. Gastric Secretion

Most studies provide evidence that mild exercise has little effect on gastric secretion or on gastric emptying. Markiewicz (1) observed little change in basal gastric secretion in healthy men riding a bicycle, but after exercise, acid secretion decreased. Lactic acid in the gastric juice increased both during and after exercise. Campbell *et al.* (2) and Ramsbottom and Hunt (3) both found a decrease in gastric acid secretion during exercise in healthy men and they, as well as Hellerbrandt and Tepper (4), observed that the decrease paralleled the quantity of exercise and not its type. Thus, jogging (motion) versus riding a bicycle ergometer (stationary) produced similar effects with comparable levels of exercise, but as the exercise load was increased to strenuous levels, further decreases in acid secretion were observed. In addition, Hellerbrandt and Tepper (4) observed a decrease in acid secretion during the restitution period. Markiewicz *et al.* (1) studied 10 patients with chronic duodenal ulcer and observed a significant increase in gastric juice volume as well as acid output during exercise with an ergometer. They exercised patients to a load that gave a constant pulse rate increase equal to 50% of the age related maximum. Values obtained during the recovery period were similar to those obtained at rest. The contrast of this finding to observations made on normal individuals is difficult to explain but could relate to differences in autonomic responses. These patients did have a higher basal acid output at rest than did the normals. This finding raises the question of whether exercise or, more appropriately, strenuous exercise in patients with active duodenal ulcer may be deleterious.

B. Gastric Emptying: Influence of Dietary Factors

It is of interest that Beaumont was the first to note that severe exercise retarded gastric emptying but that mild exercise hastened it. Hellerbrandt and Tepper (4) and Campbell *et al.* (2) using different techniques observed accelerated gastric emptying with moderate exercise but severe exhaustive exercise delayed it. The study by Fordtran and Saltin (5) indicates that exercise had little effect on gastric emptying until the working intensity exceeded 70% of the maximum oxygen uptake. Cammack *et al.* (6) observed accelerated emptying with intermittent prolonged pedalling. However, unlike the other investigators, he employed a noninvasive technique with a radioactive isotope to determine gastric emptying. Exercise has been observed to increase the delay in gastric emptying at rest which occurs following the ingestion of high volume, increased osmolality, and fatty foods. At rest, Costill and Saltin (7) observed that glucose induced a marked decrease in the rate of gastric emptying and this was particularly accentuated with high intensity exercise.

C. Intestinal Absorption

Fordtran and Saltin (5) reviewed previous studies on the influence of exercise on intestinal absorption. They cited evidence that suggested that exercise reduced blood flow to the gut and this in turn reduces active but not passive intestinal absorption. They failed to observe any influence of exercise on absorption in both jejunum and ileum to glucose, water, sodium, chloride, potassium, or bicarbonate. Williams *et al.* (8) had observed that absorption in dogs is markedly reduced when blood flow to intestinal segments is decreased below the 50% level. They suggested that exercise has a greater effect on active absorption than it has on passive absorption although the latter was reduced somewhat. Williams *et al.* (8) also observed a decrease in intestinal transit during exercise and they suggested that this finding may relate to the increased blood levels of catecholamines and corticosteroids as well as the effect of prolonged moderate exercise on mucosal blood flow. Cammack *et al.* (6), measuring breath hydrogen excretion, did not observe any significant effect of prolonged moderate exercise on intestinal absorption. Similarly, Aslaksen and Aanderrud (9) failed to find any significant differences in absorption of drugs (quinidine sulfate, sodium salicylate, and sulfadimidine) during exercise. However, Williams *et al.* (8) measured vitamin A absorption during exercise and found it decreased. The latter may represent a difference between the absorption of fat- versus water-soluble substances. Varro *et al.* (10) observed that there were critical levels of oxygen tension and blood flow that influenced intestinal absorption even of isotonic carbohydrates; although the intestine has a capacity for regulation to compensate for reduced blood flow, the decrease in oxygen supply may be the key factor.

Different sugars may be absorbed at different rates during exercise. A study by Koivisto and associates (11), employing different carbohydrates, specifically glucose and fructose with a placebo revealed that fructose produced less of a rise than glucose in blood sugar levels and therefore less of an increase in insulin. They were unable to demonstrate any difference in performance of athletes in response to different sugars. Others have shown that glucose administration prior to exercise can result in hypoglycemia during vigorous exercise.

D. Liver

Rowell *et al.* (12) point out that previous studies have demonstrated a decrease in hepatic blood flow during exercise. They estimate that a decrease of as much as 80% or more in estimated hepatic blood flow occurs in upright men during strenuous exercise. Bunch (13) found that athletes, particularly long-distance runners, may have an increased SGOT as well as some increase in bilirubin and alkaline phosphatase during and/or after exercise. He cautions against making the erroneous assumption that these changes imply liver disease.

E. Biliary Excretion

There is evidence in both man and animals that exercise may have a favorable effect on lipid metabolism, bile composition, bile flow, and excretion. This subject is reviewed by Sinko (14) who points out that, in addition to lowering cholesterol in skeletal muscle and increasing fecal excretion of cholesterol, exercise can decrease the incidence of cholelithiasis. It has been shown that as the output of cholesterol and bile acids into bile increases with exercise, there is preferential release of unsaturated fatty acids from adiopose tissue. In this regard, short bursts of physical activity repeated several times a day may be equally or more beneficial than prolonged exercise. He suggests that, to be effective, physical exercise should be regular and continuous throughout life.

II. GASTROINTESTINAL SYMPTOMS AND EXERCISE

A. Heartburn

Reflux from stomach to esophagus, the main cause of heartburn, is dependent on a number of factors but the most important of these is the lower esophageal sphincter pressure. That this can be overcome by a marked increase in intra-abdominal pressure is well known. Changes in position which straighten the angle of the esophagogastric junction may also allow reflux to occur more readily. Thus, it is not surprising that Sullivan (15), in a survey of 57 competitive runners, observed an incidence of heartburn of 10%. Cohen (16) in a study of patients with chest pain, failed to observe any effect of a stress test on the lower esophageal sphincter.

B. Chest Pain

Chest pain is another symptom that can be related to the esophagus, with or without reflux. In a study reported by Tibbling (17), 80% of patients with hiatal hernia had chest pain and in 63% it was effort related. In some, pain could be reproduced with an acid infusion test. Of the 217 patients with a positive acid test, 82% had a history of chest pain which was effort related. The author concludes, as have others, that the esophagus is a more common cause of substernal pain induced by exercise than is angina pectoris due to myocardial ischemia. Tibbling (17) also makes the point that substernal chest pain is more likely to originate from the esophagus due to reflux or esophageal motor dysfunction than it is from heart disease.

C. Nausea and Vomiting

Volpicelli (18) discusses nausea and vomiting resulting from exercise. He cites nervous tension, inhibition of gastric emptying, ingestion of improper foods before exercise, and alterations in circulation as the major causes for these symptoms. It is well known among athletes that nausea and vomiting are more apt to occur in individuals who are poorly trained than in those with adequate conditioning.

D. Diarrhea

A number of authors have documented the occurrence of diarrhea with or without colic in patients during or after exercise. Plasma motilin levels increase during exercise and perhaps the rise in this hormone accounts for or contributes to the augmented motility observed. Sullivan (15) cited an incidence of the urge or need to defecate in 30% of competitive runners. Of these, most had troublesome cramps. Cantwell (19) described several patients with similar symptoms in whom severe and even bloody diarrhea occurred. In one, operation revealed a pale and edematous bowel with small bleeding points observed on the serosa of the cecum and ascending colon. Biopsies revealed nonspecific colitis. In a 27-year-old female, gut ischemia was also thought to be the cause of her bloody diarrhea. Fogoros (20) discusses "runner's trots" as being largely crampy, periumbilical pain and diarrhea. He points out, as do others, that diarrhea plus the dehydration of running may lead to severe renal problems. He again cites gut ischemia as the major factor, particularly with poor or inadequate training.

III. INFLUENCE OF EXERCISE ON GASTROINTESTINAL DISEASE

A. Peptic Ulcer

Studies done on male and female patients with peptic ulcer by Bulvas *et al.* (21) revealed that they react to cold stimulus with more marked vasoconstriction than healthy individuals. The vasoconstriction observed in patients with duodenal ulcer was greater than those with gastric ulcer. And finally, they reported that the peripheral arteries of both men and women with duodenal ulcer, as measured by an oscillographic technique, reacted more strongly to exercise and to exercise following application of cold than did corresponding controls, and in the case of the women, in addition, to those with gastric ulcer. Also, Brandsborg *et al.* (22) observed that exercise increases fasting gastrin concentrations. They cite a relationship between the rise in serum gastrin and plasma adrenalin but it is known that many hormones will increase during exercise. Markiewicz *et al.* (1) observed increased acid output in patients with duodenal ulcer after exercise in contrast to the decrease observed in normals (see Section I,A). With regard to the gastrointestinal tract, peptic ulcer has been the center of interest of the epidemiologists. Frenkl (23) observed a lower incidence of peptic ulcer in sportsmen engaging in regular training than in individuals in the same age group abstaining from physical activity. He observed, further, that the serum of subjects well conditioned to exercise was found to reduce gastric acid secretion in rats. In a study of college students, Paffenbarger *et al.* (24) reported reduced participation in physical activity as a factor that predisposes to peptic ulceration. They found the incidence of peptic ulcer inversely related to sports participation. Those who did not participate in sports at all had an incidence rate of peptic ulceration of 18.8 per 1000 and those involved in 10 or more hours of sports participation per week had a rate of 13 per 1000 or 31% lower. Parallel findings were reported for participation in varsity athletics. Finally, in a study of the incidence of peptic ulcer in the Royal Navy, Watt (25) pointed out that peptic ulcer was highest in the sedentary groups and lower in the active groups. Four factors that they claim may be responsible for the increased incidence of peptic ulcer in their Naval personnel are (1) personality of those attracted to a seagoing life, (2) operational conditions associated with tension, (3) inactive physical activity, and (4) a diet rich in refined carbohydrates.

B. Ileostomy and Colostomy

The question of exercise in the patient with ileostomy was addressed by Pressel (26), in an interview with the well-known football player and kicker, Rolf Benirschke. He points out that an ileostomy will physically limit participation in contact sports because of the potential of trauma. However, he as a kicker does well. He stated that he skis, plays hockey, and swims and does not find that his ileostomy produces any difficulty in any of these sports. As better appliances and adhesives have been devised, more and more patients with ileostomy are engaging in vigorous sports. Golf, tennis, bowling, and jogging are other sports that patients of ours participate in without difficulty. The patient with a colostomy, particularly a left-sided pouch, has even greater freedom of activity and could probably participate in any athletic endeavor except for violent contact sports. We have known a number of patients with colostomies who have continued participation in sports after their surgery without their associates being aware of their medical problem.

C. Hepatitis

A major concern to the clinician is the influence of rest and physical activity in patients with infectious hepatitis. Chalmers *et al.* (27) pointed out that patients with hepatitis improved as rapidly when allowed to ambulate as do patients kept at strict bed rest. Relapses occurred equally among the two groups. It should be noted, however, that this was *ad lib* ambulation. Patients were allowed to stay in bed if they did not feel well enough to be up and around. Physical reconditioning during convalescence did result in some increase in symptoms, signs, and laboratory abnormalities to a small degree, but in most, this was transient in nature. The incidence of chronic disability or significant residual abnormality observed in the follow-up study was no greater for patients who were permitted *ad lib* ambulation versus those started on strenuous physical rehabilitation early in convalescence. It should be emphasized, however, that patients were never forced to stay out of bed or to perform any labor. There was no evidence that rest is not advantageous when the patient feels sick. They suggest that *ad lib* activity be carried out as soon as the serum bilirubin level has been 1.5 mg or less for 1 week. However, Krikler and Zilberg (28) and Krikler (29) reported five cases of fulminant hepatitis in patients who had taken vigorous exercise at the start or induction of their disease. This strenuous exercise, during the preicteric stage, led to death in three of the five patients. They suggested, therefore, that exercise had made mild attacks more severe and that strenuous exercise should be avoided if early hepatitis is suspected. Since this was a retrospective study, Repsher and Freehern (30) performed a controlled study on 199 Viet Nam servicemen affected with hepatitis. They encouraged strenuous exercise for approximately 3 hours/day in the recovery phase when symptoms were considered to be light. This activity did not adversely affect serum bilirubin or relapse rate. However, the subjects were previously young, healthy men and this regimen might not apply to the general population.

Swift *et al.* (31) were the first to show that exercise in patients with hepatitis, with serum bilirubins over the level of 3 mg, could prolong convalescence and even induce relapse. Levels below 3 mg did not have any effect on the course of the disease. One could conclude that vigorous exercise should be avoided in patients with hepatitis; that *ad lib* limited activity or ambulation is not contraindicated if it does not adversely affect the way the patient feels; and that once the serum bilirubin is below 1.5, mild exercise need not be precluded. A study by Frenkl and Pavlik (32) in rats indicated that exercise enhances liver enzyme induction after partial hepatectomy. However, in spite of some suggested benefits of exercise, greater care or restrictions should be advised in the older patient as well as the more seriously affected patient.

D. Inflammatory Bowel Disease

There is a lack of objective data regarding the influence of exercise on inflammatory bowel disease (IBD) but in dealing with hundreds of patients with IBD, including some well-known athletes, the following generalities would seem to apply. The patient with inactive disease has little problem in participating in most sports. However, we have observed patients with inactive disease who have had problems with diarrhea when engaged in excessive physical activity such as basketball, lacrosse, and long-distance running. In addition, competitive sports may induce emotional tension, which in the patient with IBD, can result in increased intestinal activity. In the presence of active disease, participation in sports will have to be reduced or curtailed depending on the severity of the exacerbation. Mild participation, particularly in young patients, should be encouraged if well tolerated.

E. Gastric Cancer

Stukonis and Doll (33) found some relationship between the mortality from gastric cancer and increased physical activity at work. They felt that this may relate to the fact that occupations involving heavy work require workers to eat more, and consequently they are exposed to a greater quantity of carcinogens in their food. They point out also that carcinogens may be present in greater concentrations in cheap food than in expensive food and, in particular, in foods that have been imperfectly preserved. Thus, it is not clear if this report represents a relationship of gastric cancer to exercise or to other factors.

IV. GASTROINTESTINAL DISEASES OR DISORDERS RESULTING FROM PARTICIPATION IN SPORTS

A. Neuropathy

Dancaster (34) has described neuropathy in two marathon runners. This disorder results from severe dehydration, aggravated by diarrhea, which leads to rhabdomyolysis pigmenturia.

B. Trauma

A variety of injuries to the gastrointestinal tract can result from traume induced by sports. Fixation of a segment of bowel across the spine can produce a midline injury to the intestine. The location of the injuries suggests that a shearing force between two opposing surfaces is a primary cause of intestinal injury due to blunt trauma. Baker (35) cites two instances of such a problem both resulting in perforation of the jejunum. Holt *et al.* (36) cite a similar case. Repeated references are made in the literature to injury of the pancreas resulting from blunt trauma. The damage to the pancreas may consist of anything from edema to hematoma to actual rupture of ducts of the gland. This is discussed in detail by Foley and Teele (37). Finally, water skier's enema has been described by Kaiser (38). Landing on water at high speeds in a sitting position forces water up the rectum which causes pain, cramps, desire to defecate, and can lead to bloody diarrhea.

C. Serum Hepatitis

Ringertz and Zetterberg (39) observed 568 cases of this disease over a 5-year period among cross-country trackers in Sweden. They conclude that this unusual transmission of the virus resulted from the cutting effect of sharp branches that became contaminated by a seropositive carrier and then was transferred to susceptible individuals.

As is true with other groups, hepatitis outbreaks can occur in an athletic team, particularly from contaminated water. Morse *et al.* (40) described the infection of 90 of 97 persons at risk involving the Holy Cross football team.

D. Swimmers Dysentery

A number of investigators including Baron *et al.* (41), Cabelli *et al.* (42), Koopman *et al.* (43), and Rosenberg *et al.* (44) have described a greater incidence of disabling gastrointestinal illnesses occurring in swimmers, particularly those who swim in swimming pools that may be contaminated with a high fecal coliform count. Thus, bacterial contamination of water poses a problem to such individuals and can result in dysentery.

V. CONCLUSIONS

The variability in observations reported in this chapter on the influences of exercise on gastrointestinal function, disorders, and diseases depends on population studied (young healthy athletes versus others), the type and magnitude of the exercise utilized, as well as the techniques employed in measuring responses. In general, mild to moderate exercise has little adverse affect on the gastrointestinal tract and, in some ways, improves function. Severe exercise, producing a marked reduction in splanchnic blood flow, neural responses and the release of a variety of hormones (45), may compromise a number of gastrointestinal functions. In disease states, exercise has to be tempered according to the specific disease, its severity, the age of the patient, as well as to the response experienced to the specific exercise.

REFERENCES

1. Markiewicz, K., Cholewa, M., and Lukin, M. (1979). Gastric basal secretion during exercise and restitution in patients with chronic duodenal ulcer. *Acta Hepato-Gastroenterol.* **26**, 160–165.
2. Campbell, H. M. H., Mitchell, M. B., and Powell, A. T. W. (1928). The influence of exercise on digestion. *Guy's Hosp. Rep.* **78**, 273–279.
3. Ramsbottom, N., and Hunt, J. N. (1974). Effects of exercise on gastric emptying. *Digestion* **10**, 1–8.
4. Hellerbrandt, F. A., and Tepper, R. H. (1934). Studies on the influence of exercise on the digestive work of the stomach. *Am. J. Physiol.* **107**, 355.
5. Fordtran, J. S., and Saltin, B. (1967). Gastric emptying and intestinal absorption during prolonged severe exercise. *J. Appl. Physiol.* **23**, 331–335.
6. Cammack, K. J., Read, N. W., Cann, P. A., Greenwood, B., and Hulgak, A. M. (1982). Effect of prolonged exercise on the passage of a solid meal through the stomach and small intestine. *Gut.* **23**, 957–961.
7. Costill, D. L., and Saltin, B. (1974). Factors limiting gastric emptying during rest and exercise. *J. Appl. Physiol.* **37**, 679–683.
8. Williams, J. H., Jr., Mager, M., and Jacobson, E. D. (1964). Relationship of mesenteric blood flow to intestinal absorption of carbohydrates. *J. Lab. Clin. Med.* **63**, 853–863.
9. Aslaksen, O., and Aanderud, L. (1980). Drug absorption during physical exercise. *Br. J. Clin. Pharmacol.* **10**, 383–385.
10. Varro, V., Blacho, G., Csernag, L., Jung, I., and Szarvas, F. (1965). Effect of decreased local circulation on the absorptive capacity of a small intestine loop in the dog. *Am. J. Dig. Dis.* **10**, 170–177.
11. Koivisto, V. A., Karonen, S.-L., and Nikkila, E. A. (1981). Carbohydrate ingestion before exercise: Comparison of glucose, fructose, and sweet placebo. *J. Appl. Physiol.* **51**, 793–797.
12. Rowell, L. B., Blackmon, J. R., and Bruce, R. A. (1964). Indocyanine green clearance and estimated hepatic blood flow during mild to maximal exercise in upright man. *J. Clin. Invest.* **43**, 1677–1690.
13. Bunch, T. W. (1980). Blood test abnormalities in runner. *Mayo Clin. Proc.* **55**, 113–117.
14. Sinko, V. (1978). Physical exercise and the prevention of atherosclerosis and cholesterol gall stones. *Post grad. Med. J.* **54**, 270–277.
15. Sullivan, S. N. (1981). The gastrointestinal symptoms of running. *N. Engl. J. Med.* **304**, 915.
16. Cohen, S. (1982). Personal communication.
17. Tibbling, L. (1981). Angina-like chest pain in patients with oesophageal dysfunction. *Acta Med. Scand., Suppl.* **644**, 56–59.
18. Volpicelli, N. A. (1981). Effect of sports on the gastrointestinal tract and liver. *In* "Sports Medicine" (R. Atkinson and O. Appenzeller, eds.), pp. 95–104. Urban & Schwartzenberg, Munich.
19. Cantwell, J. E. (1981). Gastrointestinal disorders in runners. *JAMA, J. Am. Med. Assoc.* **246**, 1404–1405.
20. Fogoros, R. N. (1978). Runner's trots, gastrointestinal disturbances in runners. *JAMA, J. Am. Med. Assoc.* **243**, 1743–1744.

21. Bulvas, M., Puchmeyer, V., Albrecht, V., Kotous, J., Koutousova-Stankova, A., and Gesior, R. (1978). Peripheral arterial reactivity in patients with peptic ulcers and in healthy subjects. *Cor Vasa* **20**, 292–299.

22. Brandsborg, O., Christensen, N. J., Galbo, H., Brandesborg, M., and Lorgreen, N. A. (1978). The effect of exercise, smoking and propranolol on serum gastrin in patients with duodenal ulcer and in vagotomized subjects. *Scand. J. Clin. Lab. Invest.* **38**, 441–446.

23. Frenkl, R. (1971). Humoral mechanism of ulcer resistance of the organism adapted to physical exercise. *Acta Med. Acad. Sci. Hung.* **28**, 69–73.

24. Paffenbarger, R. S., Wing, A. L., and Hyde, R. T. (1974). Chronic disease in former college students. XIII. Early precursors of peptic ulcer. *Am. J. Epidemiol.* **100**, 307–315.

25. Watt, J. (1972). The sailor's stomach. *J. R. Nav. Med. Serv.* **58**, 12–34.

26. Pressel, P. (1981). Interview with Rolf Benirschke: Ileostomate and second leading 1980 NFL Scorer. *Jet.* **8**, 22–56.

27. Chalmers, T. C., Eckardt, R. K., Reynolds, W. E., Cigerroc, J. G., Neare, N., Reiffenstein, R. W., Smith, C. W., and Davidson, C. S. (1955). The treatment of acute infectious hepatitis. Controlled studies of the effects of diet, rest, and physical reconditioning on the acute course of the disease and on the incidence of relapses and residual abnormalities. *J. Clin. Invest.* **34**, 1163–1235.

28. Krikler, D. M., and Zilberg, B. (1971). Hepatitis and activity. *Lancet* **2**, 1046–1047.

29. Krikler, D. M. (1971). Hepatitis and activity. *Postgrad. Med. J.* **47**, 490–492.

30. Repsher, L. H., and Freehern, R. K. (1969). Effects of early and vigorous exercise on recovery from infectious hepatitis. *N. Engl. J. Med.* **281**, 1393–1396.

31. Swift, W. E., Jr., Gardner, H. T., Moore, D. J., Streitfield, F. H., and Havens, W. D., Jr. (1950). Clinical course in viral hepatitis and the effect of exercise on convalescence. *Am. J. Med.* **8**, 614.

32. Frenkl, R., and Pavlik, G. (1980). A study of the enzyme inducing effect on physical exercise after partial hepatectomy in the rat. *Acta Physiol. Acad. Sci. Hung.* **55**, 313–317.

33. Stukonis, J., and Doll, R. (1969). Gastric cancer in man and physical activity at work. *Int. J. Cancer* **4**, 248–254.

34. Dancaster, C. P. (1969). Nephropathy in marathon runners. *S. P. Med. J.* **43**, 758–760.

35. Baker, B. E. (1978). Jejunal perforation occurring in contact sports. *Am. J. Sports Med.* **6**, 403–404.

36. Hot, R. W., Wold, G. J., and Franco, P. E. (1976). Rupture of the jejunum secondary to blunt trauma in a football player. *South. Med. J.* **69**, 281–285.

37. Foley, L. C., and Teele, R. L. (1979). Ultrasound of epigastric injuries after blunt trauma. *Am. J. Radiol.* **132**, 593–598.

38. Kaizer, K. W. (1980). Medical hazards of the water skiing douche. *Ann. Emer. Med.* **9**, 268–269.

39. Ringertz, O., and Zetterberg, B. (1967). Serum hepatitis among Swedish track finders. *N. Engl. J. Med.* **276**, 540–546.

40. Morse, L. J., Bryan, J. A., Change, L. W., Hurley, J. P., Murphy, J. F., and O'Brien, T. F. (1970). Holy Cross football team hepatitis outbreak. *Antimicrob. Agents Chemother.* **10**, 30–32.

41. Baron, R. C., Murphy, F. D., Breenberg, H. B., David, C. E., Bregman, D. J., Gary, G. W., Hughes, J. M., and Schonberger, L. B. (1982). Norwalk gastrointestinal illness: An outbreak associated with swimming in a recreational lake and secondary person to person transmission. *Am. J. Epidemiol.* **115**, 163–172.

42. Cabelli, V. J., Durfour, A. P., Levin, M. A., McCabe, L. J., and Hebermin, P. W. (1979). Relationship of microbial indicators to health effects at marine bathing beaches. *Am. J. Public Health* **69**, 690–696.

43. Koopman, J. S., Eckert, E. A., Greenberg, H. B., Strohn, B. C., Isaacson, R. E., and Monto,

A. S. (1982). Norwalk virus enteric illness acquired by swimming exposure. *Am. J. Epidemiol.* **115**, 173–177.

44. Rosenberg, M. L., Hazlet, K. K., Sheefer, J., Wells, J. G., and Pruneda, R. G. (1976). Shigellosis from swimming. *JAMA, J. Am. Med. Assoc.* **236**, 1849–1852.
45. Appenzeller, O., Standerfer, J., Appenzeller, J., and Atkinson, R. (1980). Neurology of endurance training. V. Endorphins. *Neurology* **30**, 418–419.

CHAPTER 14

Exercise in Renal and Hypertensive Disease

DAVID T. LOWENTHAL and SUSAN J. BRODERMAN

The William Likoff Cardiovascular Institute
Hahnemann University School of Medicine
Philadelphia, Pennsylvania

It is now well accepted that sustained elevation of blood pressure for a long enough period results in significant vascular damage throughout the body and early death from hypertensive cardiovascular disease (1–3). Lowering the blood pressure with pharmacologic agents is effective in reducing morbidity and mortality not only in patients with malignant and severe hypertension but also in patients with moderately severe and mild blood pressure elevation (4–8). Furthermore, in the absence of drug therapy, borderline hypertensives have experienced a fall in blood pressure following physical training with aerobic (isotonic) activities (9). Acute isometric exercise increases diastolic pressure but whether chronic static activity will do the same and result in fixed hypertension remains conjectural.

Since the mechanisms responsible for elevation of blood pressure are multifactorial, the therapeutic and exercise approaches to essential hypertension must remain empirical. Our challenge is to reduce elevated blood pressure effectively

Exercise Medicine: Physiological Principles
and Clinical Applications

without producing side effects that would make the therapy essentially counterproductive and to incorporate a program of physical activity which would synergistically act with drug therapy to reduce blood pressure.

I. HEMODYNAMICS OF HYPERTENSION

Although the etiology of essential hypertension remains undefined, extensive hemodynamic studies have elucidated the alterations of the circulation in these patients (10). In hemodynamic terms, the blood pressure is related both to cardiac output (the flow of blood through the general circulation) and to the resistance offered to the blood flow by the peripheral arterioles (total peripheral vascular resistance). This relationship is expressed by the formula BP = CO × TPR. The hemodynamics of hypertension change with age (Table I). Thus, arbitrarily, between the ages of 12 and 29, essential hypertension may be characterized by an elevation in heart rate and in cardiac output with a normal total peripheral resistance and an increase in the oxygen consumption of the body. It must be understood that along with this increase in cardiac output (which occurs early) there is a relative increase in total peripheral vascular resistance, but, clinically, diastolic pressure is normal. Since norepinephrine and renin may increase in borderline hypertension (genetic and labile) under conditions of exercise (11), high-salt diet (12), and mental stress (13), there may be some abnormal response within the autonomic nervous system (possibly an increase in sympathetic or a decrease in parasympathetic response). From age 30 to less than age 50, the cardiac output and heart rate revert to normal, but characteristic of fixed essential hypertension is an absolute increase in total peripheral vascular resistance and an increase in diastolic blood pressure. Beyond age 50, cardiac output may decrease with greater increases in total peripheral vascular resistance. When hypertension has become well established, the peripheral resistance is uniformly elevated in different areas of circulation, except in the kidneys where

TABLE I

Hemodynamic Changes with Age in Primary (Essential) Hypertension

Age	Changes
12–29	CO ↑, HR ↑, TPR-N; systolic ↑; diastolic-N-SI ↑.
Over 30 and less than 50	CO-N, HR-N, TPR- ↑; systolic and diastolic ↑.
Over 50	CO ↓, TPR ↑ ↑; systolic and diastolic ↑ ↑.

it appears to be slightly higher. Therefore, the kidneys probably play a fundamental role in the long-term maintenance of the hypertensive state.

The kidney is one of the most severely affected organs in essential hypertension. As the disease progresses, renal function gradually becomes impaired (14–16), and the more severe the blood pressure elevation, the more likely it is that significant renal damage will occur (17). Considerable evidence indicates that therapeutic reduction of blood pressure effectively arrests the progressive deterioration of renal function in patients with severe nonmalignant hypertension and those in the malignant phase of essential hypertension (17–20). Therefore, the patients with hypertension complicated by impairment of renal function should receive prompt and adequate antihypertensive therapy. For effective preservation of renal function, the blood pressure must remain normal both in the supine and standing positions, including appropriate cardiovascular responses to exercise, especially when on antihypertensive regimens.

Lund-Johansen (10) has critically examined the hemodynamics of exercise in trained, mildly hypertensive men.

II. HEMODYNAMICS OF HYPERTENSION DURING EXERCISE

Hypertensive patients who have trained in aerobic exercise programs have had hemodynamic studies performed on a bicycle ergometer at 300, 600, and 900 kpm/minute (Table II).

It should be noted that the heart rate response is greater in the hypertensive and is probably related to a greater underlying adrenergic sympathetic response and a higher arteriovenous oxygen difference. Simultaneously, however, there is less of an increase in stroke volume and in the cardiac index. The stroke volume tends to fall progressively with age and this is linked directly to a smaller rise in the cardiac index which likewise decreases significantly with age. Total peripheral resistance is higher at all ages and at all levels of work in the hypertensive trained individuals, thus, leading to a *greater blood pressure response* both in the systolic and diastolic components. Left ventricular stroke work is increased in both normotensive and hypertensive groups, but in the hypertensive group, it is higher with light and moderate work because of an increase in heart rate. There is no difference, however, when severe work is done, probably because of a lower stroke volume. Finally, the arteriovenous oxygen difference is significantly higher in hypertensives, as this is a safety mechanism for hypertensives to meet oxygen demands from the tissue. This arteriovenous oxygen difference increases with age. Exercise has been shown to normally increase muscle blood flow in both normotensive and hypertensive subjects (21). At rest, both muscle blood flow and resistance are increased in hypertensives, as compared to normoten-

TABLE II

Hemodynamic Effects during Dynamic Physical Activity (Trained Individuals)

Measure	Normotensive	Hypertensive
HR	↑	↑ ↑ (probably due to greater adrenergic response and higher A-V_{O_2} differences)
SV	↑ ↑	↑ (progressively falls with age and leads to subnormal cardiac output)
CI	↑ ↑	↑ (decreases significantly with age in the hypertensives)
TPR	±[a] or ↓[b]	↑ ↑ (higher at all ages and at all levels of work)
BP	↑[b]	↑ ↑ (res ipsa loquitor)
LVSW	↑	↑ (higher with light and moderate work because of ↑ hr; no difference when severe work is done because of lower SV)
A-V_{O_2}	↑	↑ ↑ ("safety mechanism" for hypertensives to meet O_2 demands from tissue, A-V_{O_2} difference increases with age)

[a] ±, no change.

[b] During aerobic activity, systolic pressure rises; diastolic pressure is either unchanged from control or it decreases.

sives, indicating that muscle blood vessels share the increased resistance, though probably to a lesser extent than the total circulation. In the upright position, muscle blood flow determined after ischemic exercise decreases in normal subjects; this change has been shown to be even more pronounced in hypertensive subjects. It may be concluded, however, that during periods of high flow after ischemic exercise, hypertensives subjects are able to decrease their resistance in the muscles that are stressed during the exercise procedure, but resistance continues to remain higher than in normotensive controls. Thus, aerobic exercise may be used synergistically, in addition to a diuretic in mildly hypertensive patients, i.e., diastolic blood pressure less than 105 mm Hg, or by itself in an attempt to reduce total peripheral vascular resistance. On the contrary, anaerobic exercises, e.g., weight lifting, hand gripping, and wrestling, are associated with increases in diastolic blood pressure (22). Such activity should be minimized and discouraged in hypertensive patients, especially if left ventricular function is compromised.

A. Biochemical Changes with Exercise

The predominant biochemical responses to dynamic physical activity involve the neuroendocrine and renin–angiotensin system. The interaction of these hormonal responses to exercise aids in the regulation of the plasma potassium concentration.

During maximal activity, norepinephrine, epinephrine (to a lesser degree than norepinephrine) (23), renin, aldosterone, and potassium concentrations are increased (24–26). The return to base line occurs within 2 hours after stopping the activity. Exercise programs that emphasize activity 4 days per week for 30–40 minutes each session can result in a reduction in plasma norepinephrine concentration (27) in association with a lower systolic pressure and heart rate. If norepinephrine is a biochemical reflector of sympathetic nervous system activity, this reduction should help explain the decrease in blood pressure and heart rate vis-à-vis an indirect decrease in renin, angiotenin II, and aldosterone. However, the vascular smooth muscle response to exercise is likely to be one of a *decrease in sensitivity rather than to absolute change in concentration.* This contention is best substantiated by the increase in plasma volume and aldosterone which occurs with exercise training (28). Does this worsen the hypertensive state? Is the vascular smooth muscle receptor more responsive and sensitive to norepinephrine than to aldosterone?

From the data of Choquette and Ferguson (9), it is apparent that blood pressure and heart rate can be reduced by exercise alone providing that the hypertensive state is "mild" or "borderline" by WHO Classification I criteria. Therefore, it is conceivable (albeit hypothetical) that the beneficial response to exercise is due to readaptation of vascular smooth muscle to catecholamines, regardless of the level of the aldosterone. One may infer that low-salt diet, relaxation, and biofeedback may accomplish the same results (29–31).

It is now well accepted that most patients with sustained hypertension have elevated blood pressure with normal cardiac output and an elevated total peripheral vascular resistance (the indicator of peripheral arterial vasoconstriction). It is desirable, from a therapeutic standpoint, to correct the hypertension by correcting the hemodynamic derangement of the disease, that is, to lower total peripheral vascular resistance and maintain cardiac output. In this way, blood flow to the vital organs and systems can be maintained.

As a protagonist speaking on behalf of the inclusion of aerobic exercise into a regimen for treating hypertension, it is imperative to cite the direct and indirect influences of the benefits of regular physical activity (32,33). These prerequisites may directly be related to a fall in blood pressure or may be (and in large degree are) catalysts that initiate a trend of events resulting in a fixed lowering of blood pressure.

1. Decrease in body weight.
2. Cessation from smoking.
3. Alteration of alcohol consumption.
4. Readaptation to mental stress leading to decreased sympathetic response to stress.
5. Improvement in sleeping habits.

6. Decreased plasma catecholamines (23,27) at same work load after a successful exercise training program, in normals and in ischemic heart disease.
7. Biochemical risk factors influenced by exercise (33): decrease LDL cholesterol; decrease triglycerides; increase HDL cholesterol.

These benefits subsequent to the exercise program (designed by an exercise M.D. or physiologist) accrue at the expense of alterations in the circulatory system during exercise which may *transiently* result in pertubations of the hypertensive state.

B. Is Exercise Beneficial in Lowering Blood Pressure?

The major dilemma confronting us today is whether exercise and/or other nonpharmacologic modalities can be used to the exclusion of drug treatment. For the past 25–30 years, we have been taught, based on VA and Public Health Service retrospective and prospective epidemiological studies (5–8), that the pharmacologic treatment of hypertension is effective in preventing or resolving target organ damage by means of lowering blood pressure. The only nonpharmacologic approach for which there are data indicating efficacy is the low-salt diet (29). However, in our society, where added salt is a well-accepted means of enhancing food flavor, the successful implementation of the low-salt regimen is fraught with meager compliance.

For the other nonpharmacologic considerations, long-term data are not yet available to suggest that exercise (9), biofeedback maneuvers (30,34), or relaxation techniques (30,35) will prevent or reverse target organ damage associated with hypertension.

C. Drug–Exercise Interaction

The therapeutic strategy for the physically active patient whose hypertension is not controlled by nonpharmacologic means is to give antihypertensive drugs that will not embarass the hemodynamic response and/or produce significant hyperkalemia.

Those agents that permit normal circulatory responses to dynamic exercise are diuretics, clonidine, methyldopa, and prazosin (Table III) (36–40). All β-adrenoceptor blocking agents blunt normal circulatory responses. Initially (25) and long-term (41), depending on dose, they can significantly increase plasma potassium over the dynamic exercise-induced increase seen with placebo. On the contrary, in diuretic-induced hypokalemic adolescents, dynamic exercise can result in an increase in serum potassium, a finding that supports the observations that total body stores of potassium are not depleted in these patients (42).

TABLE III

Hemodynamic Changes during Dynamic Physical Activity after 1 Year of Antihypertensive Therapy[a]

	HR	SI	CI	TPR	BP
Hydrochlorothiazide	sl ↑	↑	↑	↓	sl ↑
α-Methyldopa	↑	±	↑	↓	↑
Clonidine	↑	↑	↑	↓	↑
β blocker	±	sl ↑	sl ↑	↓ [b]	sl ↑
Prazosin	↑	↑	↑	↓	sl ↑

[a] The responses are related as increase, decrease, or no change as compared with those responses to antihypertensive therapy at rest. ↑, increases; ↓, decreases; ±, no significant change; sl ↑ slight increase; sl ↓ slight decrease.

[b] At rest, TPR is increased; TPR decreases with exercise but still remains above base line.

The antirenin antihypertensives, methyldopa and clonidine, do not produce untoward hyperkalemia, yet mildly suppress the exercise-induced increases in norepinephrine and renin concentration. In contrast, propranolol causes a substantial reduction in exercise-induced rises in renin, heart rate and systolic pressure but an increase in potassium greater than with placebo (24–26). The fall in rate–pressure product seen with propranolol is an excellent variable to judge myocardial oxygen consumption in patients with ischemic heart disease. Herein lies its usefulness. Pindolol, a β antagonist in part, can exert a partial agonist effect and result in a less suppressed response to exercise than other β antagonists lacking this property.

The rise in diastolic pressure induced by isometric exercise, i.e., hand grips at 30 and 50% of maximum effort, can be blocked by clonidine, metoprolol, propranolol (43), and prazosin (44). Thus, patients taking these drugs, who do heavy upper extremity labor, may be protected against untoward increases in afterload.

Table IV gives guidelines for exercise in patients with hypertension.

III. EXERCISE IN PATIENTS WITH END-STAGE RENAL DISEASE (45)

A normochromic normocytic anemia is characteristic of patients with end-stage renal disease (ESRD). Characteristically, the hemoglobin is between 7 and 8 gm% and the hematocrit between 20 and 24%. The patients generally adapt well to this anemia. The hyperdynamic circulation seen in many such patients may be related to the anemia, and when an A-V fistula is created for chronic maintenance hemodialysis, this tends to increase the cardiac work in addition to

TABLE IV

Guidelines for Exercise in Patients with Hypertension

1. Stress testing should be performed prior to starting an exercise program. The objectives are to observe BP control and response, incidence and type of arrhythmias, evidence of ischemia, and exercise capacity.
2. Emphasis should be on dynamic (aerobic) forms of activities, e.g., jogging, swimming, cycling, walking.
3. Exercise in lieu of antihypertensive drugs must not be considered a substitute form of therapy. Exercise and pharmacotherapy should be considered as synergistic components of treatment.
4. Gradual adaptation to training will permit better patient acceptance and will decrease the likelihood for injury. Toleration for extremes of ambient temperature is also related to a slow, progressive adaptation to the activity being performed.
5. Potassium supplements (Elixir of KCl, Slo-K) or potassium-sparing diuretics (amiloride, triamterene) may be necessary for patients receiving diuretics and who exercise in hot climates. Water should be considered the preferred fluid replacement.

that seen with anemia. Yet, the patients seem to adapt well to even the A-V fistula and the hemodynamic changes that accrue from its presence. Aerobic exercise has been shown to increase the hemoglobin and hematocrit concentrations (Fig. 1) as well as work load and duration of activity over an 8-week training period.

The lipid abnormality observed in renal failure resulting in an increase in triglycerides and in low density lipoproteins is due to a decrease in lipoprotein lipase. This has been related to the development of accelerated atherosclerosis. The atherosclerosis resulting from this lipid abnormality in addition to the increase in vascular resistance consequent to the hypertension may be directly related to the increased incidence of coronary artery disease and peripheral vascular disease in patients with ESRD. Dynamic physical activity has been demonstrated to result in a rise in high density lipoproteins and a fall in triglycerides.

The hypertension associated with ESRD is, in general, related to an inability to excrete salt and water. Therefore, hemodialysis and peritoneal dialysis, which remove adequate quantities of salt and water, can correct the hypertension due to volume expansion. The incidence of this type of hypertension is seen in about 70–75% of cases. The remaining cases of hypertension need pharmacologic intervention with the same classes of drugs listed above. Bilateral nephrectomy is rarely needed for the control of hypertension. In some cases dynamic physical activity can work synergistically with dialysis and/or drug therapy in reducing blood pressure.

The renal osteodystrophy begins very early as renal function begins to decrease. When serum creatinine doubles, glomerular filtration rate falls by 50%. If the decrease in phosphate excretion follows the fall in glomerular filtration,

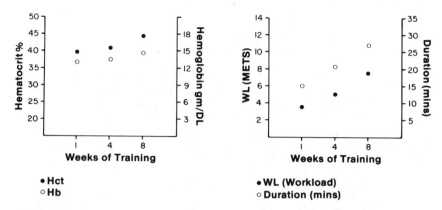

Fig. 1. Changes in hemogram, work load, and duration of activity after 8 weeks of exercise training in a dialysis patient.

then parathyroid hormone will increase and affect bone metabolism. In addition, the defect in bone metabolism is related to a decrease in the oxidative process performed by the diseased kidney, which converts 25-hydroxycholecalciferol to 1,25 dihydroxycholecalciferol. This compound is now available as an oral medication (Rocaltrol) for the control of metabolic bone disease. Phosphate binding by drugs taken to absorb phosphate within the intestinal lumen can result in restoration of calcium to normal. Weight-bearing exercises such as those done with dynamic physical activity may result in an improvement in bone volume, although adequate data are not yet available to substantiate this response.

The carbohydrate intolerance seen in ESRD is related to a defect in the peripheral utilization of insulin. In spite of high levels of insulin detected by RIA, blood glucose concentration may be high in the absence of overt diabetes mellitus. Dynamic physical activity has been shown to increase insulin receptor density and result in improved utilization of insulin and lowering of blood glucose (45,46).

In summary, based on the existing data which, albeit small in patient numbers, has been carefully obtained, there is evidence that dynamic physical activity may have a beneficial effect in ESRD similar to that in patients with normal renal function.

Table V gives guidelines for exercise in patients with ESRD.

IV. CONCLUSION

When it is clinically safe, i.e., following maximal graded stress testing where blood pressure response is determined every 2–3 minutes, an exercise prescrip-

TABLE V

Guidelines for Exercise in Patients with ESRD

1. Stress testing: see Table IV, 1.
2. Dynamic activity is preferred. However, if LV function is normal and if BP is controlled, some static (isometric) activity should be encouraged in order to improve muscle tone. Dynamic exercises, especially jogging, may be limited due to renal osteodystrophy.
3. Gradual adaptation: same principles as in Table IV. In addition, the anemia that these patients have underscores the need for gradual, progressive training.
4. It is probably wise, in all instances, to avoid potassium supplements. These patients will not be exercising to great intensities and will most likely be intolerant of extremes in ambient temperature, especially heat.
5. Fluid replacement, if necessary, *may be* more liberal if exercise is performed following a dialysis treatment. Best guide to fluid replacement should be body weight.

---

tion can be given to a patient providing the hypertensive state is "mild" and risk factors are minimal. It is certainly worth employing nonpharmacologic interventions, e.g., salt restriction, weight reduction, and advice regarding the risk factors of smoking and alcohol, in an attempt to act in concert with exercise. One must at all times remember that drug therapy is a proved modality, not without toxicity, and should be given to the patient when clinically indicated either at the inception of the exercise program or after a period of trial and lack of adherence to the nonpharmacologic maneuvers.

Finally, whether exercise will be of benefit in the early, neurogenic form of hypertension as described by Esler (47) in protecting against the development of fixed hypertension remains to be determined. It is well appreciated that mental stress (12) and isometric exercise (22) (as opposed to isotonic exercise) will provoke an increase in blood pressure in those with neurogenic or labile hypertension. Exercise of the dynamic or isotonic variety such as distance running may induce sufficient parasympathomimetic influence to decrease the neurogenic and/or adrenergic component of blood pressure control and thus, alter the evolution of fixed diastolic hypertension. Whether similar mechanisms can account for a depressor effect in patients with renal disease, many of whom have autonomic imbalance, remains fertile ground for clinical research.

REFERENCES

1. Dublin, L. J., Lotka, A. J., and Spiegelman, M. (1949). Length of Life: A Study of the Life Table, 2nd ed., Ronald Press, New York.
2. Hamilton, M., Thompson, E. N., and Wisniewski, T. K. M. (1964). The role of blood pressure control in preventing complications of hypertension. *Lancet* 1, 235.
3. Hodge, J. V., and Smirk, F. H. (1967). The effect of drug treatment of hypertension on the

distribution of deaths from various causes. A study of 173 deaths among hypertensive patients in the years 1959 to 1964 inclusive. *Am. Heart J.* **73**, 441.

4. Moyer, J. H., Heider, C., Pevey, K., and Ford, R. V. (1958). The effect of treatment on the vascular deterioration associated with hypertension, with particular emphasis on renal function. *Am. J. Med.* **24**, 177.

5. Veterans Administration Cooperative Study Group on Antihypertensive Agents (1967). Effects of treatment on morbidity in hypertension. Results in patients with diastolic blood pressures averaging 115 through 129 mmHg. *JAMA, J. Am. Med. Assoc.* **202**, 1028.

6. Veterans Administration Cooperative Study Group on Antihypertensive Agents (1970). Effects of treatment on morbidity in hypertension. II. Results in patients with diastolic blood pressures averaging 90 through 114 mmHg. *JAMA J. Am. Med. Assoc.* **213**, 1143.

7. Special communication (1977). Report of the Joint National Committee on Detection, Evaluation and Treatment of High Blood Pressure. *JAMA J. Am. Med. Assoc.* **237**, (3), 255.

8. Special report (1980). The 1980 Report of the Joint National Committee on Detection, Evaluation, and Treatment of High Blood Pressure. *Arch. Intern. Med.* **140**, 1280.

9. Choquette, G., and Ferguson, R. J. (1973). Blood pressure reduction in "Borderline" hypertensives following physical training. *Cancer Med. Assoc. J.* **108**, 699.

10. Lund-Johansen, P. (1967). Hemodynamics in early hypertension. *Acta Med. Scand.* **181**, Suppl. 482, 1.

11. Robertson, D., Shand, D. G., Hollifield, J. W. *et al.* (1979). Alterations in the responses of the sympathetic nervous system and renin in borderline hypertension. *Hypertension* **1**, 118.

12. Falkner, B., Onesti, G., and Angelakos, E. (1981). Effect of salt loading on the cardiovascular response to stress in adolescents. *Hypertension* **3**, Suppl. II, 11–195.

13. Falkner, B., Onesti, G., Angelakos, E. T., Fernandes, M., and Langman, C. (1979) Cardiovascular response to mental stress in normal adolescents with hypertensive parents. *Hypertension* **1**, 23.

14. Goldring, W., Chasis, H., Range, H. A., and Smith, H. W. (1941). Effective renal blood flow in subjects with essential hypertension. *J. Clin. Invest.* **20**, 637.

15. Talbott, J. H., Castleman, B., Smithwick, R. H. *et al.* (1943). Renal biopsy studies correlated with renal clearance observations in hypertensive patients treated by radical sympathectomy. *J. Clin. Invest.* **22**, 387.

16. Brod, J., Fenchl, V., Hejl, Z. *et al.* (1962). General and regional hypertension pattern underlying essential hypertension. *Clin. Sci.* **23**, 339.

17. Moyer, J. H., Heider, C., Pevey, K., and Ford, R. V. (1958). The effect of treatment on the vascular deterioration associated with hypertension, with particular emphasis on renal function. *Am. J. Med.* **24**, 177.

18. Reubi, F. C. (1960). The late effects of hypotensive drug therapy on renal function in patients with essential hypertension. *In* "Essential Hypertension: An International Symposium" (K. D. Bock and P. T. Cottier, eds.), p. 317. Springer-Verlag, Berlin and New York.

19. McCormack, L. J., Beland, J. E., Schneckloth, R. E., and Corcoran, A. C. (1958). Effects of antihypertensive treatment on the evolution of the renal lesions in malignant nephrosclerosis. *Am. J. Pathol.* **34**, 1011.

20. Woods, J. W., and Blythe, W. B. (1967). Management of malignant hypertension complicated by renal insufficiency. *N. Engl. J. Med.* **277**, 57.

21. Amery, A., Bossaert, H., and Verstraete, M. (1969). Muscle blood flow in normal and hypertensive subjects. Influence of age, exercise and body position. *Am. Heart J.* **78**, 211.

22. Nyberg, G. (1976). Blood pressure and heart rate response to isometric exercise and mental arithmetic in normotensive and hypertensive subjects. *Clin. Sci. Mol. Med.* **51**, 681.

23. Dimsdale, J. E., and Moss, J. (1980). Plasma catecholamines in stress and exercise. *JAMA J. Am. Med. Assoc.* **243**, 340.

24. Rosenthal, L. S., Lowenthal, D. T., Affrime, M. B., Falkner, B., and Gould, A. B. (1982). The renin—aldosterone—potassium response to methyldopa during dynamic physical activity. *Clin. Pharmacol. Ther.* **31**, 216.

25. Affrime, M. B., Rosenthal, L. S., Lowenthal, D. T., Gould, A. B., and Falkner, B. (1982). The response to single and multiple dose propranolol under the influence of maximum physical activity. *Clin. Pharmacol. Ther.* **31**, 199.

26. Lowenthal, D. T., Affrime, M. B., Rosenthal, L. S. Gould, A. B., Berruso, J., and Falkner, B. (1982). Biochemical responses to single and repeated doses of clonidine during dynamic physical activity. *Clin. Pharmacol. Ther.* **32**, 18.

27. Cooksey, J. D., Reilly, P., Brown, S., Domze, H., and Cryer, P. E. (1978). Exercise training and plasma catecholamines in patients with ischemic heart disease. *Am. J. Cardiol.* **42**, 372.

28. Maher, J. T., Jones, L. G., Hartley, L. H., Williams, G. H., and Rose, L. I. (1975). Aldosterone dynamics during graded exercise at sea level and high altitudes. *J. Appl. Physiol.* **39**, 18.

29. Morgan, T., Gilles, A., Morgan, G., Adam, W., Wilson, M., and Carney, S. (1978). Hypertension treated by salt restriction. *Lancet* **1**, 227.

30. Shapiro, A. P., Schwartz, G. E., Ferguson, D. C. E., Redmond, D. P., and Weiss, S. M. (1977). Behavioral methods in the treatment of hypertension. A review of their clinical status. *Ann. Intern. Med.* **86**, 626.

31. Grollman, A., Harrison, T. R., Mason, M. F. *et al.* (1945). Sodium restriction in the diet for hypertension. *JAMA J. Am. Med. Assoc.* **129**, 533.

32. Lowenthal, D. T., Bharadwaja, K., and Oaks, W. W. (1979). "Therapeutics Through Exercise." Grune & Stratton, New York.

33. Amsterdam, E. A., Wilmore, J. H., and DeMaria, A. N. (1977). "Exercise in Cardiovascular Health and Disease." Yorke Medical Books, New York.

34. Miller, N. E., and Dworkin, B. R. (1977). Effects of learning on visceral functions—biofeedback. *N. Engl. J. Med.* **296**, 1274.

35. Benson, H. (1977). Systemic hypertension and the relaxation response. *N. Engl. J. Med.* **296**, 1152.

36. Lund-Johansen, P. (1970). Hemodynamic changes in long-term diuretic therapy of essential hypertension. *Acta Med. Scand.* **187**, 509.

37. Lund-Johansen, P. (1973). Hemodynamic changes in long-term therapy of essential hypertension. A comparative study of diuretics, alphamethyldopa and clonidine. *Clin. Sci. Mol. Med.* **45**, 199.

38. Lund-Johansen, P. (1974). Hemodynmic changes at rest and during exercise in long-term clonidine therapy of essential hypertension. *Acta Med. Scand.* **195**, 111.

39. Lund-Johansen, P. (1974). Hemodynamic changes at rest and during exercise in long-term beta blocker therapy of essential hypertension. *Acta Med. Scand.* **195**, 117.

40. Lund-Johansen, P. (1975). Hemodynamic changes at rest and during exercise in long-term prazosin therapy for essential hypertension. *Postgrad. Med. Symp. Prazosin, 1975* p. 45.

41. Leenan, F. H. H., Coenen, C. H. M., Zonderland, M., and Maas, A. H. J. (1980). Effects of cardioselective and non-selective β-blockade on dynamic exercise performance in mildly hypertensive men. *Clin. Pharmacol. Ther.* **28**, 12.

42. Falkner, B., Lowenthal, D. T., and Affrime, M. B. (1983). The effect of exercise on diuretic-induced hypokalemia in adolescent hypertension. *Clin. Pharmacol. Ther.* (in press).

43. Virtanen, K., Jänne, J., and Frick, M. H. (1982). Response of blood pressure and plasma norepinephrine to propranolol, metoprolol and clonidine during isometric and dynamic exercise in hypertensive patients. *Eur. J. Clin. Pharmacol.* **21**, 275.

44. Lowenthal, D. T., Yarnoff, A., Affrime, M. B., Falkner, B., Saris, S., Hare, T., and Hakki, H.

(1982). The pharmacodynamic response to Prazosin using isometric exercise. *Clin. Res.* **30,** 337A.

45. Goldberg, A. P., Hagberg, J. M., Delmez, J. A., Haynes, M. E., and Harter, H. R. (1980). Metabolic effects of exercise training in hemodialysis patients. *Kidney Int.* **18,** 754.

46. Gavin, J. R., Goldberg, A. P., Hagberg, J., Delmez, J. A., Geltman, E., and Haiter, H. R. (1982). Endurance exercise training improves insulin sensitivity in uremia. *Clin. Res.* **30,** 393A.

47. Esler, M., Julius, S., Zweifler, A. *et al.* (1977). Mild high renin essential hypertension. A neurogenic human hypertension? *N. Engl. J. Med.* **296,** 405.

CHAPTER 15

Metabolic and Endocrine Disorders and Exercise

PHILIP FELIG
*Department
of Medicine
Yale University
School of
Medicine
New Haven
Connecticut*

I. INTRODUCTION

The role of exercise vis-à-vis the endocrine system has special significance in a variety of ways. First, the metabolic response to exercise involves a complex interaction of hormonal as well as neurogenic signals designed to meet the energy requirements of contracting muscle while maintaining an uninterrupted flow of substrates to other vital tissue (e.g., the provision of glucose to the brain). Second, exercise has long been advocated as a therapeutic modality in the management of the most frequently encountered endocrine disturbance of man,

305

Exercise Medicine: Physiological Principles
and Clinical Applications

namely, diabetes mellitus. Third, in some diabetics (those treated with insulin) exercise may impose hazards not usually encountered in the general population (severe symptomatic hypoglycemia). Fourth, physical training may be associated with disturbances of the hypothalamic–pituitary–gonadal axis, manifesting as menstrual disturbances and/or infertility. Finally, exercise tolerance may be markedly altered in patients with disturbances of thyroid or adrenal function.

In this chapter, the fuel–hormone responses to exercise will initially be reviewed, to provide a background for understanding the responses to and role of exercise in endocrine disease. Particular emphasis will be placed on glucoregulatory hormones and diabetes, since as noted above, exercise has received increasing attention in the management of the diabetic patient.

II. METABOLIC RESPONSE TO EXERCISE IN NORMAL MAN

The metabolic changes encountered in response to exercise in normal man may be considered in the context of the following categories: (1) fuel utilization and production; (2) hormone secretion; (3) the postexercise recovery period; (4) effects of physical training on hormone secretion and sensitivity.

A. Fuel Utilization and Production

The human is not only a collection of organ systems but is also a repository of combustible fuels. The three major body fuels are carbohydrate, stored primarily as glycogen in liver and muscle; fat, stored primarily as triglyceride in adipose tissue; and protein, present primarily as muscle tissue. As shown in Table I, fat constitutes by far the largest available source of stored calories. In contrast, carbohydrate is present in relatively limited amounts. Although protein is present in greater quantities, its oxidation would entail dissolution of muscle or parenchymal tissue. The magnitude and nature of these fuel depots thus clearly have implications for the pattern and processes of fuel turnover during exercise.

In the resting state, muscle tissue derives virtually all of its energy by utilizing fat, extracted from the bloodstream as free fatty acids (1). Stimulation of glucose

TABLE I

Body Fuel Stores in a 70-kg Man

Fuel	Tissue	Energy value (kcal)
Fat	Adipose tissue	100,000–150,000
Protein	Primarily muscle	32,000–48,000
Carbohydrate	Liver and muscle glycogen	1100

uptake by muscle may occur in the resting state by feeding a glucose meal. In fact, when a carbohydrate-containing meal is fed, muscle tissue is the major site of peripheral (extrahepatic) glucose uptake. This uptake of glucose does not, however, result in immediate glycolysis or oxidation, but is used for storage as glycogen. During recovery from exhaustive exercise, glucose uptake by resting muscle in fasted (2) or fed subjects (3) is accelerated so as to replenish muscle glycogen stores.

During exercise uptake of glucose by muscle is markedly stimulated and is rapidly converted to lactate or CO_2. The overall pattern of fuel utilization by muscle involves three phases, depending on the duration of the work performed (Fig. 1). For the first several minutes of exercise, the synthesis of ATP in muscle is largely dependent on the breakdown of stored glycogen to lactate. As exercise continues beyond 5–10 minutes, blood-borne fuels in the form of glucose and free fatty acids become increasingly important. The final phase, observed with very prolonged (greater than 2 hours) exercise, as in the case of marathoners, is characterized by decreasing dependence on blood glucose, and increasing utilization of free fatty acids. An interesting aspect of this triphasic response to exercise is the evidence indicating an ongoing role for muscle glycogen. Although glycogen utilization contributes only a small proportion of total caloric consump-

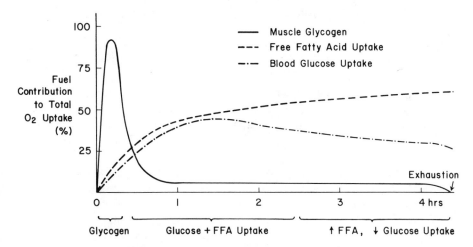

Fig. 1. Triphasic response of body fuels to acute exercise. During the first few minutes of exercise breakdown of muscle glycogen is the major source of ATP for contracting muscle. As exercise extends beyond 10 minutes, blood-borne fuels in the form of glucose and free fatty acids become increasingly important. As exercise extends beyond 90–120 min (e.g., in marathon runners), there is an increasing dependence on fat and lesser uptake of glucose. Muscle glycogen contributes a small proportion of the fuel requirements even in prolonged exercise, and its depletion is associated with exhaustion. Not shown is the small contribution of body protein breakdown to total fuel utilization in prolonged exercise (generally < 5–10% of total caloric utilization).

tion in prolonged exercise, depletion of muscle glycogen has been implicated as a key factor in the development of fatigue when exercise is performed at an intensity in excess of 70% of maximal aerobic power (4). Recent data suggest that protein catabolism also contributes to fuel utilization in prolonged exercise (5). However, protein-derived amino acids are of limited importance as a metabolic fuel since they contribute no more than 5–10% of the total caloric consumption (5).

The quantitative aspects of fuel utilization are of particular interest with respect to blood borne glucose in view of the limited stores of liver glycogen available in man (Table I) and the ongoing requirement for glucose delivery to the brain. As compared to the resting state, glucose uptake by muscle increases 7- to 40-fold, depending on the intensity and duration of the exercise performed (6). This exercise-induced stimulation of glucose uptake is not dependent on a rise in plasma insulin. In fact, glucose uptake during exercise will occur in the face of minimal amounts of insulin (2 μ/ml) (7). The clinical implication of this phenomenon is that even the poorly regulated, insulin-deficient diabetic demonstrates an increase in glucose utilization in response to exercise (8).

The marked enhancement in glucose utilization during exercise is accompanied by a simultaneous increase in glucose production. The site of this glucose release into the bloodstream is the liver (6). Exercise thus constitutes a very effective stimulus of hepatic glycogenolysis and gluconeogenesis. In fact, the highest rates of hepatic glucose production observed in circumstances of either health or disease are those encountered with intensive exercise.

During periods of exercise extending for 40–90 minutes the rate of glucose production is extremely well coordinated with the rate of glucose utilization by muscle (Fig. 2). As a consequence, there are minimal changes in blood glucose. However, with more prolonged exercise blood glucose concentrations decline, reaching values less than 45 mg/dl in as many as 30–40% of normal subjects. This reduction in blood glucose is a result of a depletion of liver glycogen stores and the failure of hepatic glucose production to keep pace with the ongoing elevated rates of glucose utilization despite an increase in hepatic gluconeogenesis (2,9) (Fig. 3). The decline in blood glucose which may be observed with very prolonged exercise in normal subjects is to be differentiated from the exercise-induced, symptomatic hypoglycemia, which may occur in insulin-treated diabetics (see Section III,A). In the normal subjects, the reduction in blood glucose occurs very gradually, is generally asymptomatic and may not interfere with exercise performance (10).

B. Hormonal Responses

The overall hormonal response to exercise may be viewed as directed primarily at providing a milieu which favors the release of glucose from the liver

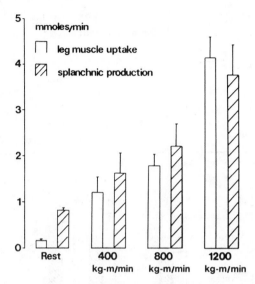

Fig. 2. Glucose utilization and production during short-term leg exercise of varying intensities. The close correspondence between the rates of glucose output from the liver (splanchnic bed) and uptake by the exercising legs allows for the maintenance of euglycemia during exercise. Based on the data of Wahren *et al.* (6).

(glycogenolysis and gluconeogenesis) and the release of fatty acids from adipose tissue (lipolysis). As shown in Table II, exercise results in a decline in plasma insulin and increased concentrations of glucagon, epinephrine, norepinephrine, cortisol, and growth hormone. The extent of these hormonal alterations is accentuated as the intensity of the exercise increases and is blunted by physical training (11,12). Since insulin is an inhibitor of glycogenolysis and gluconeogenesis whereas the other hormones shown in Table II stimulate one or both of these processes, the hormonal response provides the major stimulus to the augmentation in glucose production which characterizes exercise. In addition, an increase in activity in the splanchnic sympathetic nerves may also be a contributory factor.

The hormonal changes in exercise also favor lipolysis. Insulin is the most potent antilipolytic hormone. Consequently, a reduction in insulin coupled with elevations in catecholamines and growth hormone results in accelerated mobilization of free fatty acids.

Other hormonal changes observed with acute exercise include mild elevations in TSH and prolactin, the precise significance of which remains to be established (13). The observation that prolonged exercise results in increased plasma levels of endogenous opioid-like peptides (β-endorphin) is particularly intriguing, and has been speculated as contributing to "runner's high" (14).

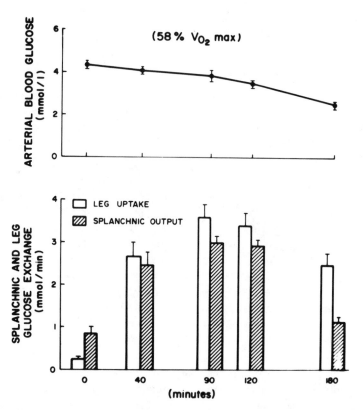

Fig. 3. Arterial blood glucose concentration and rates of splanchnic glucose production and leg glucose uptake during prolonged leg exercise at 58% of maximal aerobic power. As exercise continues beyond 90–120 minutes, hepatic glucose output fails to keep pace with glucose utilization resulting in a decline in blood glucose. The fall in hepatic glucose output presumably is a consequence of depletion of liver glycogen stores. Based on the data of Ahlborg and Felig (2).

C. Postexercise Recovery

The influence of exercise on body fuel metabolism extends to the postexercise recovery period. Increased uptake of glucose by muscle occurs during recovery, presumably as a means of repleting muscle glycogen stores (2). This augmentation in glucose uptake occurs in the face of low plasma insulin levels indicating that the post-exercise recovery period, particularly after exhaustive work, is characterized by enhanced insulin sensitivity (2,15). The effects of exercise on blood glucose homeostasis in the insulin-treated diabetic thus may persist into the recovery period.

TABLE II

Neurohumoral Responses to Exercise[a]

↓ Insulin
↑ Glucagon
↑ Cortisol
↑ Growth Hormone
↑ Epinephrine
↑ Norepinephrine
↑ Splanchnic sympathetic nerve activity

[a] The overall neurohumoral response enhances glycogenolysis, gluconeogenesis, and lipolysis in response to exercise.

D. Physical Training and the Endocrine System

The effects of physical training in altering the fuel–hormone response to acute exercise and muscle enzyme activity are discussed elsewhere in this volume in detail. Physical training also alters a variety of aspects of endocrine function in the resting state. A reduction in insulin secretion in the fasting state and in response to glucose ingestion is observed in very well-trained athletes (16), and after a period of physical training in previously sedentary subjects (17,18). Accompanying this reduction in insulin secretion is an increase in muscle sensitivity to insulin (17,18). This enhanced sensitivity in muscle may be mediated by an increase in insulin binding (19). In contrast, the liver fails to demonstrate a similar increase in sensitivity (17) and in fact shows the enzymatic consequences of hypoinsulinemia, as reflected by a fall in liver glucokinase (20). The complexity of the response by the pancreatic islets, muscle and liver to physical training may account for the varying effects of physical training on blood glucose control in the diabetic (see Section III,A).

Physical training is also associated with decreased secretion of gonadotropins and sex steroids (13,21). These changes are discussed further in Section V.

III. EXERCISE AND DIABETES

Since exercise increases glucose utilization while diabetes is characterized by an impairment in glucose utilization, it is reasonable to expect that exercise would be beneficial for the management of diabetes. In fact, exercise was recommended for the treatment of diabetes even before insulin became available. Nevertheless, in practical terms the interaction between exercise and diabetes is sufficiently complex that, depending on the circumstances, exercise may result in either an elevation or reduction of blood glucose. Furthermore, the state of our knowledge has not progressed to the point where an exercise prescription may be written in a manner analogous to management of diabetes with diet and/or insulin.

A. Blood Glucose Response to Acute Exercise

In the insulin-requiring diabetic the blood glucose response to exercise is influenced by the prior status of diabetes control as well as the timing and route of delivery of insulin. If prior to initiation of exercise, the diabetes has been very poorly controlled, as reflected by hyperglycemia in excess of 300–400 mg/dl and plasma ketones of > 2 mmoles/liter, acute exercise will result in a further rise in blood glucose (Fig. 4). In addition, exercise will result in an acceleration of already increased rates of gluconeogenesis and ketogenesis in such subjects (8). The net effect of exercise in the very poorly regulated diabetic is thus an exaggeration rather than an improvement of the diabetic state. The mechanism of this exaggeration relates to the hormonal milieu of exercise. In the insulin-deficient diabetic there is an exaggerated increase in the plasma levels of counter-regulatory hormones (catecholamines, growth hormone) (22) (Fig. 5). As a result of these hormonal increases as well as the insulin deficiency, there is an overproduction of glucose by the liver resulting in hyperglycemia (Fig. 6). These hormonal changes also result in an acceleration of ketogenesis.

In the non-insulin-dependent diabetic and in circumstances of insulin-dependent diabetes in which there is good to moderate control of blood glucose, exercise results in a reduction in blood glucose (8). In fact, the major clinical problem that may be encountered in the insulin-treated diabetic is exercise-induced hypoglycemia. This phenomenon is observed with conventional insulin administration in the form of a bolus injection of regular or modified (intermediate or long-acting) insulin in a subcutaneous site. In contrast, the continuous infusion of insulin in basal amounts by either the intravenous or subcutaneous route (as in patients treated with portable insulin pumps) is not associated with exercise-induced hypoglycemia (22–24). The mechanism of exercise-induced hypoglycemia with conventional insulin treatment thus appears to depend on the absorption of insulin from a repository site of bolus insulin injection in subcutaneous tissue resulting in plasma insulin levels that exceed normal basal concentrations. As a consequence of the hyperinsulinemia, glucose production is inhibited and glucose utilization may be exaggerated, resulting in hypoglycemia. The absorption of injected insulin may be spontaneous and related to the amount and time course of action of the administered insulin, or it may be exaggerated by exercising the injected site (25–27). However, enhanced insulin absorption by exercising the injected area has not been uniformly observed (28,29).

The development of hypoglycemia in response to exercise in the insulin-treated diabetic may not occur until the postexercise recovery period. In some

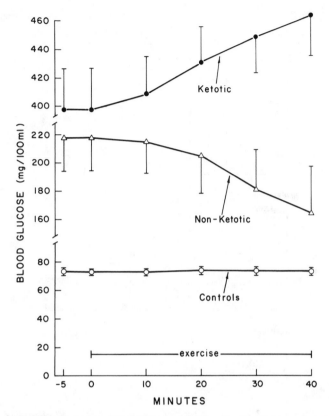

Fig. 4. Influence of the status of blood glucose control on the blood glucose response to acute exercise in insulin-dependent (Type I) diabetics. In those diabetics with marked hyperglycemia and moderate ketonemia prior to exercise, the exercise resulted in a worsening of hyperglycemia. Based on the data of Wahren *et al.* (8).

individuals this may take the form of a reduction in insulin requirement on the day following exhaustive exercise, a phenomenon that has been recognized for over 50 years (30). The mechanism of this response relates to the increase in muscle sensitivity to insulin which is observed in the postexercise recovery period (2,15), as well as spontaneous elevations in plasma insulin due to ongoing absorption from subcutaneous injection sites. The postulated events contributing to exercise-induced hypoglycemia in the insulin-treated diabetic are summarized in Fig. 7.

B. Physical Training and Diabetes

As in the case of normal subjects (18), physical training in the insulin-dependent (Type I) diabetic results in an increase in muscle sensitivity to insulin (31).

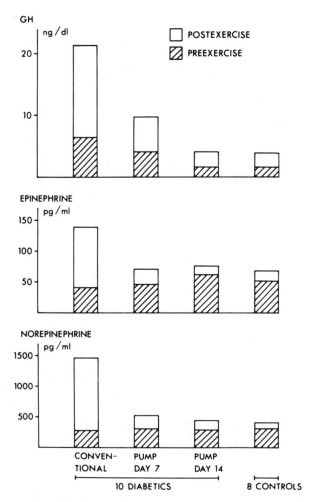

Fig. 5. The response of serum growth hormone and plasma catecholamines to acute exercise in insulin-dependent diabetics during conventional insulin treatment and after intensive management with a portable insulin infusion pump. Restoration of normal or near-normal blood glucose levels (not shown) by insulin pump treatment resulted in a lowering of the growth hormone and catecholamine response to exercise to normal values. Based on the data of Tamborlane *et al.* (22).

Furthermore, diabetics respond to physical training with adaptive increases in muscle mitochondrial enzyme activity, (e.g., succinate dehydrogenase and citrate synthase) and increases in capillarization (31). A reduction in blood cholesterol and a rise in high density lipoprotein (HDL) cholesterol has also been observed after a 16-week training program in the insulin-dependent diabetic (31).

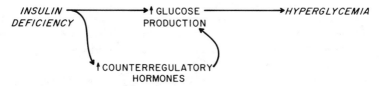

Fig. 6.   Mechanisms of exercise-induced hyperglycemia in poorly regulated insulin-dependent (Type I) diabetics.

Despite these salutary effects, physical training fails to improve overall blood glucose control in Type I diabetes when no effort is made to optimize dietary measures or insulin treatment (31). This lack of improvement may relate to the fact that although muscle sensitivity to insulin is augmented with physical training, a similar improvement is not observed in the liver. These observations underscore the fact that exercise training can only be viewed as an adjunct in the management of diabetes and not a replacement for attempts to optimize diet and insulin administration.

In the insulin-independent (Type II) diabetic variable effects of physical training on glucose tolerance have also been observed. Although plasma insulin levels are reduced and intravenous glucose tolerance has been noted to improve (32,33), inconsistent effects on oral glucose tolerance are observed (32,33). The variable nature of the impact of training on blood glucose control in Type II diabetes relates to the complexity of the effects of physical training on insulin sensitivity as well as secretion. Thus, although muscle sensitivity to insulin is improved, insulin secretion is reduced, which may in turn result in a decline in key hepatic glucoregulatory enzymes (20). The net effect of physical training on glucose tolerance in Type II diabetes thus depends on the interplay among these variables.

DURING EXERCISE:

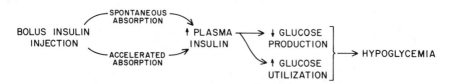

POSTEXERCISE (minutes to hours):

↑ INSULIN SENSITIVITY   +   ↑ PLASMA ⟶ ↑ GLUCOSE ⟶ HYPOGLYCEMIA
         IN MUSCLE   INSULIN   UTILIZATION

Fig. 7.   Postulated mechanisms of exercise-induced hypoglycemia in insulin-treated diabetic patients. The hypoglycemia may occur during or after the exercise.

C. Practical Considerations and Recommendations

In the insulin-dependent diabetic participating in exercise only occasionally, the possible hazards of worsening hyperglycemia or acute hypoglycemia induced by acute exercise should be recognized. If blood glucose control is very poor (fasting plasma glucose in excess of 300–400 mg/dl and ketonuria present), improvement in control of diabetes by adjustment of insulin and/or diet should be undertaken before the patient contemplates engaging in exercise.

If blood glucose control is good to moderate, the insulin-treated patient should be apprised of the possibility of exercise-induced hypoglycemia. It is not possible to predict in advance of undertaking exercise whether a given level of physical work will precipitate hypoglycemia. Certain guidelines, however, are helpful in minimizing the possibility. First, the diabetic should avoid exercise when he has not eaten for 2 or 3 hours or at times of the day when injected insulin is reaching its peak effect. Second, candy or other glucose-containing foods or beverages should be available for ingestion during the exercise if symptoms of hypoglycemia occur. Third, if on the basis of prior experience, the exercise (e.g., running or playing tennis) has provoked hypoglycemia, extra carbohydrate should be ingested prior to exercise. If hypoglycemia still recurs, a nonexercised area should be used for insulin injection and the total dose of insulin may be reduced.

A program of physical training may be encouraged in the management of insulin-dependent as well as insulin-independent diabetes, provided no contraindication exists on the basis of cardiopulmonary, orthopedic, or other considerations. Such a program can be expected to lower plasma cholesterol levels, raise HDL concentrations, and (in Type II diabetics) decrease plasma insulin. When combined with efforts at optimizing insulin and diet management, physical training will facilitate improvement in blood glucose control. In such circumstances of optimized insulin and diet management, physical training will result in a reduction in total insulin dose as compared to the sedentary state.

IV. EXERCISE AND THYROID DISORDERS

Although acute exercise fails to cause consistent changes in serum thyroxine (T_4) or triiodothyronine (T_3) (13), both hyperthyroidism and hypothyroidism are associated with reduced exercise tolerance. Decreased exercise capacity may be particularly severe in patients with thyrotoxic myopathy (34). However, even in the absence of clinical evidence of myopathy, the response to exercise is altered in thyrotoxicosis. As compared to healthy controls, hyperthyroid patients demonstrate an exaggerated increase in oxygen consumption and in heart rate for a given level of work load (35). Furthermore, the metabolic response to exercise in hyperthyroidism is characterized by an exaggerated rise in free fatty acids, lactate, and norepinephrine, and an exaggerated decline in blood glucose (35). Each of these findings may be a consequence of the deconditioning brought on with the hyperthyroid state, since the findings are the opposite of those observed with physical training (12). An additional factor contributing to the exaggerated rise in heart rate, FFA, and lactate may be the enhanced sensitivity to catecholamines associated with hyperthyroidism.

Hypothyroidism is also associated with changes in the metabolic response to exercise in addition to a decrease in work capacity. The hypothyroid state is characterized by a reduction in lipolysis and FFA utilization (36). In contrast, there is a greater dependence on blood-borne glucose and muscle glycogen in the hypothyroid state (37). Depletion of muscle glycogen may thus contribute to decreased work capacity in such patients.

V. EXERCISE AND MENSTRUAL DYSFUNCTION

Acute exercise fails to alter the plasma concentrations of the gonadotropins FSH and LH in either men or women (13,38). An increase in plasma progesterone and estradiol, however, is observed with acute exercise in women, and is proportional to the intensity of the exercise performed (38). Following physical training, these stimulatory effects of exercise on ovarian hormone concentrations are no longer observed (38). In women as well as men, exercise is also associated with an increase in plasma testosterone (13,39). These elevations in sex steroids in response to exercise are primarily a consequence of reduced hormone clearance (catabolism) rather than a result of hypersecretion (13,40,41).

Although the physiological significance of exercise-induced changes in circulating sex steroids has not been established, it is now widely recognized that physical training is associated with disturbances of menstrual function. Oligomenorrhea, amenorrhea, and delayed menarche have all been observed in well-trained athletes. Oligomenorrhea or amenorrhea has been reported in 34–60% of well-trained runners or swimmers (21,42). Such menstrual irregularities are more common as the intensity of training increases (e.g., in women running 30 miles or more per week versus women running 5–30 miles per week) (21). An additional factor increasing the frequency of oligomenorrhea or amenorrhea is the initiation of physical training prior to menarche (42). In this regard it is noteworthy that a delayed menarche (an average of 2 years or more) is observed only in those athletes who initiate training prior to the menarche (42). Thus, the delay in menarche often reported by athletes cannot be attributed to greater tendency for late maturers to choose to be athletes.

With respect to the reversibility of training-associated disturbances in menstrual function only limited observations are available. In some sports such as rowing in which there may be marked seasonal variation in activity, a resumption in menses has been observed in the off-season. In addition, there is anecdotal evidence that when oligomenorrheic or amenorrheic long-distance runners reduce or discontinue training there is a return of normal menses (21).

The hormonal pattern associated with oligomenorrhea in women athletes suggests the presence of hypothalamic–pituitary dysfunction rather than ovarian failure. Reduced concentrations of FSH and LH are observed in oligomenorrheic or amenorrheic female athletes (21). Furthermore, in those women who are having menses, serum progesterone levels are reduced during the luteal phase and FSH concentrations are low during the luteal as well as the follicular phase, suggesting the presence of anovulatory cycles (43).

Concerning the mechanisms whereby physical training may lead to disturbances in the menstrual cycle, alterations in pituitary–hypothalamic–gonadal function directly related to repeated intensive physical activity (43) and changes in body composition (lean:fat ratio) have been proposed (42). Increases in serum progesterone and testosterone associated with acute exercise could conceivably have an adverse effect on follicular development (43). Alternatively, the reduction in body fat and the failure to achieve or maintain a minimum body weight for height (representing a critical lean:fat ratio) may be responsible for disturbed menstrual function. Decreases in body fat mass have been implicated in the oligomenorrhea or amenorrhea observed in anorexia nervosa, ballet dancers, as well as athletes (42). A return of menses has been observed with weight gain even in the absence of a change in physical training (42). The contribution of adipose tissue to menstrual function may relate to its role in the aromatization of androgens, thereby acting as an extragonadal source of estrogen.

A practical consideration which derives from these observations regarding the role of fat tissue is the possible beneficial effect in premenopausal women of maintaining a high caloric intake during physical training. Although prospective data concerning such dietary intervention have not been reported, the available evidence suggests a possible beneficial effect in preventing or ameliorating disturbed menstrual function.

REFERENCES

1. Andres, R., Cader, G., and Zierler, K. (1956). The quantitatively minor role of carbohydrate in oxidative metabolism by skeletal muscle in intact man in the basal state. *J. Clin. Invest.* **35,** 671.
2. Ahlborg, G., and Felig, P. (1982). Lactate and glucose exchange across the forearm, legs and splanchnic bed during and after prolonged leg exercise. *J. Clin. Invest.* **69,** 45.
3. Maehlum, S., Felig, P., and Wahren, J. (1978). Splanchnic glucose and muscle glycogen after glucose feeding during post-exercise recovery. *Am. J. Physiol.* **235,** E255.
4. Hultman, E. (1967). Studies on muscle metabolism of glycogen and active phosphates in man with special reference to exercise and diet. *Scand. J. Clin. Lab. Invest.* **19,** Suppl. 94, 1.

5. Rennie, M. J., Edwards, R. H. T., Krywawych, S., Davie, C. T. M., Halliday, D., Waterlow, J. C., and Millward, D. J. (1981). Effect of exercise on protein turnover in man. *Clin. Sci.* **61**, 627.

6. Wahren, J., Felig, P., Ahlborg, G., and Jorfeldt, L. (1971). Glucose metabolism during leg exercise in man. *J. Clin. Invest.* **50**, 2715.

7. Berger, M., Hagg, S. A., Goodman, M. N., and Ruderman, N. B. (1976). Glucose metabolism in perfused skeletal muscle. *Biochem. J.* **158**, 191–202.

8. Wahren, J., Hagenfeldt, L., and Felig, P. (1975). Splanchnic and leg exchange of glucose, amino acids and free fatty acids during exercise in diabetes mellitus. *J. Clin. Invest.* **55**, 1303.

9. Ahlborg, G., Felig, P., Hagenfeldt, L., Hendler, K., and Wahren, J. (1974). Substrate turnover during prolonged exercise in man: Splanchnic and leg metabolism of glucose, free fatty acids and amino acids. *J. Clin. Invest.* **53**, 1080.

10. Felig, P., Ali-Cherif, M. S., Minagawa, A., and Wahren, J. (1982). Hypoglycemia during prolonged exercise in normal man. *N. Engl. J. Med.* **306**, 895.

11. Hartley, L. H., Mason, J. W., Hogan, R. P., Jones, L. G., Kotchen, T. A., Mougey, E. H., Wherry, F. E., Pennington, L. L., and Ricketts, P. T. (1972). Multiple hormonal responses to graded exercise in relation to physical training. *J. Appl. Physiol.* **33**, 602.

12. Koivisto, V., Hendler, R., Nadel, E., and Felig, P. (1982). Influence of physical training on the fuel-hormone response to prolonged low intensity exercise. *Metab. Clin. Exp.* **31**, 192.

13. Galbo, H. (1983). Hormonal and Metabolic Adaptation to Exercise." Thieme, Stuttgart.

14. Carr, D. B., Bullen, B. A., Skrinar, G. S. *et al.* (1981). Physical conditioning facilitates the exercise-induced secretion of beta-endorphine and beta-lipotropin in women. *N. Engl. J. Med.* **305**, 560.

15. Richter, E. A., Canetto, L. P., Goodman, M., and Ruderman, N. (1982). Muscle glucose metabolism following exercise in the rat. *J. Clin. Invest.* **69**, 785.

16. Lohmann, D., Liebold, F., Heilmann, W., Stenger, J., and Pohl, A. (1978). Diminished insulin response in highly trained athletes. *Metab. Clin. Exp.* **27**, 521.

17. Mondon, C. E., Dolkas, C. B., and Reaven, G. M. (1980). Site of enhanced insulin sensitivity in exercise-trained rats at rest. *Am. J. Physiol.* **239** (*Endocrinol. Metab.* **2**), E169.

18. Koivisto, V. A., DeFronzo, R., Hendler, R., and Felig, P. (1982). The difference in insulin sensitivity and metabolic response to acute exercise in trained and sedentary subjects. *In* "Diabetes and Exercise" (M. Berger, P. Christacopoulos, and J. Wahren, eds.), pp. 122–132. Huber, Bern.

19. LeBlanc, J., Nadeau, A., Boulay, M., and Rouseau-Migneron, S. (1979). Effects of physical training and adiposity on glucose metabolism and ^{125}I-insulin binding. *J. Appl. Physiol.: Respir., Environ. Exercise Physiol.* **46**, 235.

20. Zawalich, W., Maturo, S., and Felig, P. (1982). Influence of physical training on insulin release and glucose utilization by islet cells and liver glucokinase activity in the rat. *Am. J. Physiol.* **243** (*Endocrinol. Metab.*), E464.

21. Dale, E., Geriach, D. H., and Wilhite, A. L. (1979). Menstrual dysfunction in distance runners. *Obstet. Gynecol.* **54**, 47.

22. Tamborlane, W. V., Sherwin, R. S., Koivisto, V., Hendler, R., Genel, M., and Felig, P. (1979). Normalization of the growth hormone and catecholamine response to exercise in juvenile onset diabetics treated with a portable insulin infusion pump. *Diabetes* **28**, 785.

23. Zinman, B., Murray, F. T., Vranic, M., Albisser, A. M., Leibel, B. S., McClean, P. A., and Marliss, E. B. (1977). Glucoregulation during moderate exercise in insulin treated diabetics. *J. Clin. Endocrinol. Metab.* **45**, 641.

24. Champion, M. C., Shepherd, G. A. A., Rodger, N. W., and Dupré, J. (1980). Continuous subcutaneous insulin infusion in the management of diabetes mellitus. *Diabetes* **29**, 296.

25. Koivisto, V. A., and Felig, P. (1978). Effects of leg exercise on insulin absorption in diabetic patients. *N. Engl. J. Med.* **298**, 79.

26. Dandona, P., Hooke, D., and Bell, J. (1978). Exercise and insulin absorption from subcutaneous tissue. *Br. Med. J.* **1,** 479.

27. Ferrannini, E., Linde, B., and Faber, U. (1982). Effect of bicycle exercise on insulin absorption and subcutaneous blood flow in the normal subject. *Clin. Physiol.* **2,** 59.

28. Kemmer, F. W., Berchtold, P., Berger, M., Starke, A., Cuppers, H. J., Gries, F. A., and Zimmerman, H. (1979). Exercise-induced fall of blood glucose in insulin treated diabetics unrelated to alteration of insulin mobilization. *Diabetes* **28,** 1131.

29. Susstrunk, H., Morell, B., Ziegler, W. H., and Froesch, E. R. (1982). Insulin absorption from the abodomen and the thigh in healthy subjects during rest and exercise: Blood glucose, plasma insulin, growth hormone, adrenaline, and noradrenaline levels. *Diabetologia* **22,** 171.

30. Lawrence, R. D. (1926). The effect of exercise on insulin action in diabetes. *Br. Med. J.* **1,** 648–652.

31. Wallberg-Henriksson, W., Gunnarsson, R., Henriksson, J., DeFronzo, R., Felig, P., Ostman, J., and Wahren, J. (1982). Increased peripheral insulin sensitivity and muscle mitochondrial enzymes but unchanged blood glucose control in Type I diabetics after physical training. *Diabetes* **31,** 1044.

32. Saltin, B., Lindgarde, F., Houston, M., Horlin, R., Nygaard, E., and Gad, P. (1979). Physical training and glucose tolerance in middle-aged men with chemical diabetes. *Diabetes* **28,** Suppl. 1, 30.

33. Ruderman, N. B., Ganda, U. P., and Johansen, K. (1979). The effect of physical training on glucose tolerance and plasma lipids in maturity-onset diabetes. *Diabetes* **28,** Suppl. 1, 89–92.

34. Kissel, P., Hartemann, P., and Duc, M. (1965). "Les syndroms myothyroidiens." Masson, Paris.

35. Nazar, K., Chwalbinska-Moneta, J., Machalla, J., and Kaciuba-Usilko, H. (1978). Metabolic and body temperature changes during exercise in hyperthyroid patients. *Clin. Sci. Mol. Med.* **54,** 323.

36. Paul, P. (1971). Uptake and oxidation of substrates in the intact animal during exercise. *In* "Muscle Metabolism during Exercise" (B. Pernow and B. Saltin, eds.), p. 225. Plenum, New York.

37. Baldwin, K. M., Hooker, A. M., Herrick, R. E., and Schrader, L. F. (1980). Respiratory capacity and glycogen depletion in thyroid-deficient muscle. *J. Appl. Physiol.* **49,** 102.

38. Bonen, A., Ling, W. Y., MacIntyre, R. N., McGrail, J. C., and Belcastro, A. N. (1979). Effects of exercise on the serum concentration of FSH, LH, progesterone and estradiol. *Eur. J. Appl. Physiol.* **42,** 15.

39. Sutton, F. R., Coleman, N. J., Casey, J., and Lazarus, L. (1973). Androgen responses during physical exercise. *Br. Med. J.* **1,** 529.

40. Keizer, H. A., Poorhman, J., and Bunnik, G. S. J. (1980). Influence of physical exercise on sex-hormone metabolism. *J. Appl. Physiol.* **48,** 765.

41. Terjung, R. (1979). Endocrine response to exercise. *Exercise Sport Sci. Rev.* **7,** 153.

42. Frisch, R. E., Gotz-Welbergen, A. V., McArthur, J. W., Albright, T., Witschi, J., Bullen, B., Birnholz, J., Reed, R. B., and Hermann, H. (1981). Delayed menarche and amenorrhea of college athletes in relation to age of onset of training. *JAMA, J. Am. Med. Assoc.* **246,** 1559.

43. Bonen, A., Belcastro, A. N., Ling, W. Y., and Simpson, A. A. (1981). Profiles of selected hormones during menstrual cycles of teenage athletes. *J. Appl. Physiol.* **50,** 545.

CHAPTER 16

The Effects of Exercise on Genitourinary Function

DAVID T. LOWENTHAL and SUSAN J. BRODERMAN

The William Likoff Cardiovascular Institute
Hahnemann University School of Medicine
Philadelphia, Pennsylvania

Renal function and electrolyte balance during exercise may mimic pathological states, represent supernormal function, or exemplify normal physiology. This chapter will examine the relationships between kidney function, electrolyte homeostasis, and exercise.

321

Exercise Medicine: Physiological Principles
and Clinical Applications

I. RENAL HEMODYNAMICS DURING EXERCISE

In the normal resting state, 20% of the total cardiac output perfuses the kidneys. With physical exertion, the renal perfusion is diminished as blood is shunted from the splanchnic circulation to the exercising muscles. Renal plasma flow as measured by clearance of para-aminohippurate (PAH) is decreased proportionately with increasingly strenuous exercise until the maximum pulse is obtained (1). At this level of maximum exertion, renal plasma flow is decreased approximately 50% from the resting level. After heavy supine exercise, the renal plasma flow returns to normal within 1 hour.

Although renal plasma flow is decreased 50% during and immediately subsequent to heavy exercise, the reduction in the glomerular filtration rate is only on the order of 30%. As a consequence, filtration fraction is increased to approximately 25%. This relative preservation of glomerular filtration is apparently accomplished by efferent arteriolar vasoconstriction. This alteration in the renal microcirculation may have consequences on the kidney in exercise other than those on the glomerular filtration rate. It may be an important factor in the mechanism of exercise proteinuria, as will be detailed later.

The decrease in the glomerular filtration rate is maximal during exercise of moderate intensity and, unlike renal plasma flow, does not correlate with heart rate. The state of hydration during exercise can modify the change in glomerular filtration rate during exercise, with dehydration further reducing glomerular filtration rate.

With sustained repetitive exercise, such as marathon training, a new phase of alteration of the glomerular filtration rate occurs after the initial decline. Beginning at the end of a week of heavy physical exertion, the glomerular filtration rate increases to levels 20% above resting normal (2). This increase coincides with an increase in total body water and plasma volume. A causal relationship between increased plasma volume and the increase in the glomerular filtration rate probably exists, although other nonvolume factors, such as a neurogenic mechanism, may also play a part in the increase of the glomerular filtration rate.

II. THE RENIN–ANGIOTENSIN SYSTEM IN EXERCISE

Several studies (3–7) have demonstrated that plasma renin activity is significantly elevated during exercise. This has been demonstrated not only during prolonged heavy exercise in the erect posture but also during brief exercise in the supine position (7). Plasma renin and aldosterone levels rise after brief heavy exercise with both the rise in plasma aldosterone and plasma renin activity being approximately twice control values (4). The elevation in plasma aldosterone may persist for several hours to several days depending on the duration of exercise.

The maximum for the plasma renin activity is reached shortly after cessation of exercise.

The mechanism of renal activation during exertion has been the subject of some study. The administration of ethacrynic acid during supine exercise increased plasma renin activity over exercising controls (5). This finding tends to contradict the thesis that renin released during exercise is a response to diminished sodium delivery to the distal tubule. Administration of dihydralazine, which minimizes renal vasoconstriction, did not diminish exercise-induced plasma renin activity enhancement (1). Hence, renal vasoconstriction per se is not likely to be a factor initiating renin activity elevation. Some evidence does exist that the renin elevation of exercise is mediated by autonomic nervous system mechanisms. The administration of ganglionic blockers prevent renin elevation from occurring in exercising rats (8). Furthermore, it has been shown that exercising humans have prominent rises in plasma norepinephrine levels as well as plasma renin levels (6). These data are by no means conclusive but suggest that autonomic nervous system may mediate exercise-induced renin release. The rapid time course of the elevation of renin is consistent with such a neural mechanism.

III. ANTIDIURESIS DURING EXERCISE

The urine flow rate decreases during strenuous exercise such as cross-country skiing or marathon running, frequently falling below 0.5 ml per minute (1,3). The magnitude of antidiuresis not only depends on the degree of exertion but also on the state of hydration of the exercising subject. There is marked individual variation in the decrease in urine flow.

Four factors that apparently underlie the phenomenon of antidiuresis during exercise are decreased free water clearance, increased sodium reabsorption, decreased osmolar clearance, and decreased glomerular filtration rate. The factor that correlates best with diminished urine flow is the reduction in free water clearance (9). It has been suggested that enhanced antidiuretic hormone (ADH) release and/or production underlies the decrease in free water clearance. Enhanced ADH may be elicited by neurogenic factors as well as the hyperosmolality and hypovolemia which develop during exercise.

Increased sodium reabsorption is a second factor in antidiuresis during exercise. Reduction in urine sodium excretion occurs briefly after the onset of heavy exercise. As will be discussed below, it appears to occur as a result of both renin–aldosterone activation as well as other mechanisms. The decrease in osmolar clearance which occurs during exercise is not only due to the decrease in urine sodium excretion but also to the decrease in the concentration of urea, phosphate, and chloride (10). This impaired concentrating ability may be the result of impaired delivery of solute out of the proximal tubule as proximal reabsorption increases for several solutes. The fourth factor in the reduction in urine flow during prolonged heavy exercise is the reduction in the glomerular filtration rate. Although this is not always evident in the early stages of exercise, there is a significant correlation of GFR decrease in urine flow during prolonged exercise and associated dehydration (1).

IV. SODIUM BALANCE DURING EXERCISE

The net sodium balance during exercise is predominantly a function of sodium loss through sweat and urine since minimal intake occurs during exercise. As mentioned above, reduction in urine sodium excretion occurs briefly after the onset of heavy exercise. Although renin-mediated aldosterone elevation has been documented in exercise (3–5) and most probably is a factor in enhanced sodium reabsorption, the rapidity of onset of antinatriuresis at a time before aldosterone elevation can be detected suggests that an alternate mechanism is acting. Brod has suggested that a neural mechanism mediates this rapid increase in tubular sodium reabsorption (11).

The sodium concentration of sweat varies with the rate of sweat production. Although levels of sweat sodium concentration approximate 20 mEq/liter at basal condition, at maximal sweating rates sodium concentration can reach 50 mEq/liter (3). Hence, the main route of sodium loss during heavy exercise is through enhanced sweating. However, even when dehydration during exercise is as much as 6%, the reduction in total interstitial sodium is substantially less than the reduction in interstitial water (12). As a consequence, the serum sodium concentration rises on an average of 6 mEq/liter (13). Sodium concentration within exercising muscle cell water is unchanged (12).

V. CHANGES IN TOTAL BODY WATER DURING EXERCISE

A. Acute Changes

The quantitative changes in total body water during exercise are a complex combination of transmembrane movement as well as net water loss to the environment. With initiation of heavy exercise, water moves out of the vascular space into the active muscle cell, as demonstrated by muscle biopsy techniques (13). Tissue hyperosmolality generated by active metabolism initiates this movement of water out of the interstitium and plasma (12). The plasma volume is decreased and plasma osmolality is increased early in exercise. This decline plateaus within the first half hour of exercise, however, apparently as a result of the increased plasma osmolality. Further water losses are then derived from interstitial and/or intracellular spaces. At a level of approximately 6% dehydration as measured by weight loss, the plasma osmolality will rise an average of 20 mOsm/liter (12). At levels of dehydration of 3%, the bulk of the water loss comes from the interstitial space (12). At greater levels of dehydration, the intracellular space becomes the major compartment for water loss. Some of this water is released during the process of glycolysis and some is produced from oxidative reactions.

B. Chronic Changes

In chronic, repetitive heavy exertion such as marathon training, alterations occur in plasma volume, total body water, and total body sodium that are the opposite of those that occur during the acute phase of exercise. After 1 week of heavy training, total body sodium, total body water, and plasma volume are increased above resting values (3). This effect persists for several days after the cessation of exercise. This hypervolemia is the factor responsible for the so-called "athlete's anemia" since hemodilution of the red cell mass does occur.

VI. POTASSIUM BALANCE IN EXERCISE

Potassium homeostasis during exercise includes several mechanisms involving the kidneys, sweat glands, and transcellular movement. In mild exercise, a slight increase in urine potassium excretion is observed, whereas during brief heavy exercise diminished potassium excretion occurs (1). During prolonged athletic training, several environmental factors affect potassium balance. Reduction of potassium in the diet during training results in a decrease of urinary potassium excretion, although a moderate potassium body deficit may develop (approximately 70 mEq in 4 days) (3). In addition, potassium restriction per se will lead to a decrease in urine flow rate during exercise (3). Reduction of urinary potassium excretion occurs despite the elevation of circulating aldosterone levels, which by itself would favor potassium excretion.

Knochel offers evidence that heavy physical training in a hot, humid climate leads to a significant abnormality of potassium homeostasis. He demonstrated using a ^{42}K tracer method that subjects training under hot, humid conditions developed reduced total body potassium when compared with similar trainees in a cooler climate (2). The trainees in the hot climate developed total body potassium deficits of approximately 500 mEq. Potassium efflux from active muscle cells has been demonstrated by muscle biopsy techniques to occur early in acute exercise. Much of the average 13% rise in serum potassium concentration, however (14), can be accounted for by the contraction of the plasma volume as a result of the loss of plasma water. The rise in serum potassium after a marathon run is on the order of 0.5 mEq/liter, whereas after a 50-mile run (15) potassium changes suggest that potentially fatal hyperkalemia may develop in the most severe forms of physical exertion.

The homeostatic response to an acute increase in potassium during dynamic physical activity involves the release of several hormonal substances including catecholamines (16), renin (15–19), aldosterone (20–22), and glucagon (23,24). The fall in insulin (24–27) during exercise is countered by an immediate rise in insulin when the activity is stopped, resulting in a fall in potassium (27).

It has been suggested that single and multiple doses of β-adrenergic blocking agents interfere with both catecholamine effects and the renin–aldosterone axis causing an increased hyperkalemic response to exercise (28–30). This has been shown to be dose related. Methyldopa and clonidine, which are also renin-inhibiting antihypertensive drugs, are known to interfere with the sympathetic nervous system. Yet, they do not produce exercise-induced hyperkalemia disproportionate to that rise seen *de novo* or in placebo controlled studies.

VII. ALTERATIONS IN OTHER SERUM CATIONS

In contrast to sodium and potassium, serum magnesium levels are decreased after prolonged heavy exercise by approximately 0.4 mEq/liter (14). Most of the loss of magnesium from the body during exercise is through increased quantities of sweat. Magnesium concentration in sweat is about 4.5 mEq/liter and does not vary with the rate of sweat production (3). In addition, a 12% reduction in muscle magnesium concentration has been observed following exercise and denotes efflux of magnesium out of muscle cells (3). Changes in serum magnesium during exercise do not appear to be of the magnitude that would have clinical importance.

Serum calcium concentration is unchanged after heavy exertion (14). This lack of change in serum concentration probably reflects concomitant hemoconcentration and moderate calcium losses in urine and sweat. The concentration of calcium in sweat actually decreases as the quantity of sweat produced increases (3).

VIII. HEMATURIA DURING EXERCISE

There are three clinical possibilities to explain red urine (31) occurring during exercise; e.g., hematuria (RBCs), myoglobinuria, and lower urinary tract trauma. In general, the hematuria associated with exercise is microscopic. Rarely, gross hematuria is encountered. One must question whether the red color is present throughout urination or only terminally. If it occurs terminally then it is related to a bladder problem. If it occurs early and throughout the urinary stream it is more likely related to a renal parenchymal process. One must also question whether there is any dysuria, back pain, flank pain, or radiating colicky pain suggestive of calculi. If clots are present, then this virtually eliminates the likelihood that its coming from the glomeruli.

In a group of 50 male marathon runners, 7 had microscopic, and 1 had gross hematuria (32). There were no red cell casts or other formed elements. The hematuria resolved within 48 hours. The exact mechanism is not understood although the decrease in glomerular filtration rate, i.e., relative ischemia, and/or bladder trauma may be implicated.

If the urine is occult blood positive and red cells are present, then one can feel sure that the bleeding is from an anatomical source. On the other hand, if the occult blood is positive and there is an absence of red cells but free hemaglobin is present, then one is obliged to look for hemolysis. If there is occult blood-positive urine and an absence of red cells but myoglobin is present then this is presumptive evidence for rhabdomyolysis. The presence of red urine with negative occult blood tests means that there is either some disease producing pigment, i.e., ochronosis, acute porphyria, or some external process such as a drug phenazopyridine hydrochloride (Pyridium).

Following competitive ice hockey, more formed elements may be found such as epithelial cells, leukocytes, hyaline, or granular casts, all of which are cleared within 48 hours after the game (33).

When hematuria persists and/or is associated with red blood cell casts this implies a renal parenchymal disease, most likely glomerular. On the other hand, if gross hematuria, an infrequent occurrence after running, is noted then one should consider bladder trauma (34,35). Cystoscopically, there is focal mucosal injury owing to repeated trauma of the posterior bladder wall against the prostatic base. Lesions are either ecchymoses or frank contusions. They are situated on the interureteric bar, the posterior half of the rim of the internal meatus, and the posterior wall in which position there is seen "mirroring" of the trigonal lesions. This has not been documented as yet in women whose urinary pelvic anatomy is different than the male. One speculation for the problem relates to the fact that an empty bladder while running may lead to contusions due to exertional forces and intra-abdominal pressure producing repeated impact of the flaccid wall of the bladder against the bladder base. The fact that there is a decrease in urine flow may help contribute to the empty bladder syndrome and consequent contusion development. On the other hand, at one time the bladder may be full and no problems will occur and yet in the same runner in an empty bladder state the lesion may appear significant.

IX. EXERCISE HEMOGLOBINURIA

It is almost a century since Fleischer described hemoglobinuria occurring subsequent to a prolonged march (36). Since then, several cases of hemoglobinuria occurring subsequent to running or marching for a prolonged distance on hard surfaces have been reported. Repetitive traumatic exercise of the upper extremities, such as karate or congo drumming, have also been reported to result in hemoglobinuria (37). The syndrome of exercise hemoglobinuria is characterized by the voiding of urine darkened by its content of hemoglobin subsequent to the inciting exercise. In addition, evidence of intravascular hemolysis is present, namely, elevated serum-free hemoglobin, methemalbuminemia, and decreased serum haptoglobin. In addition, the urinalysis frequently reveals granular casts suggesting that some tubular injury may be sustained. Cases of acute renal failure resulting from exercise hemoglobinuria are exceptional but have been reported (38).

There have been some studies of exercise hemoglobinuria which support the thesis that hemolysis is the result of mechanical trauma to erythrocytes while they circulate through the plantar vessels during hard impact on hard surfaces. Davidson compared the hemolysis of blood from both patients suffering from exercise hemoglobinuria and control subjects (39). The blood from both the control and patient groups showed greater hemolysis when running was done on a hard surface, although blood from the patient suffering from exercise hemoglobinuria showed relatively greater hemolysis on both surfaces. Spicer (40) showed that cases suffering from march hemoglobinuria had a low grade hemolytic state with the minor trauma of normal activity. Routine laboratory tests of erythrocyte fragility in these patients are normal, however. A particular susceptibility of erythrocytes to hemolysis cannot be excluded. It should be noted that running on soft surfaces as well as the use of properly padded soles can substantially reduce the occurrence of exercise hemoglobinuria in susceptible individuals.

X. PROTEINURIA RELATED TO EXERCISE

The occurrence of increased urinary excretion of protein during exercise has been known for a century, yet the etiology of this phenomenon remains uncertain. Castenfors describes total protein excretion after prolonged heavy exercise rising threefold to 150 mg/g creatinine excreted (41). The magnitude of proteinuria during exercise is small. Only about 20% of exercising subjects tested reach a level of proteinuria that can be detected by usual clinical tests. After short, heavy exertion, protein excretion returns to normal within 1 hour, while after prolonged exercise proteinuria persists as long as 10 hours (41).

The analysis of the composition of the protein excreted in the urine during exercise reveals that albumin accounts for approximately 45% and the remainder consist of α-, β-, and γ-globulins. The average molecular weight of the protein excreted is on the order of 50,000–60,000. There is a great deal of individual variation in the protein excretion, and in a few cases the predominant protein excreted were globulins.

The occurrence of proteinuria during exercise could be the result of either (1) enhanced glomerular filtration of protein; (2) diminished reabsorption by the proximal tubule; or (3) enhanced secretion of protein distally. The composition of the constituents of urinary protein in exercise is consistent with an origin as filtered plasma protein. Although Tamm–Horsfall protein has been observed to be increased (42), this increase is too small to account for the proteinuria of exercise.

The integrity of proximal tubular reabsorptive function during strenuous exercise has been assessed by measurement of excretion of glucose, α-amino acids, and the low molecular weight enzyme ribonuclease. These substances are normally reabsorbed in significant quantities in the proximal tubule, and their normal excretion rate during exercise support the notion that proximal tubular reabsorption is intact at this time (41).

The observed increase in plasma renin activity during exercise raises the possibility that alterations in the renin angiotensin system may be a factor in exercise proteinuria. Castenfors was unable to demonstrate a correlation between urine protein excretion and plasma renin activity during exercise, although such a relation was present before exercise was begun (41). This apparent inconsistency may be understood if renin–angiotensin activation is but one of several factors that modify renal hemodynamic changes during exercise and indirectly alter protein excretion. Norepinephrine and other vasoconstrictive substances may contribute to hemodynamic changes and proteinuria in the exercising human.

Perhaps the mechanism of exercise proteinuria may best be understood in light of the recent knowledge of the hydrodynamic forces across the glomerular membrane. Studies by Brennan (43) and Bohrer (44) show that when there is an elevation of the filtration fraction, the glomerular–capillary flow rate can be diminished while the single nephron glomerular filtration rate is unchanged, and that such changes can result in an increase in the concentration of plasma protein along the glomerular wall. Enhanced glomerular passage of plasma protein can subsequently occur without an alteration in membrane permeability characteristics or structure.

In fact, angiotensin II has been shown to produce proteinuria in an experimental model (44). In addition, a number of other vasoactive substances which can elevate filtration fraction may also result in increased protein excretion.

Exercise proteinuria may be the result of increased production of vasoactive substances, including angiotensin, which alter glomerular microhemodynamics and raise filtration fraction. Proteinuria then ensues through alterations of convective forces rather than a change in the glomerular membrane.

Occult diabetic nephropathy may become overt during exercise (45). Insulin-dependent diabetics who have had their disease for more than 10 years and who have no evidence of nephropathy may produce large quantities of nonselective proteinuria following dynamic exercise. Infusions of lysine may provoke a similar response (46).

Thus, a large quantity, i.e., >1000 mg proteinuria, which is slow to clear following exercise should point to underlying parenchymal disease, probably glomerular.

XI. RHABDOMYOLYSIS AND ACUTE NEPHROPATHY AS A CONSEQUENCE OF SEVERE EXERCISE

Knochel and associates (47) and other investigators (48) have offered evidence that exercise in a hot, humid environment is a significant cause of rhabdomyolysis and acute renal failure. This is an unusual occurrence in athletes and appears to be confined to poorly trained subjects suddenly undergoing heavy exertion particularly in hot, humid climates.

A fundamental concept in the pathogenesis of heat–exercise-induced rhabdomyolysis is the occurrence of potassium deficiency. As noted above, potassium deficits may develop during heavy training in hot, humid climates. Knochel, in experiments with laboratory dogs, shows that the efflux of potassium out of contracting muscle cells appears to provide an important vasodilatory effect on those vessels supplying the active muscles (49). Furthermore, the study showed that potassium deficiency diminished the potassium release and blunted the increase in blood flow produced necrosis of muscle cells. If an analogous mechanism is functional in the human, hypokalemia and potassium depletion may render exercising subjects particularly prone to muscle injury.

Potassium deficiency may mediate or predispose to muscle injury by an additional mechanism. The muscles of potassium-depleted laboratory animals show an abnormal glycogen content. Since glycogen is an important fuel source for the exerting muscle, a glycogen deficiency may predispose muscle cells to injury during exercise.

When muscle cells lyse, myoglobin is liberated into the circulation and subsequently filtered at the glomerulus. Although myoglobin per se is nontoxic to renal tubular cells, it is metabolized to hematin, a breakdown product toxic to tubular cells (50). The conversion of myoglobin to the hematin byproduct is enhanced in an acidic environment. The urine of the exercising subject usually has a pH of less than 5.0 and hence will be predisposed to the conversion of hematin.

Rhabdomyolysis may result in the release of yet another nephrotoxic substance into the circulation. As has long been noted, serum uric acid levels can be markedly elevated after exercise (51). Injured muscle cells release purines into the circulation and the uric acid is the metabolic end product. Since uric acid must compete with lactic acid for excretion and the lactate levels will be elevated during exercise, impaired excretion of uric acid combines with increased production of uric acid to lead to dangerously high levels of uric acid in the renal interstitial fluid. Furthermore, the acid pH of the urine would favor precipitation of uric acid in the tubule and interstitium, which can produce acute renal failure if the uric acid levels of the interstitium exceed critical levels.

The occurrence of acute rhabdomyolysis in acute renal failure is exceptionally uncommon in the well-trained athlete. It may be that the enhanced glomerular filtration previously described is a factor that provides a measure or protection from these potentially nephrotoxic substances released by muscle injury. In addition, the well-trained athlete may sustain significantly less muscle injury during the same degree of exertion. The clinical syndrome of exercise-induced acute rhabdomyolysis and acute renal failure is predominantly limited to untrained subjects, such as military recruits, who suddenly undergo heavy exertion. A hot, humid climate is also an important predisposing factor for this clinical phenomenon.

XII. CONCLUSIONS

The changes that occur in renal function and fluid and electrolyte balance in acute exercise appear to be counterbalanced by changes that occur during the repetitive heavy exertion that occurs during physical training. The fall in glomerular filtration, total body water, and total body sodium appears to be counterbalanced by the rise of these factors during repetitive exercise. These adaptations appear to be a fundamental part of the "training" process.

Alterations in the renin–aldosterone–angiotensin system appear to be part of the physiological adaptation to exercise but may also account for some of the "abnormalities," such as proteinuria, seen in subjects undergoing heavy exertion. Maintenance of relatively normal water and electrolyte balance appears to be important in prevention of untoward effects of heavy exercise on the kidney, namely, rhabdomyolysis and subsequent acute renal failure.

Exercise hemoglobinuria appears to be related to traumatic sheering forces of hard surfaces, but may be confined to particularly susceptible individuals.

REFERENCES

1. Castenfors, J. (1967). Renal function during exercise. *Acta Physiol. Scand.* **70,** Suppl. 293, 1.

2. Knochel, J. P. (1977). Potassium deficiency during training in the heat. *Ann. N.Y. Acad. Sci.* **170**, 175.

3. Costill, D. L. (1977). Sweating: Its composition and effects on body fluids. *Ann. N.Y. Acad. Sci.* **170**, 160.

4. Bozovic, L., Castenfors, J., and Piscator, M. (1967). Effect of prolonged heavy exercise on urinary protein excretion and plasma renin activity. *Acta Physiol. Scand.* **70**, 143.

5. Castenfors, J. (1967). Effect of ethacrynic acid on plasma renin activity during supine exercise in normal subjects. *Acta Physiol. Scand.* **70**, 215.

6. Chodahons, K., Nazas, K., Mocial, B. *et al.* (1975). Plasma catecholamines and renin activity in response to exercise in patients with essential hypertension. *Clin. Sci. Mol. Med.* **49**, 511.

7. Collier, J. G., Keddie, J., and Robinson, B. T. (1975). Plasma renin activity during and after dynamic and static exercise. *Cardiovasc. Res.* **9**, 323.

8. Bozovic, L., and Castenfors, J. (1967). Effect of ganglionic blocking on plasma renin activity in exercising and pain-stressed rats. *Acta Physiol. Scand.* **71**, 253.

9. Castenfors, J. (1967). Renal clearance and urinary sodium and potassium excretion during supine exercise in normal subjects. *Acta Physiol. Scand.* **70**, 207.

10. Refsan, N. E., and Stroinic, S. B. (1975). Relationship between urine flow, glomerular filtration and urinary solute concentration during prolonged heavy exercise. *Scand. J. Clin. Lab. Invest.* **35**, 775.

11. Brod, J. (1964). Die Nieren, Physiologie, Klinische Physiologie und Klinik." VEB Verlag Volk, Berlin.

12. Costill, D. L., Cote, R., and Fink, W. (1970). Muscle water electrolytes following varied levels of dehydration in man. *J. Appl. Physiol.* **40**(1), 6.

13. Bergstan, J. (1962). Muscle electrolyte in man. Determination by neutron activate analysis on needle biopsy specimen. *Scand. J. Clin. Lab. Invest.* **18**, 16.

14. Rose, L. I., Carroll, D. R., Lore, S. L. *et al.* (1970). Serum electrolyte changes after maraton running. *J. Appl. Physiol.* **29**, (4), 449.

15. McKechni, J. K., Leary, W. P., and Jourbet, S. M. (1967). Some electrocardiographic and biochemical changes recorded in marathon runners. *S. Afr. Med. J.* **41**, 722.

16. Kotchen, T. A., Hartley, L. A., Rice, T. W., Mongey, E. H., Jones, L. G., and Mason, J. W. (1971). Renin, norepinephrine and epinephrine responses to graded exercise. *J. Appl. Physiol.* **31**, 178.

17. Aurell, M., and Vikgren, P. (1971). Plasma renin activity in supine muscular exercise. *J. Appl. Physiol.* **31**, 839.

18. Bonelli, J., Waldhäusl, W., Magometschnigg, D., Schwarzmeier, J., Korn, A., and Hitzenberger, G. (1977). Effect of exercise and of prolonged oral administration of propranolol on hemodynamic variables, plasma renin concentration, plasma aldosterone and c-AMP. *Eur. J. Clin. Invest.* **7**, 337.

19. Fasola, A. F., Martz, B. L., and Helmer, O. M. (1966). Renin activity during supine exercise in normotensives and hypertensives. *J. Appl. Physiol.* **21**, 1709.

20. Adler, S. (1970). An extrarenal action of aldosterone on mammalian skeletal muscle. *Am. J. Physiol.* **218**, 616.

21. Davis, J. O., Urquhari, J., and Higgins, J. T., Jr. (1963). The effects of alteration of plasma sodium and potassium concentration on aldosterone secretion. *J. Clin. Invest.* **42**, 597.

22. Maher, J. T., Jones, L. G., Hartley, L. H., Williams, G. H., and Rose, L. I. (1975). Aldosterone dynamics during graded exercise at sea level and high altitude. *J. Appl. Physiol.* **39**, 18.

23. Lavine, R. L., Lowenthal, D. T., Gellman, M. D., Klein, S., Recant, L. R., and Rose, L. I. (1980). The effect of long distance running on plasma immunoreactive glucagon levels. *Eur. J. Appl. Physiol.* **43**, 41.

24. Santeusanio, F., Faloona, G. R., Knochel, J. R., and Unger, R. H. (1973). Evidence for a role of endogenous insulin and glucagon in the regulation of potassium homeostasis. *J. Lab. Clin. Med.* **81**, 809.

25. Himi, N., Morgenstern, I., Davidson, M. B., Bonorris, G., and Miller, A. (1973). Role of insulin in the transfer of infused potassium to tissue. *Horm. Metab. Res.* **5**, 84.

26. Lavine, R. L., Lowenthal, D. T., Gellman, M. D., Klein, S., Vloedman, D., and Rose, L. I. (1978). Glucose, insulin and lipid parameters in 10,000m running. *Eur. J. Appl. Physiol.* **38**, 301.

27. Pruit, E. D. R. (1970). Plasma insulin concentrations during physical work at near max O_2 uptake. *J. Appl. Physiol.* **29**, 155.

28. Affrime, M. B., Rosenthal, L. S., Lowenthal, D. T., Gould, A. B., and Falkner, B. (1982). The response to single and multiple dose propranolol under the influence of maximum physical activity. *Clin. Pharmacol. Ther.* **31**, 199.

29. Carlsson, E., Fellenius, E., Lundborg, P., and Svensson, L. (1978). β-adrenoceptor blockers, plasma potassium and exercise. *Lancet* **2**, 424.

30. Lennen, F. H. H., Coenen, C. H. M., Zonderland, M., and Mass, A. H. J. (1980). Effect of cardioselective and non-selective β-blockade on dynamic exercise in mildly hypertensive men. *Clin. Pharmacol. Ther.* **28**, 12.

31. Berman, L. B. (1977). When the urine is red. *JAMA, J. Am. Med. Assoc.* **237**, 2753.

32. Siegel. A. J., Hennekens, C. H., Solomon, H. S., and Van Boeckel, B. (1979). Exercise-related hematuria. *JAMA, J. Am. Med. Assoc.* **241**, 391.

33. Fletcher, D. J. (1977). Athletic pseudonephritis. *Lancet* **1**, 910.

34. Blacklock, N. J. (1977). Bladder trauma in the long-distance runner: 10,000 meters hematuria. *Br. J. Urol.* **49**, 129.

35. Blacklock, N. J. (1979). Bladder trauma in the long-distance runner. *Am. J. Sports Med.* **7**, 239.

36. Fleischer, R. (1881). Ueber eine nene form von hemoglobinuria bein menshen. *Klin. Wochenschr.* **47**, 691.

37. Caro, X. J., Sathetlard, P. W., Mitchel, D. B. *et al.* (1975). Traumatic hemoglobinuria associated with congo drums. *West. J. Med.* **123**, 141.

38. Pollard, T. D., and Weiss, I. W. (1970). Acute tubular necrosis in a patient with march hemoglobinuria. *N. Engl. J. Med.* **283**, 803.

39. Davidson, R. J. (1964). Exertional hemoglobinuria: A report of three cases with studies on the hemolytic mechanism. *J. Clin. Pathol.* **17**, 536.

40. Spicer, A. J. (1970). Studies on March hemoglobinuria. *Br. Med. J.* **1**, 115.

41. Castenfors, J., Mossfeld, F., and Piscator, M. (1967). Effect of prolonged heavy exercise on renal function and urinary protein excretion. *Acta Physiol. Scand.* **70**, 194.

42. Patel, R. (1964). Urinary casts in exercise. *Australas. Ann Med.* **13**, 170.

43. Brennan, B. M., Bohrer, M. P., Boylis, C. *et al.* (1977). Determinants of glomerular permeability: Insight derived from observation in vivo. *Kidney Int.* **12**, 229.

44. Bohrer, M. P., Dean, W. M., Robertson, C. R. *et al.* (1977). Mechanism of angiotensin II—induced protein in the rat. *Am. J. Physiol.* **2**, F13.

45. Mogensen, C. E., Vittinghus, E., and Sølling, K. (1979). Abnormal albumin excretion after two provocative renal tests in diabetes: Physical exercise and lysine injection. *Kidney Int.* **16**, 385.

46. Mogensen, C. F., and Sølling, K. (1977). Studies on renal tubular protein reabsorption . Partial and near complete inhibition by certain amino acids. *Scand. J. Clin. Lab. Invest.* **37**, 477.

47. Knochel, J. P., Dotin, N. H., and Hamburger, R. J. (1974). Heat stress, exercise and muscle effects on urate metabolism and renal function. *Ann. Intern. Med.* **81**, 321.

48. Schrier, R. W., Henderson, H. S., Tischer, C. C. *et al.* (1967). Nephropathy associated with heat stress and exercise. *Ann. Intern. Med.* **67**, 356.

49. Knochel, J. P., and Schlein, E. M. (1972). On the mechanism of rhabdomyolosis in potassium depletion. *J. Clin. Invest.* **51,** 1750.
50. Knochel, J. P., and Carter, N. W. (1976). The role of muscle cell injury in the pathogenesis of acute renal failure after exercise. *Kidney Int.* **10,** 558.
51. Cathcart, E. P., Kernanny, E. L., and Leather, J. B. (1908). On the origin of endogenous uric acid. *Q. J. Med.* **1,** 416.

CHAPTER 17

Psychological Aspects
of Exercise

RONALD M. LAWRENCE

Department of Psychiatry
University of California School of
Medicine
Los Angeles, California

I. INTRODUCTION

As of July 1981 Sachs and Buffone (1) listed over 700 references on psychological considerations in exercise including exercise as psychotherapy, exercise addiction, and the psychology of running. The number of papers being published in this area is increaseing at an exponential rate; by 1983 there will be over 1000 publications available. Early studies examined small groups of subjects and were not well designed. Later studies dealt with larger groups of subjects and were also better planned. However, we still have a long way to go toward matching the large population studies of exercise effects on the cardiovascular and pulmonary systems. The unique problems that arise in studying the psyche are inherent in the complex nature of the brain versus the lesser complexity of the heart and lungs. Understanding the complexity of the brain was called by the great psychologist, William James, "The ultimate of ultimate problems" (2). However,

Exercise Medicine: Physiological Principles
and Clinical Applications

the decade of the 1980s should bring forth data relating exercise and mental function comparable to data produced during the 1970s exploring the cardiovascular realm.

The primary form of exercise used to treat depression, anxiety, and phobias is running. Most therapeutic approaches are based on running therapy for several reasons, among which are the comparative ease with which the doctor can quantify the exercise prescription and also the fact that the early therapists were runners themselves. However, other forms of endurance exercise, such as swimming, bicycling, mountain climbing, or rowing, can induce similar physiological and psychological effects (3).

Exercise addiction was probably first explored by psychiatrist William Glasser who wrote the best selling book "Positive Addiction" (4). Concomitant with addiction is exercise euphoria or the exercise high. Even though the degree of exercise euphoria varies from subject to subject, the basic mechanisms seem to be similar in most runners. These topics will be discussed in detail later. Effects opposite to exercise euphoria may also occur with exercise. Exercise-induced depression is known to result from overtraining or overexertion. Too much of a good thing can create a state of exhaustion in any of the body systems including the brain.

It should be emphasized that the use of exercise to treat mental disorders is empiric even though exercise has been recognized for its beneficial effects on the psyche for over a century. Personal or anecdotal information abounds. The early Greeks recognized that vigorous exercise will produce certain positive effects on the mental development of young athletes. "Mens sana in corpore sano" was written by Homer who recognized the veracity of the mind–body relationship. An early paper by Gutin (5) heralded the beginning of modern exploration of exercise and mental health but well-organized studies did not begin to produce useful data until about 1970. Therefore, psychologic exercise therapy is still in an early stage of development regarding psychobiological mechanisms. At the present time, concepts on basic processes need to be modified every 2–3 years, but the concept of exercise's influence on the psyche has been well established.

II. DEPRESSION AND ANXIETY

To date, none of the studies using exercise treatment for depression has taken into consideration a categorical analysis of depression based on the Diagnotics and Statistical Manual (DSM III) (6). Grades of severity are based for the most part on scores of such accepted tests as the self-rating Zung Depression Inventory, Symptom Checklist-90 (SCL-90), Minnesota Multiphasic Personality Inventory (MMPI), D (Depression) Score, and similar psychological testing instruments.

Depression is a global term encompassing a spectrum ranging from mild, normal, and fleeting everyday "blues" through normal grief; then extending to the abnormal range to include moderate depression and, at the far end of the spectrum, the major depressions of the psychotic-endogenous type. Griest *et al.* (7,8) have stated that running as a treatment for depression shares many features with other medical treatments. It has been effective for some cases of mild or moderate depression but not all. He felt that if there was any secret to his patient's success it was that they tried to run every day in such a way that they desired to run again the next day. Based on studies to date, the category of depression best helped by exercise is still unclear. Mild to moderate depression from whatever etiology seems to be helped by exercise (7). Therefore, the physician would be safe in advising the patient who exercises that after a suitable time, usually 3 weeks, he may expect an alleviation of depression. More severe depression might be helped if such patients can be provided with a supervised exercise program, since therapeutic dynamics applied to mild or moderate depression should apply equally to more severe depression. Griest and associates (7) found that running was at least effective as time limited or time unlimited psychotherapy in alleviating the symptoms of depression and target complaints for individuals with mild to moderate depression (6).

Patients may show immediate exercise effects in lessening depressive symptomatology but a minimum of 3 weeks should be considered before such an effect is noted. Exercise should be performed in a graded fashion as is done with cardiovascular patients. A supervisory program is preferred especially since boredom and overuse may cause the patient to become an early dropout. Running has become the easiest mode of therapy to use, although other aerobic exercise of equal caloric expenditure can be substituted. The aerobic point system of Cooper (9) provides a simple method to compare exercise modes.

The beneficial effects of exercise are explained on several theoretical bases at present. They include biochemical, physiological, neurophysiological, psychoanalytic, meditative or consciousness alteration, hypnotic, religious, and psychological. Large muscle groups activity, because of the associated blood flow changes and muscular enhancement, is considered important in exercise therapy. Brown *et al.* (10) have advanced the concept that mental depression may represent a primary movement disorder. Mathew *et al.* (11) have shown that marked decreases in regional cerebral blood flow correlated significantly with depth of depression as measured by the Hamilton Depression Scale. Their work leads one to speculate that increasing regional cerebral blood flow may indeed help alleviate depression. Exercise is known to increase cerebral blood flow (12). Although the exact mechanism for cerebral blood flow reduction in depressed persons is unclear, Gur (13) reported that regional blood flow measurements can differentiate depressed patients from normal control subjects and abnormal blood flow normalizes after successful treatment.

III. PREVIOUS STUDIES

Brown et al. (10) studied psychological correlates of self-selected exercise regimens maintained for 10 weeks in depressed and normal subjects. His results indicated a significant improvement in various affective states measured by adjective check lists and the Zung depression scale. Physical activity schedules in his study largely consisted of jogging 3–5 times per week.

It has been hypothesized that neurotransmitters, specifically catecholamines (norepinephrine and dopamine) and indoleamines (largely serotonin) are involved in naturally occurring human depression (14). Jones and Smith (15) noted that brisk exercise can stimulate norepinephrine release. According to Smith and Jones, British researchers believe that a simple 10-minute exercise session 3 times a week could relieve depression.

Other data (16,17) have been provided concerning increased release of catecholamines and indoleamines through exercise. These studies suggest that 5-hydroxyindoleacetic acid (5-HIAA), homovanillic acid (HVA) and 3-methoxy-4,4-hydroxyphenylethylene glycol (MHPG), the major metabolites of serotonin, dopamine, and norepineprhine, respectively, may be involved in the exercise effect on brain function. Barchas and Freedman (18) had rats swim to exhaustion and found that brain serotonin levels decreased 20%. Changes in the levels of the two amines were seen to be time related. Elevated serotonin was seen immediately after exercise, and returned to preexercise levels within 2 hours; norepinephrine did not return to normal for 6 hours. Brown et al. (19) studied the role of endurance training and high-fat diet on two neurotransmitters (norepinephrine and 5-HT-serotonin) in three separate areas of the female rat brain. In most brain areas, NE and 5-HT levels were significantly greater among exercise–normal diet and exercise–fat diet, compared to both sedentary groups.

Other have demonstrated that MHPG levels drop when depression is induced in rats (20). The same researchers also found close parallels between MHPG levels in the rats' brains and those in the urine of certain types of depressed human patients, whereas in other types of depression the researchers found high MHPG levels. An important unanswered question is which depressive disorders have increased or decreased levels of MHPG.

Data from studies on catecholamine levels in depressed patients have been inconclusive and inconsistent. Post et al. (21) thought that this variability in results might be related to degree of activity. They examined the differences in spinal catecholamines of inactive and active depressed patients. Their results suggest that experimentally induced increases in psychomotor activity significantly elevate the cerebrospinal fluid levels of 5-HIAA, HVA, and MHPG.

The reduction of anxiety and depression using running therapy has been explored extensively by Morgan and associates (22–42). They did not confirm a reduction of anxiety or depression in all subjects. In one study, they found that 6 weeks of exercise did not elicit a significant reduction in depression for most of the subjects. However, for subjects who demonstrated a measureable depression initially, some improvement was noted. Subjects who exercise on a treadmill did not exhibit reduced levels of anxiety or depression when compared with a control group of normal individuals. Morgan, however, has reported consistent reductions in anxiety state with acute physical activity.

IV. EXERCISE ADDICTION

Whether addiction to exercise relates to psychological or biochemical causes remains a moot question. Certainly exercise addiction as a valid phenomenon has been accepted especially if one defines addiction as "the condition of being addicted (to a habit); habitual inclination" (43). The importance of recent work on the opiate-like peptide neurontransmitters raises questions about neurochemical mediators contributing to biochemical addiction. However, the more likely etiological basis of addiction lies with the psychological factors ranging from benign compulsion to sadomasochistic tendencies (44–54).

The problem of exercise induced anxiety and depression is a very real one today. It represents one end of the spectrum of behavioral changes induced by exercise which range from the beneficial to deleterious. The transition from benefit to detriment varies for each individual and is dependent on a multitude of factors ranging from previous training to genetic constitution. With more participants in endurance exercise, the number of exercise-induced psychological problems is increasing. Sometimes, in an attempt to overcome untoward mental feelings, more exercise is undertaken with a worsening of the condition and a vicious cycle develops. Some authors (55) have viewed the problem of overtraining from a preexisting or preexercise psychic propensity to primary affective disorders. Colt *et al.* (55) demonstrated a high prevalence of affective disorders in female runners and a similar (though statistically insignificant) trend in male runners. He hypothesized that these runners were motivated to continue running by the mood-improving actions of running. These investigators raised several important questions:

1. Is the addictive propensity of running related to its antidepressant effect possibly via a unifying "monoamine hypothesis?"
2. What happens to the personalities of athletes who stop exercising? Do they become depressed?
3. Is increased prevelance of depression among the aged related to decreased activity?
4. Is running as pleasurable to persons of normal mood as it is to those with disturbances of mood?

Little (56–58) proposed that the athlete's neurosis is a deprivation crisis and reports a not uncommon psychological etiology associated with the sudden development of neurotic symptoms (anxiety, depression, etc.) in males of apparently robust premorbid personality. It is characterized, according to Little, by a "striking absence of disturbed interpersonal relations." Therefore, the therapist should be familiar with the possibility of neurotic symptoms following athletic deprivation or cessation (59). Sudden stopping of an athletic program should be discouraged especially with endurance exercises (running, swimming, bicycling, etc.). Tapering off or gradual reduction of activity should be encouraged, where possible, over a period of weeks. Acute injury may make this impossible but the doctor should be alert to the potential psychological symptomatology and be prepared to intervene either pharmacologically or with other supportive mechanisms until the adaptive phase is over. Rarely, the mental status may become so disturbed as to lead to suicide or at least to overt or occult attempts to suicide. The author has one case, dating from 1967, of an inveterate amateur tennis player who played 4–5 hours daily and who, when deprived of his exercise for 2 weeks, become pathologically depressed and attempted suicide. On resuming his vigorous tennis workouts the depression lifted. Here an alternate form of strenuous exercise, such as a stationary bicycle, might be a helpful adjunct to drug therapy. This case has been published in detail previously (60).

V. PHOBIAS

The treatment of agoraphobia and situational phobias with running therapy was explored by Orwin (61,62) in the early 1970s. His conclusions enforce the concept that physical activity itself rates high as a treatment for phobias that frequently defy other forms of therapy. Orwin's work was substantiated by Muller and associates (63) in treating a case of elevator phobia, which might be classified as a subdivision of agoraphobia. The treatments consist of recognized controlled exercise regimens performed on a chronic frequent schedule of at least three times weekly.

VI. EXERCISE EUPHORIA

Exercise euphoria or exercise high has been the subject of numerous papers (45–53). In addition, it has been casually discussed in papers dealing with other aspects of exercise (64–67). The value of this response in maintaining subjects in an ongoing exercise program is well appreciated.

Appenzeller (68) discusses some of the biochemical factors involved in exercise euphoria (see Chapter 10). The phenomenon or pseudophenomenon of addiction closely relates to the euphoric state. This euphoria has been described as a feeling of religious ecstasy (60–69), a feeling related to a sexual orgasm (69), a tranquil meditative state (44), or assumption of right brain (creative hemisphere) dominance even if ever so briefly. Mandell's (70) concept of "The Second Second Wind" leads him to speculate that exercise euphoria results from activating the serotonergic (or other amines) system so far that, given an exquisite sensitivity to its own transmitter (serotonin turning off serotonin cells) (71,72), the system is inhibited and both hemispheric temporal lobe limbic structures are released completely, rather than changing their bilateral distribution or inhibition. He feels that the effect is imitated by LSD. He postulates other ways of achieving this state "beyond pain, hunger,thirst, anger, or depression: Transcendent" such as by quieting the brain and its sensory driving of the raphe system (73,74).

The effect of the exercise high or euphoria, however, can also be viewed as possibly detrimental. It can drive the athlete into an overuse or stress state, which is not only potentially physically harmful but also psychologically destructive. It may create a reckless state and the athlete should be warned not to view himself as invincible while so intoxicated. Kostrubala (75) considers endurance athletes to be subject to delusions of extreme capabilities and invincibility.

VII. EXERCISE NEUROSIS AND STRESS REDUCTION

Exercise induced anxiety is a much wider problem than recognized. Much of this anxiety is based on unrealistic athletic goals or training schedules, which lead to distortions in conceptions of self, body image, or schema. Critchley (76) alludes to this when he states that a striking lack of correspondence may be encountered in the discrepancy between the true appearance of the anatomy as obvious to everyone around, and the notion which the individual himself entertains. The two may be entirely different. Although exercise is well known for its stress reducing properties (64–67), it is also known to be an effective producer of stress especially in overuse syndromes (56–58). Mechanisms for stress reduction abound in the literature (77,78) and those relating to stress causation have been adequately explored; these include physical as well as psychological etiologies (64–67).

VIII. CONCLUDING REMARKS

Suffice it to say that exercise regimens should be tailored specifically for each individual, considering not only the physiological characteristics involved but the mental state as well. To this end, administration of a broad based psychometric test such as the Minnesota Multiphasic Personality Index (79) to each patient is advisable to study any areas of psychological dysfunction prior to undertaking an exercise program. The MMPI is a self-administered test taking little, if any, of the physician's time and it can either be scored by office personnel or inexpensively by outside psychological service organizations, a list of which can be provided by the American Psychiatric Association or the American Psychological Association. The test can also be used to monitor the psychological progress of the subject especially in the event of future problems with the psyche.

From the psychological point of view, a 5 day per week exercise schedule is usually the most effective one for most individuals (7,8). However, this, too, must be individually evaluated. Some people do better with an every other day schedule and a few do better with a daily schedule. Only by empirically evaluating the subject on at least a monthly basis can the final program be deduced. A brief 15-minute office interview can establish which regimen is best from the psychological viewpoint. Questions relating to a sense of well-being and a review of a daily diary to explore levels of energy, enthusiasm, and activity can offer the practitioner guidelines for program adjustment.

Kostrubala (80) in his now classic book "The Joy of Running" broadly discusses the use of running therapy. His impetus resulted in the formation of the International Association of Running Therapists (IART). He also relates the training of such a running therapist in a 1978 paper (81).

Running and exercise programs are discussed and offered widely in the popular literature from Fixx's "The Complete Book of Running" (82) to more recent works by Cantu et al. (83). All of them appear to be variations on commonly accepted themes dating back to the early 1970s and adequately proved by cardiovascular–respiratory research explored elsewhere in this volume.

Exercise effects on the mind are beneficial overall except when done to excess. The responsibility of the therapist is to learn where enough ends and where excess begins.

REFERENCES

1. Sachs, M. H., and Buffone, G. W. (1981). "Bibliography: Psychological Considerations in Exercise, Including Exercise as Psychotherapy, Exercise Dependence (Exercise Addiction) and the Psychology of Running." Université du Québec à Trois-Rivières, Quebec, Canada (available from the first author).
2. James, W. (1910). "The Principles of Psychology." Holt, New York.
3. Snyder, E. E., and Spreitzer, E. A. (1974). Involvement in sports and psychological well-being. *Int. J. Sport Psychol.* **5** (1), 28–39.
4. Glasser, W. (1976). "Positive Addiction." Harper, New York.
5. Gutin, B. (1966). Effect of increase in physical fitness on mental ability following physical and mental stress. *Res. Q.* **37**, 211–220.

6. "Diagnostic and Statistical Manual" (1980). 3rd ed. (DSM-III). Am. Psychiatr. Assoc., Washington, D.C.

7. Griest, J. H., Klein, M. H., Eischens, R. R., Faris, J., Gurman, A. S., and Morgan, W. P. (1978). Running through your mind. *J. Psychosom. Res.* **22,** 259–294.

8. Griest, J. H. *et al.* (1978). *Behav. Med.* **5,** 19–24.

9. Cooper, K. H. (1968). "Aerobics." Bantam Books, New York.

10. Brown, R. S., Ramirez, D. E., and Taub, J. M. (1978). *Physician Sports Med.* **6**(12), 34–37, 40–41, 44–45.

11. Mathew, R. J., Meyer, J. S., Semchuk, K. M., Francis, D., Mortel, K., and Claghorn, J. L. (1980). Regional cerebral blood flow in depression: A preliminary report. *J. Clin. Psychiatry* **41**(12), Sect. 2, 71–72.

12. Meyers, J. S., and Schade, J. P. (1972). "Cerebral Blood Flow." Elsevier, Amsterdam.

13. Gur, R. (1982). *Clin. Psychiatry News.*

14. Akiskal, H., and McKinney, T. (1975). Research in depression. *Arch. Gen. Psychiatry* **32,** 285–305.

15. Jones, S., and Smith, T. (1979–1980). Impression of running/jogging and their effect on mental health. *Psychology, Q. J. Hum. Behav.* **16,**(4), 21–24.

16. Edington, D. W., and Edgerton, V. R. (1976). "The Biology of Physical Activity." Houghton, Boston, Massachusetts.

17. Morehouse, L., and Miller, A. T., Jr. (1971). "Physiology of Exercise." Mosby, St. Louis, Missouri.

18. Barchas, J., and Freedman, D. (1963). Brain amines: Responses to physiological stress. *Biochem. Pharmacol.* **12,** 1232–1235.

19. Brown, B. S., Payne, T., Kim, C., Moore, G., Krebs, P., and Marting, W. (1979). Chronic response of rat in brain norepinephrine and serotonin levels to endurance training. *J. Appl. Physiol.* **46,**(1), 19–23.

20. Tracing the Chemistry of Depression (1980). *Sci. News* **117,**(6), 247.

21. Post, R. M., Kotin, J., Goodwin, F. K., and Gordon, E. K. (1973). Psychomotor activity and cerebrospinal fluid amine metabolities in effective illness. *Am. J. Psychol.* **130,**(1), 67–72.

22. Morgan, W. P. (1968). Psychological considerations. *J. Phys. Educ. Recreation* **39,** 26–28.

23. Morgan, W. P. (1969). Physical fitness and emotional health: A review. *Am. Corrective Ther. J.* **23,** 124–127.

24. Morgan, W. P. (1969). A pilot investigation of physical working capacity in depressed and nondepressed psychiatric males. *Res. Q.* **40,** 849–861.

25. Morgan, W. P. (1969). Selected physiological and psychomotor correlates of depression in psychiatric patients. *Res. Q.* **39,** 1037–1043.

26. Morgan, W. P. (1970). Physical fitness correlates of psychiatric hospitalization. *In* "Contemporary Psychology of Sport" (G. S. Kenyon, ed.). The Athletic Institute, Chicago, Illinois.

27. Morgan, W. P. (1970). Physical working capacity in depressed and non-depressed females: A preliminary study. *Am. Corrective Ther. J.* **24,** 14–16.

28. Morgan, W. P. (1972). Sport psychology. *In* "The Psychomotor Domain" (R. N. Singer, ed.). Lea & Febiger, Philadelphia, Pennsylvania.

29. Morgan, W. P. (1973). Influence of acute physical activity on state anxiety. *Proc., Nat. Coll. Phys. Educ. Assoc. Men, 76th Annu. Meet.*

30. Morgan, W. P. (1974). Exercise and mental disorders. *In* "Sports Medicine" (A. J. Ryan and F. L. Allman, Jr., eds.), Chapter 31. Academy Press, New York.

31. Morgan, W. P. (1976). Psychological consequences of vigorous physical activity and sport. *In* Academy Papers: Beyond Research—Solutions to Human Problems" (M. G. Scott, ed.). Am. Acad. Phys. Educ., Iowa City, Iowa.

32. Morgan, W. P. (1978). The mind of the marathoners . *Psychol. Today* **11**(11), 38–40, 43, 45–46, 49.
33. Morgan, W. P. (1979). Anxiety reduction following acute physical activity. *Psychiatr. Ann.* **9**, 36–45.
34. Morgan, W. P. (1980). Psychological benefits of physical activity. *In* "Exercise, Health and Disease" (F. J. Nagle and H. J. Montoye, eds.). Thomas, Springfield, Illinois.
35. Morgan, W. P., Brown, D. R., and Raven, P. B. (1981). Interaction of anxiety, perceived exertion, and dyspnea in the person-respirator interface. *Med. Sci. Sports Exercise* **13**(2), 73.
36. Morgan, W. P., and Costill, D. L. (1972). Psychological characterics of the marathon runner. *J. Sports Med. Phys. Fitness* **12**, 42–46.
37. Morgan, W. P., and Horstman, D. H. (1976). Anxiety reduction following acute physical activity. *Med. Sci. Sports* **8**,62 (abstr.).
38. Morgan, W. P., Horstman, D. H., Cymerman, A., and Stokes, J. (1979). Use of exercise as a relaxation technique. *J. S. C. Med. Assoc.* **75**, 596–601.
39. Morgan, W. P., and Pollock, M. L. (1977). Psychologic characterization of the elite distance runner. *Ann. N. Y. Acad. Sci.* **301**, 382–403.
40. Morgan, W. P., and Pollock, M. L. (1978). Physical activity and cardiovascular health: Psychological aspects. *In* "Physical Activity and Human Well-Being" (F. Landry and W. A. R. Orban, eds.). Symposia Specialists, Inc., Miami, Florida.
41. Morgan, W. P., Roberts, J. A., Brand, F. R., and Feinerman, A. D. (1970). Psychological effect of chronic physical activity. *Med. Sci. Sports* **2**, 213–217.
42. Morgan, W. P., Roberts, J. A., and Feinerman, A. D. (1971). Psychologic effect of acute physical activity. *Arch. Phys. Med. Rehabil.* **52**(9), 422–425.
43. Webster's New Twentieth Century Dictionary (1963). 2nd ed. Library Guild, New York.
44. Solomon, E. G., and Bumpus, A. K. (1978). The running meditation response: An adjunct to psychotherapy. *Am. J. Psychother.* **32**, 583–592.
45. Sachs, M. L. (1978). Exercise addiction. *Racing South.* **1**,(3), 14–16.
46. Sachs, M. D. (1980). On the trail of the runner's high. A descriptive and experimental investigation of characteristics of an elusive phenomenon. Doctoral Dissertation, Florida State University, Tallahassee (unpublished).
47. Sachs, M. D. (1980). The runner's high. *Pap. 3rd Annu. Psychol. Running Semin. Cornell Univ. Med. Coll.* Eric Doc. No. ED 191-832.
48. Sachs, M. L. (1981). Running addiction. *In* "The Psychology of Running" (M. H. Sachs and M. L. Sachs, eds.), pp. 116–126. Human Kinetics Publ., Champaign, Illinois.
49. Sachs, M. L., and Pargman, D. (1979). Addiction to running: Phenomenon or pseudophenomenon. *Pap., Int. Cong. Phys. Educ. 1979.*
50. Sachs, M. L., and Pargman, D. (1979). Commitment and addiction to regular running. *Pap., Annu. Conv. Am. Alliance Health, Phys. Educ. Recreation* Abstracts, Res. Pap. 1979 AAHPER Conv., p. 141.
51. Sachs, M. L., and Pargman, D. (1979). Personality and the addicted runner. *Pap., Int. Congr. Phys. Educ., 1979.*
52. Sachs, M. L., and Pargman, D. (1979). Running addiction: A depth interview examination. *J. Sport Behav.* **2**, 143–155.
53. Sachs, M. L., and Pargman, D. (1980). On the trail of the runner's high. *Pap., Annu. Conv. Am. Alliance Health, Phys. Educ. Recreation Dance* Abstracts, Res. Pap. 1980 AAHPERD Conv., p. 80.
54. Epstein, J. (1981). Running and other vices. *In* "Psychology of Running" (M. Sacks and M. Sachs, eds.), pp. 176–185. Human Kinetics Publ., Champaign, Illinois.
55. Colt, E. W. D., Dunner, D. L., Hall, K., and Fieve, R. (1981). A high prevalence of affective

disorder in runners. "Psychology of Running" (M. H. Sachs and M. L. Sachs, eds.), pp. 234–248. Human Kinetics Publ., Champaign, Illinois.

56. Little, J. C. (1966). Physical prowess and neurosis. M.D. Thesis, University of Bristol (unpublished).

57. Little, J. C. (1969). The athlete's neurosis—a deprivation crisis. *Acta Psychiatr. Scand.* **45,** 187–197.

58. Little, J. C. (1979). Neurotic illness in fitness fanatics. *Psychiatr. Ann.* **9**(3), 49–51, 55–56.

59. Baekeland, F. (1970). Exercise deprivation: Sleep and psychological reactions. *Arch. Gen. Psychiatry* **22,** 365–369.

60. Lawrence, R. M. (1979). The psychology of sports competition. *In* "Therapeutics Through Exercise" (D. Lowenthal, K. Bharadevaja, and W. Oaks, eds.), pp. 103–111. Grune & Stratton, New York.

61. Orwin, A. (1973). The running treatment: A preliminary communication on a new use for an old treatment (physical activity) in the agoraphobia syndrome. *Br. J. Psychiatry* **122,** 175–179.

62. Orwin, A. (1974). Treatment of a situational phobia—a case for running. *Br. J. Psychiatry* **125,** 95–98.

63. Muller, B., and Armstrong, H. E. (1975). A further note on the 'running treatment' for anxiety. *Psychother.: Theory, Res. Pract.* **12,** 385–387.

64. Dienstbier, R. A. (1978). Running and personality change. *Today's Jogger* **2,**(1), 30–33, 48–49.

65. Dienstbier, R. A. (1980). Long-term changes in stress tolerance in runners. *Pap., 3rd Annu. Psychol. Running Semin., 1980.*

66. Dienstbier, R. A. (1981). An historical perspective and current theory on the psychology of exercise. *Pap., Midwest Symp. Exrcise Ment. Health, 1981.*

67. Dienstbier, R. A., Crabbé, J., Johnson, G. O., Thorland, W., Jorgensen, J. A., Sadar, M. M., and Lavelle, D. C. (1981). Running and changes in stress tolerance, mood, and temperament indicators: A bridge to exercise and personality change. *In* "The Psychology of Running" (M. H. Sachs and M. L. Sachs, (eds.), pp. 192–210. Human Kinetics Publ., Champaign, Illinois.

68. Appenzeller, O., and Schade, D. R. (1980). Neurology of endurance training. V. Endorphins. *Neurology* **30,** 418–419.

69. Spino, M. (1976). "Beyond Jogging." Celestial Arts, Millbrae, California.

70. Mandell, A. J. (1979). The second second wind. *Psychiatr. Ann.* **9**(3), 57, 61–63, 66–69.

71. Aghajanian, G. K., and Wange, R. Y. (1978). Physiology and pharmacology of central serotonergic neurons. *In* "Psychopharmacology: A Generation of Progress" (M. A. Lipton, A. DiMascio, and K. F. Killam, eds.). Raven Press, New York.

72. de Montigny, C., and Aghajanian, G. K. (1978). Tricyclic antidepressants: Chronic treatment increase responsitivity to rat forebrain neurons to serotonin. *Science* **202,** 1303–1306.

73. Mandell, A. J. (1981). The second second wind. *In* "The Psychology of Running" (M. H. Sachs and M. L. Sachs, ed.), pp. 211–223. Human Kinetics Publ., Champaign, Illinois.

74. Mandell, A. J. (1977). Some old and new theories in biochemical psychiatry. *In* "The Impact of Biology on Psychiatry" (E. S. Gershon, R. H. Belmaker, and S. S. Kety, eds.). Plenum, New York.

75. Kostrubala, T. (1981). Running: The grand illusion. *In* "The Psychology of Running" (M. H. Sachs and M. L. Sachs, eds.), pp. 92–98. Human Kinetics Publ., Champaign, Illinois.

76. Critchley, M. (1979). Corporeal awareness: Body-image. *In* "The Divine Banquet of the Brain," p. 99. Raven Press, New York.

77. Schafer, W. (1978). "Stress, Distress and Growth." Respir. Action, Davis, California.

78. Albinson, J. G. (1979). Fitness through recreation in the industrial setting. *Rec. Res. Rev.* **6,**(4), 70–73.

79. Minnesota Multiphasic Personality Inventory (M.M.P.I.) (1943, 1970). The Psychological Corp., New York.
80. Kostrubala, T. (1976). "The Joy of Running." Lippincott, Philadelphia, Pennsylvania.
81. Kostrubala, T. (1978). The training of a running therapist. *Med. Sport (Basel)* **12,** 111–115.
82. Fixx, J. F. (1977). "The Complete Book of Running." Random House, New York.
83. Cantu, R. C. (1982). "Sports Medicine in Primary Care." Collamore Press, D. C. Heath Co., Lexington, Massachusetts.

CHAPTER 18

Medical Aspects of Diving

ALFRED A. BOVE
*Cardiovascular Division,
and Department of
Physiology
Mayo Foundation
Rochester, Minnesota*

OTTO APPENZELLER
*Departments of Neurology and
Medicine
University of New Mexico
School of Medicine
Albuquerque, New Mexico*

I. INTRODUCTION

The sport of scuba diving has become a popular recreation for more than two million trained sport divers. This population, like its counterparts in military and commercial diving, is subject to a set of diseases not commonly encountered in medical practice.

The unique stresses imposed on the human organism by the underwater environment require special knowledge of hyperbaric physiology, effects of oxy-

Exercise Medicine: Physiological Principles
and Clinical Applications

gen at high pressures, carbon monoxide and carbon dioxide intoxication, and marine toxicology. In addition, the physician must understand the relationship of various chronic diseases to the sport of diving since some chronic diseases can cause lethal complications when combined with the underwater diving environment. This chapter briefly reviews the physics and physiology of the underwater environment and provides guidelines for advising patients who wish to undertake the sport of scuba diving.

II. PHYSIOLOGY OF THE UNDERWATER ENVIRONMENT

The underwater environment imposes an increase in ambient pressure on the body as well as exposure to cold, exercise, emotional stress, increased oxygen partial pressure, the possibility of carbon dioxide and carbon monoxide toxicity, hypoxia, marine envenomation, drowning, and traumatic injuries.

III. PRESSURE EFFECTS

Increased pressure has three possible consequences. First, according to the physics of compressible gases, the volume of the gas held in a nonrigid container is inversely proportional to the pressure. This principle, sometimes called Boyle's law (1) is expressed as $PV = $ constant. As an individual submerges underwater, pressure will increase by one atmosphere (14.7 psi, 760 mm Hg) for every 33 feet of depth in seawater. A closed air space subjected to these pressure changes will be forced to contract on descent and expand on ascent. Gas spaces in the body that are not in equilibrium with the ambient pressure will undergo deformation with ultimate injury to tissue. Such spaces are the lungs, middle ear, the paranasal sinuses, and, less commonly, the gastrointestinal tract and small gas pockets sequestered beneath dental fillings. In addition, the artificial space created inside a face mask can be affected by pressure and cause injury to facial structures. Changes in ambient pressure which occur on descent or on ascent can cause alterations in the volume of these spaces which if not properly vented will ultimately cause injury. The most common disorder in diving is injury to the middle ear because of unbalanced pressure across the tympanic membrane (2–4). This illness, entitled ''middle ear squeeze,'' occurs on descent in the water when the eustachian tube does not properly vent the middle ear space. As pressure increases, the tympanic membrane is displaced inward until ultimately hemorrhage in the middle ear occurs. Further descent will cause tympanic membrane rupture. Blood in the middle ear will act as a culture medium for bacterial growth, and acute otitis media often results. In addition, vertigo from a sudden inrush of cold water through a ruptured tympanic membrane can confuse a diver underwater and cause spatial disorientation. This occurrence in an inexperienced diver can result in panic and drowning. The influx of contaminated water into the middle ear adds to the likelihood of acute otitis media. Treatment of middle ear squeeze involves antibiotics to prevent infection, decongestants to provide adequate middle ear drainage, and expectant treatment of ruptured tympanic membrane. Individuals with middle ear squeeze should not dive until the ear is completely healed, all fluid is absent, and there is no tear or perforation in the tympanic membrane. Eustachian tube function can be tested by observing motion of the tympanic membrane with an otoscope during a Valsalva maneuver. Inability to equalize middle ear pressure is a contraindication to diving. Similar mechanical effects will cause hemorrhage in the paranasal sinuses when sinuses are not properly vented to the pharynx (5,6). The diver notices epistaxis underwater. Treatment of sinus squeeze involves antibiotics and decongestants. The mild epistaxis that may be noted following sinus squeeze usually clears spontaneously and the only important complication is an acute sinusitis subsequent to the episode of diving. The interesting observation by divers with sinus squeeze of green blood in their face mask is valid since red light is absent below 15–20 feet, and blood then appears brown or green.

A less common, but more serious injury to the ear occurs when the diver performs a Valsalva maneuver during descent underwater. This maneuver is performed in order to force air into the middle ear and equilibrate pressure across the tympanic membrane. Occasionally, the high pressures developed in the venous system and spinal fluid during a Valsalva maneuver will cause a round-window rupture with loss of endolymph and a sudden abnormality in vestibular and auditory function (7). Treatment of round-window rupture is surgical, and individuals who have sustained round-window rupture should be advised to give up diving.

A. Pulmonary Barotrauma

Although middle ear squeeze is the most common diving illness, the most serious is pulmonary barotrauma with subsequent cerebral air embolism. Gas expansion in the lungs during ascent from an underwater excursion using a pressurized air supply usually is compensated by appropriate exhalation of air through an open airway. Occasionally, on ascent a diver may panic and breath hold. The results of breath holding on ascent is expansion of gas in the lung with stretching, then tearing of lung tissue, damage to alveolar membranes, and rupture of blood vessels in the lung (1,8,9). In addition, pneumothorax, mediastinal, and subcutaneous emphysema may complicate the lung injury.

A common complication of pulmonary barotrauma is entry of air into the arterial system with cerebral or cardiac air embolism (8–10). Cerebral air embolism is manifest by sudden onset of neurological symptoms upon surfacing. These symptoms may include blindness, focal motor and sensory deficits, seizures, unconsciousness, apnea, cardiac arrhythmias, or cardiac arrest. Occasionally mild cases may manifest only behavioral abnormalities. Pulmonary barotrauma with arterial air embolism has a high mortality, and requires immediate treatment (1,10,11). In spite of stringent medical standards and the ability to treat pulmonary barotrauma within seconds of the onset of symptoms, in Navy submarine escape training where trainees ascend rapidly from 100 feet underwater while exhaling, the incidence of pulmonary barotrauma is 1 in 2000 and death from air embolism, although rare, still occurs in this setting (11). Treatment of arterial gas embolism involves immediate recompression in a hyperbaric chamber and application of hyperbaric oxygen, and requires the skills of a physician trained in undersea and hyperbaric medicine in addition to the use of a hyperbaric chamber for therapy. Clinical experience has demonstrated that delays between onset of symptoms and recompression treatment are associated with an increased likelihood of permanent residual neurological injury (9). Treatment of cerebral air embolism which does not incorporate recompression is unsuccessful; thus, any person with strokelike symptoms developing upon ascent from diving with a compressed air supply should be referred immediately to a hyperbaric chamber facility for treatment. Pneumothorax, mediastinal, and subcutaneous emphyzema when unassociated with arterial gas embolism do not require recompression therapy (1). Pneumothorax is treated as any other pneumothorax with aspiration of air from the chest when cardiopulmonary functions compromised. Mediastinal and subcutaneous emphyzema are treated expectantly with some success being achieved by breathing 100% oxygen at surface pressure. Cerebral air embolism occurring from cardiac or cranial surgery should also be treated with recompression (12).

B. Decompression Sickness

A second important aspect of increased environmental pressure in diving is decompression sickness (DCS). There is a spectrum of injury in this illness (Table I) which can mimic a variety of other disorders (13–16). The disease develops on ascent from depth when a diver does not follow established procedures for returning to the surface, which are designed to prevent effervesence of dissolved inert gas (nitrogen). The formation of free gas in the body has several consequences (17–20). First, free gas entering the vascular system from the peripheral tissues will transit the veins and cause pulmonary vascular obstruction (18,19). When the free gas volume is large and significant pulmonary obstruction occurs, a classical syndrome (chokes) is described (1,13,16). This syndrome is manifest by chest pain, dyspnea, and cough. Often associated with free gas in the blood and tissue injury from expanding gas bubbles is activation of acute inflammation (21,22). The inflammatory response results in altered vascu-

TABLE I

Classification of Decompression Sickness

Type I: Pain only decompression sickness
Limb or joint pain
Itch
Skin rash
Fatigue
Type II: Serious decompression sickness
Central nervous system disorder
Pulmonary (chokes)
Systemic (hypovolemic shock)
Inner ear/vestibular

lar permeability, which allows fluid to leak into the interstitial tissues of the systemic and pulmonary vascular beds (20,21,23). In severe cases, pulmonary edema can occur and hypovolemia with significant plasma loss and hemoconcentration will result (23–25). With severe decompression sickness, endothelial damage to blood vessel occurs (25), significant focal regions of tissue ischemia are evident, and a frequent target organ is the spinal cord in man (26–28). A common manifestation of DCS in divers is evidence of spinal cord dysfunction usually at levels below the diaphragm (1,27). Symptoms include paraesthesias, muscle weakness, paralysis of the lower extremities, bowel or bladder incontinence, urinary retention, and sexual impotence. In massive cases of sudden ascent from deep depths (blowup) usually found in commercial diving exposures, a massive decompression sickness syndrome can occur with both cerebral and spinal neurological symptoms, unconsciousness, hypovolemic shock, pulmonary edema, and a high mortality rate (9,29).

A less serious type of DCS is manifest by minor pains in the extremities and joints (14,16,30). Symptoms of local joint pain are often confused with pain from injuries and the diagnosis of decompression sickness may be missed (Table II). In some populations a high incidence of aseptic bone necrosis is found in divers who have experienced decompression sickness of the joints in the distant past, or who have experienced deep, prolonged dives in commerical operations (31,32) and in Caisson workers (32). A rare but important symptom or decompression sickness is sudden acute neurological hearing loss or vestibular dysfunction. Decompression sickness of this type usually occurs from deep, prolonged commercial diving exposures, and if untreated, will result in permanent deafness.

TREATMENT OF DECOMPRESSION SICKNESS

It is not the intent in this chapter to detail the treatment of DCS. This therapy requires extensive knowledge of the use of hyperbaric chambers and hyperbaric

TABLE II

Frequency of Decompression Sickness Symptoms in
100 Cases[a]

Symptom	Percentage of all DCS Symptoms
Skin itch	4
Headache	11
Fatigue/malaise	13
Bone/joint pain	54
Spinal/back pain	11
Spinal/neurological	22
Respiratory	21

[a] From Edmonds et al. (11).

oxygen for therapy (1,14,33), and is usually relegated to specialists in diving and hyperbaric medicine. It is of utmost importance to understand that an individual complaining of any joint pain syndrome or neurological abnormality following a diving exposure requires consultation with a diving medicine expert and recompression treatment in a hyperbaric chamber. Symptoms of DCS may appear up to 24 hours following exposure (Table III). Many tragic mistreatments have resulted in permanent brain and spinal cord injury or death because of misdiagnosis by uninformed physicians. This occurrence is unfortunate since information and advice about diving accidents are available from several sources by telephone.* Since there are only a few centers in the United States which can provide expert consultation in this area, it is wise to learn of the treatment facilities available in specific regions of the United States and other countries. Persons suspected of having a diving related accident involving neurological abnormalities should not be retained in a hospital without hyperbaric treatment facilities since prolonging the delay between onset of symptoms and recompression treatment increases the risk of permanent neurological injury (9,27).

Because the presence of bubbles in blood and tissues activates the inflammatory process (21,25,34,35) a number of adjunctive treatments with various drugs have been developed recently. Individuals with neurological DCS or arterial gas embolism will benefit from adequate fluid therapy to prevent hemoconcentration, use of intravenous steroids to inhibit cerebral or spinal cord edema, and antiplatelet agents to prevent platelet aggregation by bubble surfaces in the blood (21). In cases of massive DCS, disseminated intravascular coagulation develops

---

*At the present time, the National Oceanographic and Atmosphere Administration (NOAA) supports a nationwide emergency consultation system for diving accidents. This system is centered at the F. G. Hall Laboratory of Hyperbaric Medicine at Duke University Medical Center, Durham, North Carolina, and can be contacted by calling 919/684–8111.

TABLE III

Time of Onset of Decompression Sickness Following Diving[a]

Cummulative percentage	Time of onset
50	30 minutes
85	1 hour
95	3 hours
99	6 hours
100	12–24 hours

[a] From U.S. Navy Diving Manual (1).

(34) and anticoagulation may be useful (21,22,36). Individuals with permanent neurological injury from decompression sickness or air embolism often require physical therapy to regain normal or near normal musculoskeletal function. Unlike traumatic cord injury or stroke, neurological injury from decompression sickness or air embolism, when properly treated, often results in complete or nearly complete recovery of function.

It is sometimes difficult to distinguish between severe decompression sickness and cerebral air embolism. Indeed these two conditions may coexist when a diver who has been underwater for a prolonged period of time ascends rapidly and develops pulmonary barotrauma. Because treatment of both illnesses is similar, that is, recompression in a hyperbaric chamber, hyperbaric oxygen, and adjunctive drug therapy, it is less important to make a precise diagnosis and more important to institute therapy with recompression, hyperbaric oxygen, and pharmacologic agents. Decompression sickness usually develops sometime after diving. Symptoms may develop within minutes of ascent or may be late, appearing 12–24 hours after a dive has been completed. On the other hand, pulmonary barotrauma with arterial gas embolism occurs immediately upon ascending and often produces unconsciousness upon surfacing. Unattended individuals who become unconscious in this manner will commonly drown.

C. Inert Gas Narcosis

The third pressure effect that may result in serious problems in diving is inert gas narcosis (nitrogen narcosis). This syndrome results from breathing air at depths greater than 100 feet in seawater (37–39). The symptoms are similar to alcohol inebriation and can range from loss of fine motor control and high order mathematical skills to bizarre and inappropriate behavior, improper response to emotional stress, hostility, loss of coarse as well as fine motor control, and unconsciousness. Symptoms become increasingly evident as depth increases from 100 feet. At 200–250 feet, severe symptoms occur; at depths of 300–400 feet, unconsciousness occurs due to the general anesthetic effect of nitrogen at this depth. In deep commercial and military diving, helium replaces nitrogen as the inert gas, and narcosis does not occur. In sport scuba diving, depths of 200–250 feet are attainable but not recommended. The usual depth limit using scuba gear is 130 feet. Some individuals, however, are more susceptible to nitrogen narcosis than others and may manifest severe symptoms at 130–150 feet. Fatigue, heavy work, and cold water can augment the narcotic effects of nitrogen. Treatment requires removing the diver from the increased pressure environment. Symptoms disappear immediately upon surfacing and often there is amnesia for the events that occurred below. The greatest danger from nitrogen narcosis is to the scuba diver who insists on exceeding recommended depth limit. As depth increases, judgment and motor skills diminish, and more than one diver was last seen by his partner swimming downward beyond 200 feet with no evidence of distress, oblivious of the lethal consequences of his action. Narcotic effects of nitrogen are prevented by using helium–oxygen mixtures for breathing, or by adhering to safe depth limits. Oxyhelium mixtures are not readily available to sport divers but are commonly used in commercial diving below 150 feet. Thus, sport scuba divers should be instructed to limit diving depths to 130 feet to avoid narcosis. Persons found to be exceptionally susceptible to nitrogen narcosis must limit diving to shallower depths where no symptoms are evident.

IV. COMMON MEDICAL DISORDERS AND DIVING

Although sport scuba diving has become a popular pastime in the United States and other areas of the world, limitations must be imposed on patients with certain chronic illnesses because of adverse interaction with the diving environment. Disorders that produce sudden unexpected unconsciousness are contraindications to diving. These include epilepsy, insulin-dependent diabetes melitus, and recurrent cardiac arrhythmias. Individuals with these disorders place themselves and others at significant risk for lethal underwater accidents because of the possibility of unconsciousness deep underwater with inability to maintain adequate ventilation and loss of locomotion. Many multiple deaths have occurred when other divers attempt to assist an unconscious diver and inadvertently lose their own air supply and drown.

Another important diving problem is maintenance of airway patency. Inability to adequately empty all areas of the lungs can result in pulmonary barotrauma. Because asthma produces difficulty in normal lung emptying due to airway obstruction, it is possible for an individual with asthma to have focal airway obstruction and develop local pulmonary barotrauma and arterial gas embolism because of air trapping in segments of the lung, even though proper breathing technique is practiced on ascent. Asthmatics requiring treatment or who demonstrate bronchospasm on pulmonary examination should not dive. Many diving medicine specialists feel that individuals with an asthmatic history even in the remote past should not dive because of the demonstrated hypersensitivity of airways in these individuals. The diving environment requires breathing of cold dry air, with occasional water aspiration, and the possibility of heavy exercise and severe emotional stress. All these factors may enhance the possibility for acute bronchospasm underwater, the development of severe dyspnea, and expanded lung volume. Often panic follows the development of these symptoms and irrational behavior associated with panic underwater results in ultimate drowning. Because the asthmatic is at risk for pulmonary barotrauma and arterial gas embolism and because the environment is conducive to the development of bronchospasm underwater, it is generally recommended that individuals with symptomatic asthma, clinically detectable asymptomatic asthma, or individuals wih a recent past history of asthma who at present are asymptomatic without medical treatment should not dive.

A unique and interesting problem arises in individuals with atrial or ventricular septal defects of the heart who wish to dive. It has been shown in several studies that certain diving exposures, although producing no symptoms of decompression sickness, will produce small amounts of free gas in the venous system (silent bubbles) which become trapped in the lung and exhaled with no consequence (40–42). In individuals with atrial or ventricular septal defects, the possibility of paradoxical arterial embolism is present and these individuals should be advised not to dive. Another consideration for individuals with chronic illness who seek advice on diving, is the interaction of the exercise needed for diving, with the chronic illness. Thus, patients with symptomatic coronary disease, heart failure, chronic severe anemia, and other disorders that significantly limit exercise capacity or in which exercise can have adverse consequences should be advised not to dive. The diving environment is such that the need for sudden severe exercise is unpredictable, and safe diving dictates that individuals be in good physical condition and be able to withstand relatively high work loads for brief periods of time in order to avoid diving accidents. Inability to sustain moderately high levels of exercise due to chronic illness puts a diver at risk for serious injury or death and these individuals should be advised against diving.

Diving is also contraindicated in individuals with chronically perforated tympanic membranes, unilateral neurological deafness, previous history of spinal cord decompression sickness with residual neurological findings, in patients with history of spontaneous pnemothorax, with pulmonary cysts or blebs, or patients who have had significant chest surgery with scarring and deformity of the lung. Patients on drugs which significantly suppress sympathetic function such as β blockers, ganglionic blockers, and any other autonomic blocking antihypertensive agent, will have limited capacity for exercise; in these patients exercise capacity should be tested prior to undertaking diving. It is also advised that pregnant females avoid diving until completion of pregnancy (43). This advice is based on studies suggesting that inert gas kinetics in the fetus may be different than the mother and decompression sickness may occur in the developing fetus while the mother has no symptoms (43). In addition, the hyperbaric oxygen exposure associated with diving may cause tissue injury in the fetus (44–46). Because of these considerations, it is advisable for pregnant women to avoid diving until pregnancy and delivery are complete.

V. MARINE INJURIES

Many sport scuba divers pursue their sport in tropical waters where exposure to marine toxins and dangerous marine animals is possible. Injuries from marine life range from skin rashes secondary to contact with corals, sea nettles, jellyfish, and other invertebrates to injuries from large marine animals such as stingrays or moray eels, and contact with poisonous fish such as scorpion or lion fish. Divers may also be poisoned by various toxic marine organisms which are ingested as food.

Marine invertebrates of the Coelenterate family cause stings by depositing many small nematocysts on skin which makes contact with the marine organism (47). The resultant symptoms can include mild skin itch and burning (most jellyfish) severe erythema and vesicular eruptions with pain and intense itching (fire coral), systemic anaphalactic-like reactions with vascular collapse (Portugese man-of-war), and sudden, rapid respiratory failure and cardiac arrest (deadly sea wasp of Australia). Treatment of the cutaneous component of these reactions includes topical ammonia solution, alcohol, papain to destroy remaining nematocysts, use of topical steroids, and systemic antihistamines. Severe systemic reactions may require ventilatory support, treatment of shock, volume replacement, and systemic steroids.

Injuries from sea urchins cause deposition of broken spines in subcutaneous or deeper tissues. These spines are proteinaceous and delicate. Often efforts at surgical removal results in fragmentation of the embedded spine in the tissues. Surgical debridement, however, should be undertaken for deeply embedded spines. The usual result of penetration by these spines is a local inflammation. Superficial spines can be crushed by pummeling the area (47). If the injury is painful, local anesthesia should be given. The fragments will usually be absorbed in about 1 week.

Spines of stingrays can be driven deep into skin, and reports of penetration into bone are available (47). Treatment is surgical debridement and antibiotics.

Injury from large marine animals (sharks, moray eels) although extremely rare, should be treated surgically. These injuries always result in contaminated wounds, requiring careful debridement and antibiotic therapy.

Ingestion of poisonous or toxic marine animals produces several illnesses. Ciguatera poisoning is a common and serious intoxication resulting from ingestion of flesh of large tropical fish contaminated with the toxin. The toxin is common in the Caribbean, South Pacific, and Indian Ocean. Symptoms include paresthesias of lips, tongue, and extremities, nausea, vomiting, myalgia, and muscular weakness. More severe neurological disturbances may also occur. Mortality is thought to be 12% in fully developed cases (47). Symptoms may last for months to years. Treatment is supportive. Prevention requires knowledge of the safe edible fish in a given area, and is best determined by inquiring of people native to the area. Other disorders such as scombroid poisoning and paralytic shellfish poisoning, although potentially lethal, are usually less severe, and recovery occurs spontaneously. If ingestion of a marine poison is suspected or if early symptoms are noted, stomach evacuation or induced vomiting should be carried out as soon as possible. Careful observation of the victim is necessary since occasional severe poisoning will result in respiratory failure and require supportive therapy until recovery occurs. There is no definitive treatment for these marine intoxications.

Although injury, envenomation, or poisoning by marine animals is uncommon in most medical practice, the increase in travel to tropical areas of the world for vacation and recreation may result in an encounter with one of these illnesses anywhere in the world.

This brief review of diving medicine is intended to provide familiarization with the most common of the associated disorders. More detail can be found in texts on this topic (1,10,11,48–50) and recent advances are detailed in a recent symposium (51).

REFERENCES

1. "U.S. Navy Diving Manual" (1979). NAVSEA 0994-LP-001-9010. Navy Department, Washington, D.C. (distributed by Best Bookbinders, Carson, California).
2. Farmer, J. C. (1977). Diving injuries to the middle ear. *Ann. Otol., Rhinol., Laryngol.* **86,** suppl. 36, 1–20.
3. Fields, J. A. (1958). Skindiving, the physiological and otolaryngological aspects. *Arch. Otolaryngol.* **68,** 531–541.
4. Jarrett, A. S. (1961). Reversed ear syndrome and the mechanism of barotrauma. *Br. Med. J.* **2,** 483–486.
5. Campbell, P. A. (1944). Aerosinusitis—its cause, course, and treatment. *Ann. Otol. Rhinol. Laryngol.,* **53,** 291–301.
6. Fagan, P., McKenzie, B., and Edmonds, C. (1976). Sinus barotrauma in divers. *Ann. Otol., Rhinol., Laryngol.* **85,** 64–65.

7. Freeman, P., and Edmonds, C. (1972). Inner ear barotrauma. *Arch. Otolaryngol.* **95,** 556–563.
8. Schaeffer, K. E., McNulty, S. P., Carey, C. R., and Liebow, A. A. (1958). Mechanism in development of interstitial emphysema and air embolism on decompression from depth. *J. Appl. Physiol.* **13,** 15–29.
9. Davis, J. C. (1979). "Treatment of Serious Decompression Sickness and Arterial Gas Embolism," Publ. No. 34. Undersea Medical Society, Bethesda, Maryland.
10. Miles, S., and Mackay, D. E. (1976). "Underwater Medicine" Lippincott. Philadelphia, Pennsylvania.
11. Edmonds, C., Lowry, C., and Pennefather, J. (1981). "Diving and Subquatic Medicine." Diving Medical Center, Momsan, N.S.W. Australia.
12. Bove, A. A., Clark, J. M., Simon, A. J. and Lambertsen, C. J. (1982). Successful therapy of cerebral air embolism with hyperbaric oxygen at 2.8 ATA. *Undersea Biomed. Res.* **9,** 76–80.
13. Elliott, D. H., Hallenbeck, J. M., and Bove, A. A. (1974). Acute decompression sickness. *Lancet* **2,** 1193–1199.
14. Workman, R. D. (1968). Treatment of bends with oxygen at high pressure. *Aerosp. Med.* **39,** 1076–1083.
15. Edmonds, C., and Thomas, R. (1972). Medical aspects of diving. *Med. J. Aust.* **2,** 1300–1304.
16. Erde, A., and Edmonds, C. (1975). Decompression sickness: A clinical series. *J. Occup. Med.* **17,** 324–328.
17. Elliott, D. H., and Hallenbeck, J. M. (1975). The Pathophysiology of Decompression Sickness. *In* "The Physiology and Medicine of Diving and Compressed Air Work" (P. B. Bennett and D. H. Elliott, eds.), pp. 436–455. Williams & Wilkins, Baltimore, Maryland.
18. Bove, A. A., Hallenbeck, J. M., and Elliott, D. H. (1974). Circulatory responses to venous air embolism and decompression sickness in dogs. *Undersea Biomed Res.* **1,** 207–220.
19. Neuman, T. S. Spragg, R. G., Wagner, P. D., and Moser, K. M. (1980). Cardiopulmonary consequences of decompression sickness. *Respir. Physiol.* **41,** 143–155.
20. Bove, A. A., Hallenbeck, J. M., and Elliott, D. H. (1974). Changes in blood and plasma volume in dogs during decompression sickness. *Aerosp. Med.* **45,** 49–55.
21. Bove, A. A. (1982). The basis for drug therapy in decompression sickness. *Undersea Biomed. Res.* **9,** 91–112.
22. Philp, R. B. (1974). A review of blood changes associated with compression-decompression: Relationship to decompression sickness. *Undersea Biomed. Res.* **1,** 117–150.
23. Cockett, A. T. K., and Nakamura, R. M. (1964). A new concept in the treatment of decompression sickness. *Lancet* **1,** 1102–1103.
24. Barnard, E. E. P., Hanson, J. M., Rowtar-Lee, N. A., Morgan, A. G., Polak, A., and Tidy, D. R. (1966). Post decompression shock due to extravasation of plasma. *Br. Med. J.* **2,** 154–155.
25. Levin, L. L., Stewart, G. J., Lynch, P. R., and Bove, A. A. (1981). Blood and blood vessel wall changes induced by decompression sickness in dogs. *J. Appl. Physiol.* **50,** 944–949.
26. Hallenbeck, J. M., Bove, A. A., and Elliott, D. H. (1965). Mechanisms underlying spinal cord damage in decompression sickness. *Neurology* **25,** 308–316.
27. Nix, W. A., and Hope, H. C. (1980). Central nervous system damage after decompression accidents. *Dtsch. Med. Wochenschr.* **105,** 302–305.
28. Haymaker, W., and Johnson, A. D. (1955). Pathology of decompression sickness. *Mil. Med.* **117,** 285–306.
29. Norman, J. N., Childs, C. M., Jones, C., Smith, J. A. R., Ross, J., Riddle, G., MacIntosh, A., McKie, N. I. P., MacCauley, J. I., and Fructus, X. (1979). Management of a complex diving accident. *Undersea Biomed. Res.* **62,** 209–216.
30. Gelding, F. C., Griffiths, P. D., Hempleman, H. V., Paton, W. D. M., and Walder, D. N. (1960). Decompression sickness during construction of the dartford tunnel. *Br. J. Ind. Med.* **17,** 167–180.

31. Elliott, D. H. (1971). Decompression Inadequacy in Aseptic Bone Necrosis of Divers. *Proc. Roy. Soc. Med.* **64,** 1278–1280.
32. McCallum, R. I., and Walder, D. N. (1966). Bone lesions in compressed air workers. *J. Bone J. Surg., Br. Vol.* **48B,** 207–235.
33. Behnke, A. R., Shaw, L. A., Messer, A. C., Thompson, R. M., and Motley, E. P. (1936). The circulatory and respiratory disturbances of acute compressed air illness and the administration of oxygen as a therapeutic measure. *Am. J. Physiol.* **114,** 526–533.
34. Philp, R. B., Schacham, P., and Gowdey, C. W. (1971). Involvement of platelets and microthrombi in experimental decompression sickness: Similarities with disseminated intravascular coagulation. *Aerosp. Med.* **42,** 494–502.
35. Martin, K. J., and Nichols, G. (1972). Observations on platelet changes in man after simulated diving. *Aerosp. Med.* **43,** 827–830.
36. Reeves, F., and Workman, R. D. (1971). Use of heparin for the therapeutic/prophylactic treatment of decompression sickness. *Aerosp. Med.* **42,** 20–23.
37. Behnke, A. R., Thompson, R. M., and Motley, E. P. (1935). The psychologic effects from breathing air at 4 atmospheres pressure. *Am. J. Physiol.* **112,** 554–558.
38. Davis, F. M., Osborne, J. P., Baddele, A. D., and Graham, I. M. F. (1972). Diver performance, nitrogen narcosis and anxiety. *Aerosp. Med.* **43,** 1079–1082.
39. Ackles, K. N., and Fowler, B. (1971). Cortical evoked response and inert gas narcosis in man. *Aerosp. Med.* **43,** 1181–1184.
40. Spencer, M. P. (1976). Decompression limits for compressed air determined by ultrasonically detected blood bubbles. *J. Appl. Physiol.* **40,** 229–235.
41. Spencer, M. P., and Clarke, H. E. (1972). Precordial monitoring of pulmonary gas embolism and decompression bubbles. *Aerosp. Med.* **43,** 762–767.
42. Gardette, B. (1979). Correlation between decompression sickness and circulating bubbles in 232 divers. *Undersea Biomed Res.* **6,** 99–107.
43. Fife, W. P. (1980). "Effects of Diving on Pregnancy," Publ. No. 36. Undersea Medical Society, Bethesda, Maryland.
44. Clark, J. M. (1974). The toxicity of oxygen. *Am. Rev. Respir. Dis.* **10,** 40–50.
45. Assali, N. S., Kirschbaum, T. H., and Dilts, P. V. (1968). Effects of hyperbaric oxygen on uteroplacental and fetal circulation. *Circ. Res.* **22,** 573–588, 1968.
46. Ferm, V. H. (1964). Teratogenic effects of hyperbaric oxygen. *Proc. Soc. Exp. Biol. Med.* **116,** 975–976.
47. Halstead, B. W. (1980). "Dangerous Marine Animals." Cornell Maritime Press, Centreville, Maryland.
48. Strauss, R. H. (1976). "Diving Medicine." Grune & Stratton, New York.
49. Davis, J. C., and Hunt, T. K. (1978). "Hyperbaric Oxygen." Undersea Medical Society Press, Bethesda, Maryland.
50. Bennett, P. B., and Elliott, D. H. (1975). "The Physiology and Medicine of Diving and Compressed Air Work." Williams & Wilkins, Baltimore, Maryland.
51. Bachrach, A. J., and Matzen, M. M. (1981). "Underwater Physiology VII. Proceedings of the Seventh Symposium on Underwater Physiology." Undersea Medical Society, Bethesda, Maryland.

CHAPTER 19

Prescribing Exercise Programs

ALBERT M. PAOLONE

*Department of Physical
Education
Temple University
Philadelphia, Pennsylvania*

I. INTRODUCTION

The advice to a patient that, "you should get more exercise," although well intended, will likely go unheeded. Patients who are the least likely to follow such advice are those for whom an increase in physical activity is most necessary. However, if a physician wrote a prescription for exercise in the same way that he would write a prescription for medication or some other therapeutic intervention, then the likelihood of compliance would be increased.

The case for the judicious use of physical exercise as a preventive, interventive, and rehabilitative medical therapy is strong and seems to be increasing in strength as more scientific literature is published concerning the relationship between increased physical activity and reduced risk of coronary heart disease

Exercise Medicine: Physiological Principles
and Clinical Applications

(CHD). Two thousand years ago Hipprocrates said "exercise strengthens; while inactivity wastes." It is likely that people believed him even though he had little or no hard evidence to support his claim. Scientific support for this belief began with epidemiological studies in the early 1950s by Morris and associates (15) who documented a lower incidence of myocardial infarction (MI), quicker recover from MI, and fewer deaths from all causes in the more physically active conductors than among the drivers of the buses in the London transit system. Since these early reports many better controlled studies (4,9,10,16–18,25) have corroborated the findings of Morris *et al.* (15). Although a causal relationship has not been established between exercise and prevention of coronary heart disease, strides have been made from purely statistical evidence toward a cause and effect tie. Recently, the first evidence of beneficial effects of exercise in preventing CHD in primates has appeared in the scientific literature (12). In this study two groups of monkeys were fed atherogenic diets. One group was exercised and the other was not. Coronary artery narrowing and sudden death were observed only in the nonexercised monkeys. Exercise was associated with substantially reduced atherosclerosis, larger hearts, and wider coronary arteries, thus reducing the degree of luminal narrowing.

Evidence also exists that some risk factors commonly associated with increased incidence of coronary heart disease can be favorably affected by exercise. Thus, the strategy of intervening with an exercise regimen to reduce blood pressure (2,3,19), improve the blood lipid profile (6,8,13,14), reduce body weight (3,19), and perhaps ameliorate the deleterious effects of emotional stress (2) seems worthwhile.

The rehabilitative benefits of regular exercise for post MI and post coronary bypass surgery patients have been well documented and include improved functional capacity (23,24), deterred depression, (11), perhaps a reduced risk of subsequent infarction (20–22), and enhanced collateral coronary circulation (5).

The advice from most proponents of regular exercise including the American Heart Association and the American College of Sports Medicine usually includes a recommendation to see a physician before undertaking a program of vigorous exercise.

If the physician finds no contraindications to vigorous exercise after medical screening, then the consultation should provide an exercise prescription for the patient. The prescription must address a recommended type of exercise, an intensity level at which to train, a recommendation concerning frequency of training, and a prescribed duration for each training session. The prescription must also include some provision for a return visit to follow up the initial recommendations with an evaluation of progress and modification of the prescription.

In the absence of this prescriptive response by the physician to the patient who seeks exercise advice, the patient's perception of how to exercise is vague.

Inadequate and perhaps unsafe exercise experience will follow, with very little likelihood of continued compliance.

II.   MEDICAL SCREENING

Before writing the prescription for exercise the physician must make the decision concerning the degree of medical screening necessary for the patient.

According to the American College of Sports Medicine (ACSM) guidelines (1), if an individual is asymptomatic, less than 35 years of age, has no evidence or history of cardiovascular disease, is without risk factors for CHD, and has had a medical evaluation during the previous year, no medical clearance is necessary prior to an increase in physical activity level. Furthermore, a person of any age with the same characteristics who is habitually active may alter his activity habits without medical clearance, but should seek advice from a knowledgeable physician or exercise specialist. These persons may have an exercise stress test administered by a technician for the purpose of determining exercise capacity and the writing of an exercise prescription.

Previously sedentary individuals who are 35 years and older, those with risk factors for CHD (cigarette smoking, hypertension, EKG abnormalities, or hyperlipidemia), known disease, and/or symptoms should have a complete medical evaluation and exercise stress test prior to a significant increase in physical activity level. Symptomatic patients with a recent change in disease status must be treated with caution, and a physician should be involved in the stress test and exercise prescription.

A.   Evaluation for Medical Clearance

The evaluation for medical clearance should include:

1. A comprehensive medical history including family history, personal medial history, and current health habits. Special emphasis should be placed on history of chest pain, arrhythmia, and other forms of cardiovascular disease.
2. A physical examination with special emphasis on identifying health problems that would be contraindications to exercise or exercise testing, including orthopedic or neurological considerations.
3. Evaluation of resting blood pressure.
4. Laboratory studies including a blood chemistry screen plus hematology, urinalysis, and pulmonary function if lung disease is suspected.
5. A resting 12 lead electrocardiogram.
6. An exercise stress test.

The physical examination and laboratory studies should be obtained within 1 month of the exercise test. Physician approval for the exercise test should be secured and the test should be administered according to the following procedures and meet the stated specifications:

1. An immediate pretest history should be taken which focuses on recent symptoms and current medication. This is in addition to the comprehensive history taken earlier.
2. It is most convenient to record the resting 12 lead EKG at this time in physician supervised tests. (The resting tracing should be read prior to beginning of the test.)
3. The EKG lead system that is to be monitored during the test should be recorded at base line in both the test posture and the recovery posture.
4. Pretest blood pressure should be recorded in both the test posture and the recovery posture.
5. The target end point of the test should be volitional exhaustion (maximum test) or at least 90% of age predicted maximum heart rate. Of course the test may be terminated at any time for abnormal findings.
6. Each test stage should be 3 minutes in duration so that a measure of steady state heart rate is obtained at the various work levels.
7. Blood pressure and EKG should also be recorded at every test stage. The EKG should be continuously monitored.
8. Heart rate, blood pressure, and EKG should be monitored and recorded each minute during recovery until all measures are stable (9 minutes is sufficient in most cases).

A critical part of the screening procedures is the interpretation of the exercise electrocardiogram as positive or negative for ischemic heart disease. In most cases persons found to have an ischemic response will be excluded from participation or at least be placed on a conservative regimen.

B. The Exercise Stress Test

An exercise stress test that meets the criteria stated above is an essential tool in guiding the development of a proper exercise prescription. The use of the procedure in the diagnosis of CHD has come under some degree of criticism because of its low predictive accuracy, particularly in an asymptomatic test population. However, the value of the stress test extends far beyond the presence or absence of ischemic S-T or T-wave changes and includes evaluation of the

1. Exercise capacity of the patient.
2. Appropriateness of the heart rate and blood pressure response to graded exercise.
3. Presence or absence of exercise induced arrhythmias.

4. Peripheral vascular response to exercise.
5. Pulmonary response to exercise.
6. Subjective response of the patient to graded and intense exercise.

In instances where the stress test is not administered or supervised by the physician who will be advising the patient concerning the exercise regimen, the thoroughness of the laboratory report is critical. A complete exercise stress test laboratory report must include the:

1. Preexercise heart rate and blood pressure in both the exercise posture and the recovery posture.
2. Maximum exercise level achieved and the energy cost of the maximum work load.
3. Heart rate and blood pressure at each stage of the test.
4. Heart rate and blood pressure during recovery (at least every other minute).
5. Any EKG abnormalities noted on the preexercise recording, at any test stage and during recovery.
6. Any symptoms and the test stage at which they appeared.
7. Reason for termination of the test, e.g.,
   a. Target achieved
   b. Symptoms
   c. Volitional exhaustion
   d. EKG findings
8. Test interpretation as positive or negative for ischemia.

The complete data base provided to the physician by the recommended screening procedures must be utilized to advise the patient concerning a safe and appropriate exercise regimen. The medical history and physical examination will help to identify limiting conditions, which may contraindicate certain types of exercise, whereas the personal history will identify risk factors that may be amenable to modification by exercise. The exercise history will guide the physician in recommending a type of exercise with which the patient has prior experience and competence.

An essential element of the stress test report for use in writing of the exercise prescription is the energy cost of the highest work load completed by the patient, as well as the energy cost of each stage of the test. This information will allow an appropriate exercise intensity to be recommended which can be implemented using any of a variety of exercise modalities.

III. QUANTIFYING ENERGY COST

The energy cost of exercise may be quantified in a number of ways and related to the exercise rate during the various stages of the exercise stress test. If the test modality is bicycle ergometry the work rate is measured in kilopond meters per minute (KPM/minute) or in watts (joules/minute); if the test is performed on a treadmill the work rate is measured in speed and percent grade. However, the energy cost for the patient of each test stage may be quantified in terms of the oxygen cost in liters per minute, milliliters per kilogram of body weight per minute, or the caloric cost of the work in kilocalories. The oxygen cost of each exercise level may be represented as multiples of the cost of sitting at rest, known as metabolic equivalents (METs). One MET equals approximately 3.5 ml/kg/minute of oxygen consumed, the cost of sitting at rest, with higher work levels represented in multiples of this value. For example, the oxygen consumption of work costing 10 METs would be approximately 35 ml/kg/minute.

Since MET values reflect the energy cost per unit of body weight and the absolute cost of treadmill work varies with body size, the MET cost of a given speed and grade of treadmill work will be the same for all body weights. For example, the absolute oxygen cost of walking at 3 miles per hour up a 5% grade will be about 1890 ml/minute for a 100-kg person and 945 ml/minute for a 50-kg person, but the ml/kg/minute will be the same at 18.9, which equals 5.4 METs. Bicycle ergometry, however, does not involve moving one's body weight but rather moving the wheel a given distance against a resistance load over time. The external work done will be the same for all body sizes and so the absolute oxygen cost will also be the same. The relative energy cost then must be corrected for body size. For example, the absolute oxygen cost of bicycle work at 300 KPM/minute is approximately 900 ml (600 ml to do the external work plus the 300 ml cost of sitting rest). This O_2 cost represents 18 ml/kg/minute or 5.1 METs for a person weighing 50 kg but only 9 ml/kg/minute or 2.6 METs for the person weighing 100 kg.

The MET values of different exercise rates are based on the oxygen consumed at any given rate. However, O_2 consumption is often not measured during the stress test so the MET cost of the test stages must be estimated. One source for making these estimations is provided by the ACSM (1).

IV. THE EXERCISE PRESCRIPTION

Four factors must be considered in the exercise prescription: (1) the *type* of exercise to be recommended, (2) the *frequency* of training sessions, (3) the *duration* of each session, and (4) the *intensity* of the work level.

The information base provided by the medical screening concerning age, health status (risk factors and symptomatology), current state of conditioning and functional capacity, and physical activity interests and skills will form the basis for the prescription.

A. INTENSITY

The first issue addressed should concern the intensity of effort that is safe and appropriate for achieving beneficial effects of exercise. In prescribing a given intensity of effort two factors are considered: the peak level of effort that should not be exceeded and the average level for each exercise session, not including warm-up and cool-down phases. Both the peak and average intensity levels must be based on the functional capacity of the patient as determined by the exercise stress test. Functional capacity is the value in METs or the oxygen consumption for the highest exercise intensity level completed (1) on a maximal stress test. A maximal stress test is a test in which the predetermined end point is either maximal oxygen consumption ($\dot{V}O_2$ max), maximum heart rate, or volitional exhaustion.

When some percentage of age predicted maximum heart rate is the pre-determined end point the functional capacity can be extrapolated from the last work stage completed. For example, if the predicted maximal heart rate is 200 beats per minute (BPM) and the test target heart rate of 90% of 200 BPM is achieved at a work load of 8 METs, then the max functional capacity may be estimated from the equation: 8 METS = 90% of maximal functional capacity; or 8/.90 = maximal functional capacity in METs. The extrapolation to maximal functional capacity is only appropriate for healthy, asymptomatic patients with no significant risk factors and an uneventful test. The peak exercise intensity level prescribed, however, should not exceed the work level actually achieved on the exercise test. If the exercise test is terminated early because of some abnormal finding or response then the functional capacity of the patient is the last work level completed.

The peak intensity level prescribed should be 90% of the functional capacity in METs and the average intensity level for the exercise session should be 60–70% of functional capacity. The average level may be increased to 80% of functional capacity after 3 months of uneventful and uninterrupted training.

For persons with initially low functional capacities (5 METs or lower) who may not be able to sustain physical effort at the prescribed level for a sufficient duration, a sliding scale (1) can be used to determine the average exercise intensity. The scale uses 60% as a base to which is added the functional capacity in METs to arrive at the training percentage. If the functional capacity is 5 METs then the average exercise intensity will be 60% + 5 or 65% of functional capacity. The sliding scale allows the average intensity to be weighted for the relative functional capacity or exercise tolerance of the patient. The peak will remain at 90%. The average intensity does not necessarily have to be achieved by continuous steady-state work but may be achieved by an interval schedule, so that in order to exercise at an average intensity level of 6 METs an equal amount of time may be spent doing work costing 5 METs and 7 METs for an average of 6 METs. The peak level, however, should not be exceeded.

The MET prescription should be controlled and monitored by the heart rate response to the prescribed work level. The expected heart rate for the prescribed MET cost can be determined by plotting the heart rate for each stage of the exercise test against the MET cost of the stage (Fig. 1). The expected heart rate of the patient for work at any percentage of the functional capacity in METs may then be read from the plotted graph. The prescription will provide the value in METs of 70 and 90% of the functional capacity (representing average and peak training intensities, respectively) and the heart rate corresponding to these levels. For persons with low functional capacity the sliding scale may be used for determination of the average level. The prescribed intensity levels can be easily monitored by taking the pulse for 10 or 15 seconds immediately after an exercise bout and multiplying by 6 or 4 for a conversion to a minute rate.

When the proper MET levels for the patient are determined from the exercise test data these values may then be translated into actual work levels utilizing a variety of exercise modalities, e.g., cycling ergometry, walking, jogging, running, graded treadmill walking or running, outdoor cycling, skiing, and recreational sports and games. Tables of approximate metabolic cost of a variety of activities have been developed (Table I) for this purpose. The heart rate targets which correspond to the MET levels prescribed represent a control for factors which may alter the energy cost of a given activity, such as variations in terrain,

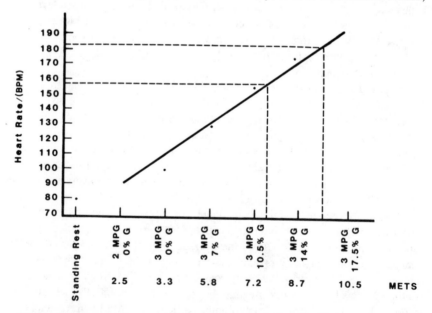

Fig. 1. Heart rate response (BPM) plotted against the MET cost of stages of exercise stress test. Functional capacity, 10.5 METs; average intensity, 7.4 METs, heart rate, 158 BPM; peak intensity, 9.5 METs, heart rate, 182 BPM.

TABLE I

Approximate Metabolic Cost of Activities[a]

	Occupational	Recreational
1½–2 METs[b] 4–7 ml O$_2$/min/kg 2–2½ kcal/min (70-kg person)	Desk work Auto driving[c] Typing Electric calculating machine operation	Standing Walking (strolling 1.6 km or 1 mile/hr) Flying[c], motorcycling[c] Playing cards[c] Sewing, knitting
2–3 METs 7–11 ml O$_2$/min/kg 2½–4 kcal/min (70-kg person)	Auto repair Radio, TV repair Janitorial work Typing, manual Bartending	Level walking (3.2 km or 2 miles/hr) Level bicycling (8.0 km or 5 miles/hr) Riding lawn mower Billiards, bowling Skeet,[c] shuffleboard Woodworking (light) Powerboat driving[c] Golf (power cart) Canoeing (4 km or 2½ miles/hr) Horseback riding (walk) Playing piano and many musical instruments
3–4 METs 11–14 ml O$_2$/min/kg 4–5 kcal/min (70-kg person)	Brick laying, plastering Wheelbarrow (45.4 kg or 100 lb load) Machine assembly Trailer-truck in traffic Welding (moderate load) Cleaning windows	Walking (4.8 km or 3 miles/hr) Cycling (9.7 km or 6 miles/hr) Horseshoe pitching Volleyball (6-man noncompetitive) Golf (pulling bag cart) Archery Sailing (handling small boat) Fly fishing (standing with waders) Horseback (sitting to trot) Badminton (social doubles) Pushing light power mower Energetic musician
4–5 METs 14–18 ml O$_2$/min/kg 5–6 kcal/min (70-kg person)	Painting, masonry Paperhanging Light carpentry	Walking (5.6 km or 3½ miles/hr) Cycling (12.9 km or 8 miles/hr) Table tennis Golf (carrying clubs)

(continued)

TABLE I (*Continued*)

	Occupational	Recreational
		Dancing (foxtrot)
		Badminton (singles)
		Tennis (doubles)
		Raking leaves
		Hoeing
		Many calisthenics
5–6 METs 18–21 ml O_2/min/kg 6–7 kcal/min (70-kg person)	Digging garden Shoveling light earth	Walking (6.4 km or 4 miles/hr) Cycling (16.1 km or 10 miles/hr) Canoeing (6.4 km or 4 miles/hr) Horseback ("posting" to trot) Stream fishing (walking in light current in waders) Ice or roller skating (14.5 km or 9 miles/hr)
6–7 METs 21–25 ml O_2/min/kg 7–8 kcal/min (70-kg person)	Shoveling 10/min (4.5 kg or 10 lb)	Walking (8.0 km or 5 miles/hr) Cycling (17.7 km or 11 miles/hr) Badminton (competitive) Tennis (singles) Splitting wood Snow shoveling Hand lawn mowing Folk (square) dancing Light downhill skiing Ski touring (4.0 km or 2½ miles/hr) (loose snow) Water skiing
7–8 METS 25–28 ml O_2/min/kg 8–10 kcal/min (70-kg person)	Digging ditches Carrying 36.3 kg or 80 lb Sawing hardwood	Jogging (8.0 km or 5 miles/hr) Cycling (19.3 km or 12 miles/hr) Horseback (gallop) Vigorous downhill skiing Basketball Mountain climbing Ice hockey Canoeing (8.0 km or 5 miles/hr) Touch football Paddleball

(*continued*)

TABLE I (*Continued*)

	Occupational	Recreational
8–9 METs 28–32 ml O$_2$/min/kg 10–11 kcal/min (70-kg person)	Shoveling 10/min (6.4 kg or 14 lb)	Running (8.9 km or 5½ miles/hr) Cycling (20.9 km or 13 miles/hr) Ski touring (6.4 km or 4 miles/hr) (loose snow) Squash racquets (social) Handball (social) Fencing Basketball (vigorous)
10 plus METs 32 plus ml O$_2$/min/kg 11 plus kcal/min (70 kg person)	Shoveling 10/min (7.3 kg or 16 lb)	Running: 6 mph = 10 METs 7 mph = 11½ METs 8 mph = 13½ METs 9 mph = 15 METs 10 mph = 17 METs Ski touring (8 + km or 5 + miles/hr) (loose snow) Handball (competitive) Squash (competitive)

[a] Reprinted from S.M. Fox, J. P. Naughton, and P. A. Gorman, (1972). Physical activity and cardiovascular health. III. The exercise prescription; frequency and type of activity. *Mod. Concepts Cardiovasc. Dis.* **41**:6. Includes resting metabolic needs.

[b] 1 MET is the energy expenditure at rest, equivalent to approximately 3.5 ml O$_2$/kg body weight/minute.

[c] A major excess metabolic increase may occur due to excitement, anxiety, or impatience in some of these activities, and a physician must assess his patient's psychological reactivity.

temperature and humidity, wind, clothing worn, altitude, and differences in individual efficiency in performing the exercise tasks.

The patient's heart rate response, if maintained at the proper level corresponding to the prescribed percentage of functional capacity as determined from the graph, will ensure that the prescribed energy expenditure is achieved regardless of the intervening factors listed above. Furthermore, variations in the patient's sleeping and eating habits, emotional state, and general state of health will be reflected in the heart rate response and, therefore, will be accounted for.

Alternative methods of prescribing intensity by heart rate alone, utilizing straight percentages of the actual or age predicted maximal rate, are much less satisfactory. A straight percentage of maximum heart rate, or of the heart rate at functional capacity, will not correspond to the heart rate at the same percentage of functional capacity in METs. In Case Study 1, for example, the heart rate at

70% of functional capacity in METs (7.2 METs) is 157 BPM. If 70% of the maximal heart rate were utilized, the heart rate prescription would be 70% of 190 BPM or 133 BPM. Data from Hellerstein *et al.* (7) indicate that a given percentage of maximum heart rate does not correspond to the same percentage of maximal oxygen consumption. The relationship is very close at work loads approching maximum but deviates considerably from a perfect relationship at lower work loads. For this reason prescribing intensity on the basis of a percentage of maximum heart rate will usually result in an intensity level well below the desired intensity in METs. It is also very difficult to measure true maximal heart rate, and age predicted values suffer from a wide range of error.

An acceptable method of prescribing intensity by heart rate is to determine the average heart rate to be achieved during conditioning by multiplying the range between the resting rate and the maximum rate by the same percentage used to determine the exercise intensity in METs and then adding the product to the resting rate.

For example:

Maximum heart rate (BPM)	= 190
Resting heart rate =	−60
Range	= 130
Conditioning intensity = 70%	× .70
	91
Resting heart rate	+ 60
Average training heart rate	= 151

The case studies presented later will serve to exemplify the use of exercise stress test data to determine the appropriate exercise intensity component of the exercise prescription.

B. Duration

Each exercise session must include a warm-up phase, a training stimulus phase, and a cool-down phase. The warm-up should last from 5–8 minutes— longer for older persons and persons with low functional capacities—and should involve stretching and flexibility exercises as well as mild rhythmic, large muscle group activities. This latter warm-up activity will elicit a gradual rise in oxygen consumption and elevate the heart rate toward the desired training stimulus level. The cool-down phase represents a tapering off period which allows the body systems to return gradually to the preexercise state. The patient should remain mildly active during this period which should last from 5 to 10 minutes for unconditioned individuals and can be shorter for highly fit people in whom recovery will be accelerated. The mild activity during the cool-down period prevents pooling of blood in the active tissues and maintains venous return and cardiac output at an acceptable level until peripheral vascular beds close down, thus preventing a precipitious drop in mean arterial blood pressure. The cool down activity should continue until heart rate has returned to below 100 BPM.

The training stimulus phase of the exercise session is the period during which energy output is elevated to the target range of 70–90% of functional capacity. The duration of this phase of the session is inversely related to the intensity of the effort. The training effect is a function of the interaction of intensity and duration. Normally, the higher the intensity level, the shorter the duration necessary to elicit beneficial changes in exercise capacity. In the first few weeks of training with intensity levels of 60–70% of functional capacity, duration should be 15–30 minutes. If a normal response is observed with no complications, the duration should then be increased to as much as 45 minutes. Duration must be increased to the desired length before changes in intensity level are recommended. The interaction of intenstiy and duration, if appropriately manipulated, should allow the patient to recover completely within 1 hour after an exercise session.

Patients with low functional capacity and thus low exercise tolerance as well as patients with exertional angina may be limited to training stimulus periods as short as 5–10 minutes, whereas patients with weight control problems should exercise for longer durations (45–60 minutes) with low initial intensity levels. Exercise of long duration can make a significant contribution to control of body weight by maintaining energy output at elevated levels for several hours per week.

C. Frequency

The frequency of exercise sessions for most patients should be three to four times per week with an alternate day schedule being most acceptable. For persons with low functional capacity (below 5 METs) who will have difficulty maintaining the prescribed intensity level for an acceptable duration, daily sessions with 10–15-minute training stimulus periods should be recommended. Patients with exertional angina, patients recovering from myocardial infarction, and coronary bypass surgery patients may be limited to 5-minute training stimulus periods and, therefore, should exercise several times per day. When the exercise tolerance of these patients is increased so that longer durations of effort are tolerated, frequency may be reduced.

Patients with weight control problems should exercise 5–7 days per week at intensity levels that can be maintained for 45–60 minutes. Seven hours per week of exercise costing 3 METs can result in significant weight loss over the course of 1 year with no reduction in caloric intake. A person weighing 100 kg (220 lb) walking at 3 mph will utilize oxygen at 1.05 liters/minute, a rate equivalent to approximately 5 kcal/minute. If this work rate is maintained for 1 hour per day, 2100 kcal/week or 109,200 kcal/year will be utilized. At 3500 kcal per pound of body fat this amount of exercise will result in a 31.2 pound weight loss. This calculation does not include the additional energy cost of the elevation in metabolism for a period of time after each exercise session which is difficult to estimate but may add considerably to the cost of the exercise alone.

D. Type of Exercise

The type of activity should be prescribed on the basis of specific conditions or limitations of the patient (orthopedic problems, elevated blood pressure, obesity, etc.), the availability of specialized equipment, and the patient's particular interests. The activity chosen, however, should use large muscle groups, be rhythmical and aerobic in nature and be capable of being sustained for 15–60 minutes. Suggested activities include walking, jogging, running, swimming, bicycling, rowing, cross-country skiing, and various endurance game-type activities (basketball, racquetball, tennis, soccer). The overriding consideration in the selection of a type of exercise is improvement of cardiorespiratory endurance with muscular strength and endurance as a secondary objective.

The initial exercise prescription should specify an exercise modality, the intensity of which can be easily controlled and maintained. The work rate of such activities as walking, jogging–running, and cycling can be easily prescribed in terms of distance per unit time and there will be little individual variability in the energy cost in METs. This type of activity will allow the uninitiated exerciser to control the effort level, and experience a level of consistency in physiological response. This consistency in level of exertion that the patient learns to expect in response to a given work rate can then be transferred to other activities, the energy cost of which are not so readily prescribed. Activities such as aerobic dancing, sports, and recreational games are desirable because of the enjoyment provided and the resultant motivation to continue regular exercise habits. This type of activity should not be prescribed, however, until the patient's sense of proper level of exertion is developed enough to avoid overexertion as a result of emotional involvement in the competitive nature of the activity.

Many leisure and occupational tasks require lifting or holding a constant load. Since the strain induced and the pressor response elicited appear to be functions of the percentage of maximum voluntary force exerted, the enhancement of muscular strength and endurance will allow the patient to perform these tasks with less strain and elevation of blood pressure. The work of the heart is determined to a great extent by the afterload (arterial pressure) against which it is working, and thus there is clearly a need to avoid high loads on small isolated groups in conditioning programs for adults where high cardiac work loads are undesirable.

Muscular strengthening activities when included should involve dynamic low tension, high repetition activities. Prolonged static holds or repetitious high tension movements of a total body straining type such as water skiing, wrestling, heavy digging, or snow shoveling should be avoided, particularly for patients with reduced cardiac function.

Flexibility activities can also be of value in reducing the incidence of low back syndrome and should be incorporated as a part of the warm-up phase of each exercise session. Static stretching of the low back and hamstrings are the most important flexibility activities and should be done after a mild rhythmic warm-up of large muscle groups as in slow running in place, slow jogging, or moderate paced walking.

E. Case Study Examples

The following case studies will serve to exemplify the use of exercise stress test data in writing an exercise prescription (cases 1, 2, and 3). Case 1 represents a maximal test with a predetermined end point of volitional exhaustion; case 2, a test terminated early because of a hypertensive response to exercise; case 3, a test terminated early because of cardiac symptoms and abnormal EKG findings. In all three cases functional capacity of the patient represents the MET cost of the last test stage completed. Prescriptions for each patient are presented along with the stress test data, and are based on the relationship between heart rate and MET cost of the various test stages (see Fig. 1).

The patients in cases 2 and 3 should be in professionally supervised programs at least for the first 6 months of their exercise experience at which time effects of the program should be reevaluated by a follow-up exercise stress test. The patient in case 1 could also benefit initially from participation in a supervised program until he learns to monitor his work intensity and develops a sense of perceived exertion.

The patient in case 1 should be referred to a community preventive program whereas the patients in cases 2 and 3 should be referred to a more strictly controlled interventive program. The characteristics of these types of programs along with a description of a cardiac rehabilitation program follow. In some cases there may be overlap between the preventive and interventive programs and between the rehabilitative and interventive programs.

Case 1

An asymptomatic, 35-year-old male with no significant risk factors for coronary heart disease, and a previously sedentary lifestyle, has the following response to a treadmill exercise stress test. Physical examination is normal. Body weight = 60 kg.

METs		HR	BP	EKG	Symptoms
	Standing rest	80	126/78	___	_____
2.5	2 MPH/0% G	90	120/80	___	_____
3.3	3 MPH/0% G	100	120/80	___	_____

5.8	3 MPH/7.0% G	130	140/70	_____	_____
7.2	3 MPH/10.5% G	155	160/65	_____	_____
8.7	3 MPH/14% G	175	180/60	_____	_____
10.5	3 MPH/17.5% G	190	200/60	_____	_____

Test terminated because of volitional exhaustion
Functional capacity = 10.5 METs at a heart rate of 190 beats/minute.
EKG negative for ischemia.

Exercise Prescription.
Intensity (see calculations at end of case)
  Peak = 9.5 METs, HR = 182
  Average = 7.4 METs, HR = 158
Duration: 15–30 minutes, training stimulus phase only
Frequency: 3–4 days per week on an alternate day schedule
Type: rhythmic large muscle group activities, e.g., jogging, stationary cycling,
  outdoor cycling
Work rate: Jogging, 5 mph
  Stationary cycling, 600 KPM/minute
  Outdoor cycling, 12 mph
Progression: after 4–6 weeks of uneventful activity, recreational games may be
  incorporated, e.g., singles tennis, basketball, and soccer, and the MET cost of
  the work must be increased to maintain initial average training heart rate.
Objectives: to increase functional capacity.
Calculation of prescribed intensity
  Peak = 90% of functional capacity (0.90 × 10.5 METs = 9.5 METs). The
  heart rate corresponding to 9.5 METs is calculated by interpolation between
  the rates at 8.7 and 10.5 METs using the following formula.
$$(9.5 - 8.7)/(10.5 - 8.7) = 0.44$$
$$0.44(190-175) = 6.6 + 175 = 181.6$$
  Average = 70% of functional capacity (0.70 × 10.5 METs = 7.4 METs).
  Calculation of corresponding heart rate:
$$(7.4 - 7.2)/(8.7 - 7.2) = 0.13$$
$$0.13(175 - 155) = 2.6 + 155 = 157.6$$

Case 2

An obese, 45-year-old male who smokes 1.5 packs of cigarettes per day, has
the following exercise stress test (treadmill) response. Physical examination is
otherwise normal. Body weight = 100 kg.

METs		HR	BP	EKG	Symptoms
	Standing rest	88	160/90	_____	_____
2.5	2 MPH/0% G	95	160/90	_____	_____
4.3	3 MPH/2.5% G	110	165/96	_____	_____

5.4	3 MPH/5.0% G	135	180/100	_____	_____
6.4	3 MPH/7.5% G	155	250/110	0.05 mV	_____
				S-T seg.	
				dep.,	
				0.08	
				seconds	

Test terminated because of systolic blood pressure of 250 mm Hg.
Functional capacity = 6.4 METs at a heart rate of 155 beats/min
EKG negative for ischemia.

Exercise Prescription
Intensity (see calculations at end of case)
  Peak = 5.8 METs, HR = 143
  Average = 4.2 METs, HR = 109 (66% of functional capacity)
Duration: 30–45 minutes
Frequency: 5–7 days per week
Type: rhythmic large muscle group activities controlled on ergometric devices
  (treadmill or cycle ergometer)
Work rate: 3 mph, 2.5% grade on treadmill, 600 KPM/minute on cycle ergome-
  ter.
Progression: after 4–6 weeks of uneventful activity the duration will be increased
  to maintain the initial average training heart rate.
Objectives: (a) to increase body caloric expenditure, for weight reduction.
        (b) to increase functional capacity.
        (c) to reduce resting blood pressure.
Calculation of prescribed intensity:
  Peak = 90% of functional capacity (0.90×6.4 METs = 5.8 METs). The
    heart rate corresponding to 5.8 METs is calculated by interpolation between
    the rates at 5.4 and 6.4 METs using the formula:
$$(5.8 - 5.4)/(6.4 - 5.4) = 0.40$$
$$0.40(155 - 135) = 8 + 135 = 143$$
  Average = 66% of functional capacity (0.66×6.4 METs = 4.2 METs).
    Calculation of corresponding heart rate:
$$(4.2 - 2.5)/(4.3 - 2.5) = 0.94$$
$$0.94 (110 - 95) = 14.1 + 95 = 109.1$$

Case 3

An asymptomatic 48-year-old male who smokes 1 pack of cigarettes per day,
has a positive family history for coronary heart disease and has the following
response to a treadmill exercise stress test. Subsequent coronary angiogram
shows single vessel coronary disease. Body weight = 76 kg.

METs		HR	BP	EKG	Symptoms
	Standing rest	75	140/100		
2.5	2 MPH/0% G	80	135/90		
3.3	3 MPH/0% G	88	135/90		
5.8	3 MPH/7.0% G	120	140/90	.1 mV S-T seg. dep., 0.08 seconds	Slight dyspnea
7.2	3 MPH/10.5% G	150	185/100	couplet of PVCs, 0.15 mV S-T seg. dep., 0.08 seconds	Severe dyspnea

Test terminated because of couplet of PVCs and dyspnea.
Functional capacity = 7.2 METs at a heart rate of 150 beats/minute.
EKG positive for ischemia.

Exercise Prescription
Intensity (see calculations at end of case)
    Peak = 6.5 METs, HR = 135
    Average = 4.8 METS, HR = 107 (67% of functional capacity)
Duration: 15–20 minutes
Frequency: 4–5 times per week
Type: rhythmic large muscle group activities controlled on ergometric devices
    (treadmill or cycle ergometer)
Work rate: walking at 3.5 mph, 2.5% G or 450 KPM/minute on a cycle
    ergometer
Progression: after 4–6 weeks of uneventful activity the duration will be increased
    to 25–35 minutes and the work rate increased to maintain the initial average
    training heart rate.
Objectives: (a) to increase functional capacity so that a greater work capacity
                will be achieved before symptoms appear.
            (b) to reduce the double product at all submaximal work rates.
Calculation of prescribed intensity:
    Peak = 90% of functional capacity (0.90 × 7.2 METs = 6.5 METs). The
        heart rate corresponding to 6.5 METs is calculated by interpolation between
        the rates at 5.8 and 7.2 METs using the formula:

$$(6.5 - 5.8)/(7.2 - 5.8) = 0.50$$
$$0.50(150 - 120) = 15 + 120 = 135$$

Average = 67% of functional capacity (0.67×7.2 METs = 4.8 METs).

Calculation of corresponding heart rate:

$$(4.8 - 3.3)/(5.8 - 3.3) = 0.60$$
$$0.60(120 - 88) = 19.2 + 88 = 107.2$$

F. Program Characteristics

1. PREVENTIVE EXERCISE PROGRAM

1. For asymptomatic, clinically normal adults with no significant risk factors.
2. Can be relatively unstructured and utilize a wide variety of activities including recreational sports and games.
3. Can be individually undertaken and relatively unsupervised.
4. Reevaluation and assessment can be infrequent.
5. Can have a greater cosmetic emphasis and include resistive exercise, isometrics, and other muscle-toning activities.
6. Conducted by community recreation agencies, YMCA's, YMHA's, health spas, company recreation personnel.

2. INTERVENTIVE EXERCISE PROGRAM

1. Serves asymptomatic persons with significant risk factors for coronary heart disease (no one with documented coronary heart disease or positive stress test).
2. Must be structured to provide for strict control of work intensity.
3. Must be designed for individual limitations and modifications of risk factors such as obesity, high blood pressure, diabetes, smoking, emotional stress.
4. Sessions should be supervised at least in the early phase.
5. Participants must be trained in monitoring techniques.
6. Less emphasis on cosmetic effects.
7. Frequent assessment and reevaluation.
8. Participants should be under a physician's care.
9. Detailed emergency procedures must be defined and rehearsed.
10. Conducted by hospitals, commercial rehabilitation clinics, YMCA groups, health spas with specially trained personnel, college and university physical education departments, certain companies for employees.

3. CARDIAC REHABILITATION PROGRAM

1. Serves post-myocardial infraction, documented coronary heart disease, symptomatic angina pectoris, post coronary bypass surgery patients, and patients with positive stress tests.

2. Must be structured to provide strict control of work intensity, which is checked frequently and in some cases monitored continuously.
3. All sessions supervised by trained exercise leaders with medical personnel on site.
4. Frequent assessment and reevaluation.
5. Patients must be referred by a physician.
6. Exercise prescription reviewed and endorsed by a physician.
7. Competition avoided.
8. Emergency equipment must be on site and detailed procedures defined and rehearsed.
9. Conducted by hospitals, commercial rehabilitation clinics, YMCA groups, health spas with specially trained personnel, college and university physical education departments.

V. SUMMARY

Regular, individually prescribed exercise may contribute to the reduction of the risk of coronary heart disease and favorably affect the recovery from myocardial infarction and coronary bypass surgery. To ensure the appropriateness of the exercise regimen and increase the likelihood of patient compliance, an exercise prescription should accompany the physician's recommendation to the patient to increase his physical activity habits. The prescription should be formulated from a data base that includes a medical history, physical examination and laboratory studies (when indicated), and an exercise stress test, and include a recommended intensity level, duration, frequency, and type of exercise. The intensity level should be prescribed in METs and controlled by heart rate. Prescription by heart rate alone is less accurate. Patients at risk should be referred to supervised programs.

REFERENCES

1. American College of Sports Medicine (1980). "Guidelines for Graded Exercise Testing and Exercise Prescription." Lea & Febiger, Philadelphia, Pennsylvania.
2. Blumenthal, J. A., Williams, R. S., Williams, R. B., Jr., and Wallace, A. G. (1980). Effects of exercise on the Type A (coronary prone) behavior pattern. *Psychosom. Med.* **42,** 289–296.
3. Boyer, J. L., and Kasch, F. W. (1970). Exercise therapy in hypertensive men. *JAMA, J. Am. Med. Assoc.* **211,** 1668–1671.
4. Brunner, D., and Manelis, G. (1960). Myocardial infarction among members of communal settlements in Israel. *Lancet* **2,** 1049–1050.
5. Hakkila, J. (1955). Studies on the myocardial capillary concentration in cardiac hypertrophy due to training. *Am. Med. Exp. Biol. Fin.* **33,** Suppl. II, 7-80.
6. Hartung, G. H., Foreyt, J. P., Mitchell, R. E., Vlasek, I., and Gotto, A. M., Jr. (1980).

Relation of diet to high-density-lipoprotein cholesterol in middle-aged marathon runners, joggers, and inactive men. *N. Engl. J. Med.* **302**, 357–361.

7. Hellerstein, H. K., and Ader, R. (1971). Relationship between per cent maximal oxygen uptake (% MAX VO2) and per cent maximal heart rate (% MHR) in normals and cardiacs (ASHD). *Circulation* **44**, Suppl. 2, 76 (abstr.).

8. Holloszy, J. O., Skinner, J. S., Toro, G., and Cureton, T. K. (1964). Effects of a six month program of endurance exercise on the serum lipids of middle-aged men. *Am. J. Cardiol.* **14**, 753–760.

9. Kahn, H. A. (1963). The relationship of reported coronary heart disease mortality to physical activity of work. *Am. J. Public Health* **53**, 1058–1067.

10. Kannel, W. B. (1967). Habitual level of physical activity and risk of coronary heart disease: The Framingham study. *Can. Med. Assoc. J.* **96**, 811–812.

11. Kavanaugh, T., Shephard, R. J., Tuck, J. A., and Qureshi, S. (1977). Depression following myocardial infarction: The effects of distance running. *Ann. N.Y. Acad. Sci.* **301**, 1029–1038.

12. Kramsch, D. M., Aspen, A. J., Abramowitz, B. M., Kreimendahl, T., and Hood, W. B., Jr. (1981). Reduction of coronary atherosclerosis by moderate conditioning exercise in monkeys on an atherogenic diet. *N. Engl. J. Med.* **305**, 1483–1489.

13. Lehtonen, A., and Viikari, Jo (1978). Serum triglycerides and cholesterol and serum high-density lipoprotein cholesterol in highly physically active men. *Acta Med. Scand.* **204**, 111–114.

14. Martin, R. P., Haskell, W. L., and Wood, P. D. (1977). Blood chemistry and lipid profiles of elite distance runners. *Ann. N.Y. Acad. Sci.* **301**, 346–360.

15. Morris, J. N., Heady, J. A., Raffle, P. A. B., Roberts, C. G., and Parks, J. W. (1953). Coronary heart-disease and physical activity of work. *Lancet* **2**, 1053–1057.

16. Morris, J. N., Kagan, A., Pattison, D. C., Gardner, M. J., and Raffle, P. A. B. (1966). Incidence and prediction of ischaemic heart-disease in London busmen. *Lancet* **2**, 553–559.

17. Paffenbarger, R. S., Jr., Laughlin, M. E., Gima, A. S., and Black, R. A. (1970). Work activity of longshoremen as related to death from coronary heart disease and stroke. *N. Engl. J. Med.* **282**, 1109–1114.

18. Paffenbarger, R. S., Jr., Wing, A. L., and Hyde, R. T. (1978). Physical activity as an index of heart attack risk in college alumni. *Am. J. Epidemiol.* **108**, 161–175.

19. Paolone, A. M., Lewis, R. R., Lanigan, W. T., and Goldstein, M. J. (1976). Results of two years of exercise training in middle-aged men. *Physician Sports Med.* **4**, 72–77.

20. Rechnitzer, P. A. (1979). The effects of training: Reinfarction and death—an interim report. *Med. Sci. Sports* **11**, 382.

21. Rechnitzer, P. A., Pickard, H. A., Paivio, A. U., Yuhasz, M. S., and Cunningham, D. (1972). Long-term follow-up study of survival and recurrence rates following myocardial infarction in exercising and control subjects. *Circulation* **45**, 853–857.

22. Rechnitzer, P. A., Sangal, S., Cunningham, D. A., Andrew, G., Buck, C., Jones, N. L., Kavanaugh, T., Parker, J. O. Shephard, R. J., and Yuhasz, M. S. (1975). A controlled prospective study of the effect of endurance training on the recurrence rate of myocardial infarction: A description of the experimental design. *Am. J. Epidemiol.* **102**, 358–365.

23. Rechnitzer, P. A., Yuhasz, M. S., Pickard, H. A., and Lefcoe, N. M. (1965). The effects of a graduated exercise program on patients with previous myocardial infarction. *Can. Med. Assoc. J.* **92**, 858–860.

24. Skinner, J. S., Holloszy, J. O., and Cureton, T. K. (1964). Effects of a program of endurance exercises on physical work: Capacity and anthropometric measurements of fifteen middle-aged men. *Am. J. Cardiol.* **14**, 747–752.

25. Taylor, H. L., Klepetar, E., Keys, A., Parlin, W., Blackburn, H., and Puchner, T. (1962). Death rates among physically active and sedentary employees of the railroad industry. *Am. J. Public Health* **52**, 1697–1707.

Index